Choices

REALISTIC ALTERNATIVES IN CANCER TREATMENT

MARION MORRA & EVE POTTS

AVON
PUBLISHERS OF BARD, CAMELOT AND DISCUS BOOKS

CHOICES: REALISTIC ALTERNATIVES IN CANCER TREATMENT is
an original publication of Avon Books. This work has
never before appeared in book form.

AVON BOOKS
A division of
The Hearst Corporation
959 Eighth Avenue
New York, New York 10019

To our wonderful supportive family
who made it possible for us to write this book
and to the many cancer patients and their families
who inspired us with their courage and their need for

information

Preface

At last, a comprehensive book about cancer, written in lay terms for people with cancer, their families and friends.

For most people, the word cancer remains plagued with fear and misconceptions. The fear is usually of the unknown, and the misconceptions are often a result of lack of information, inadequate information or misinformation. This book presents accurate, up-to-date, cross-referenced material on all aspects of cancer diagnosis and treatment. It contains specific current facts to which patients and their families are entitled, so that they may understand their illness, ask appropriate questions, receive clarification and, hopefully, cope with problems more effectively.

The quality of the information which doctors, nurses and other health professionals present to their patients and the amount of time they can spend with them and their families varies greatly. This book is meant to be a resource so that those involved can absorb the material at their own speed. It fills the gap between the material available in medical textbooks—which often is difficult for the lay person to understand—and the information presently printed in the press—which many times is premature and incomplete. This book will be an assurance and a guide to the most modern diagnoses and treatments available in this rapidly changing field.

Joseph M. Bertino, M.D., Chief of the Section of Medical Oncology and American Cancer Society Professor of Medicine and Pharmacology, Yale University School of Medicine

Mary Kathryn Knobf, R.N., Oncology Nurse-Clinician, Section of Medical Oncology, Yale University School of Medicine

To the Cancer Patient

There are so many practical things you need to know when the diagnosis is cancer—yet most of us are so gripped with fear of the verdict that practical considerations are often lost in emotional chaos. This book is designed to unlock some of the fears.

It is important for you to know that cancer is a different disease today than it was even ten years ago. Though no miracle cure has been found, it is a fact that many advances have been made in treatments. Cancer is no longer considered an incurable disease. Recoveries are being made. The future now exists for many cancer patients who would not have had a future ten years ago. Because the explosion of information has been so rapid, much of it has been slow in sifting down to the consumer.

What we have tried to do in this book is to cover every facet of cancer care, making it possible for you and your family to have enough information to ask intelligent questions that will give you the answers you need to know so that you can be a partner with your health-care team in making decisions. We have tried to limit the use of medical jargon and to translate information into understandable terms. The book is designed to be used as a reference. Make use of the index. Take notes when your doctor gives you information, so you can check things out in the book and get a better understanding of what is happening. Naturally, the book is not designed to take the place of your doctor but to supplement what he tells you and to guide you in asking the questions you need to know in order to get the best care.

The fact that you have cancer is irreversible and unchangeable. The way you and your family handle that fact makes the real difference in what happens to you.

If we can leave you with just one piece of good advice it would be: *Ask, ask, ask, and ask again.* Don't take anything for granted and don't be put off by medical jargon or a doctor who doesn't want to talk. Remember—you are a consumer and are entitled to answers to your questions.

Contents

CONTENTS (continued)

CONTENTS *(continued)*

List of Illustrations

Acknowledgments

To list all of the people, books and sources such as magazine articles, original scientific writings, pamphlets, oncology seminars, and medical textbooks which made it possible for us to write this book would be an almost impossible task. We do want to thank publicly all those from whom we learned, especially the writings of the National Cancer Institute and the American Cancer Society and the many doctors, patients, and families kind enough to share their experiences, problems, and questions with us. We gained special insight from Shirley Mead and Betty Sheffer, two good friends who died of cancer, who made us most aware of the need for real answers to patients' questions.

Two of our colleagues deserve extra-special thanks—Tish Knobf, one of the country's most experienced cancer nurses, and Joe Bertino, a world-renowned cancer researcher as well as an experienced and sensitive oncologist, who gave us many hours of their scarcest commodity, time. We thank them for their invaluable, continuing, and personal involvement in helping us to avoid medical pitfalls in our writing.

We thank the members of our family for their encouragement and their assistance from beginning to end—especially Bob Potts and Abby, Amy, Matt, and Mark, for putting up with late dinners, early mornings, and short tempers; Mollie Donovan, our other sister, for help in layout, art, and typing and for encouragement; and Ann and Gil Maurer, for their guidance. We thank our mother, who brought us up to believe that we could accomplish any task we felt we wanted to do, and our father, who did not live to see this book completed, but who would have been very proud.

Though it is through the help of many, many people that this book came to be, we alone take responsibility for any possible errors or misinterpretations.

chapter 1

Facing the Diagnosis

As Hubert Humphrey said: "The day I found out I had cancer was the worst day of my life."

It is a normal reaction—and one of the first questions that comes to mind is "How long will I live?" The answer, of course, is that no one really knows. And the answer is exactly the same for all of us—*whether or not we have cancer.*

There is hope for every patient. Some patients with cancer are cured at once, by surgery, chemotherapy and radiotherapy. Some are never cured, but are controlled so that they can expect to live for many years. Some treatments—such as those which give you hair loss and nausea or remove a limb or a breast—seem to some to be worse than the illness itself. Some treatments prolong life for no more than a few months. But the fact is that with the proper attention, no patient needs to suffer. You can have cancer and still enjoy life.

Prepare for a host of nagging feelings. You will probably experience all of them to a greater or lesser degree. Check off those that match your own most intensely.

- I don't want to die.
- I can't believe this is happening to me.
- I feel as though I've been thrown off a cliff.
- This is the loneliest experience of my life.
- No one else can know how I feel.
- Maybe it will all go away.
- It couldn't be cancer because no one in my family ever had cancer.
- If it really is cancer, what will it mean to my life?

1

- I don't know how to tell my family.
- What if the doctor says I have to go to the hospital right away?
- People will treat me differently if they find out I have cancer.
- I'm afraid.
- I'm going to be in a lot of pain.
- This is a challenge to be met and I know I can beat it.
- Why me? Why couldn't it be someone else?
- I don't want to lose my breast (or lung or leg).

Coping with the Diagnosis of Cancer

Once you suspect you have cancer, you can live in fear. Or you can learn to live with the facts and you can begin to do positive things. Knowing the facts and facing them takes a lot of the scare away.

Here are a few basics for starters. Check them and see how many actually coincide with your own thinking.

- The fact that you may have cancer cannot be changed. The time that is most important in decision-making is right now— at the very beginning—when numerous alternatives are open to you.
- Demand to know all the alternatives. If you make a decision to go ahead with surgery without sufficient testing or a second opinion, you limit the possibility for other alternatives right from the very start. Often, unless you remain calm and in control, a decision is made for you by circumstances that will take it out of your control. Learning all you can about your case and the alternatives means you can control the way your illness is handled.
- Make sure you have the *right* doctor. The kind of treatment you get depends on how much your doctor knows about your specific disease.
- As a cancer patient, you must be an activist. You must become a partner with your doctors in the fight so that you can live your life in the way that is best for you.
- You can't cope with cancer by denying you have it. You can cope with it by learning as much as you can about what is happening to you.

- Hope is not the same as denying. Denying you have cancer closes your mind and your resources to all the possibilities that exist for you. You shut off your inner abilities to deal with what is real. Denial closes the doors. Hope opens the channels for action.

- None of us knows how long he or she will live. A patient with breast cancer, diagnosed early, who is receiving adequate treatment may live longer than a patient with heart disease.

- Without any doubt, the very worst time you will experience is at the beginning, when the diagnosis is first presented to you. At that moment, cancer becomes an inescapable fact for you. That is the time when you must mobilize yourself and your resources to plan your future intelligently.

- If at all possible, a second opinion is an absolute must at the start before submitting to *any* cancer treatment of *any* kind. This is not to suggest that the diagnosis you were given is not correct or that the suggested treatment might not be the best. It is only to say that you deserve the right to have the doctor's diagnosis reconfirmed and alternative treatments explored and explained to you.

- In some cases, a second pathological opinion is a good idea. The pathology report is the basis on which all future decisions will be made, and although some cancers are pathologically diagnosed without any question, you need to check and ask about it.

- You, as a cancer patient, are a consumer. As a consumer you have the right to ask questions just as you would as a consumer of any other product. However, you need to learn what questions to ask, what the terminology means, what possibilities exist. You have to set your mind to facing the fact that you have cancer—but you must also realize that if you have all the information at hand, you will greatly increase your chances for different treatment that might lead to a cure.

- One of the most important things to remember is that there are cancer specialists (called oncologists) who see many cancer patients every day. If you have cancer, your primary care should be under the direction of a specialist who spends most of his time dealing with cancer.

- Choose your plan of action and take time to make sure your decisions are informed ones. Carefully take notes whenever talking with the doctor, radiologist, physical therapist, nurse.

- Bring a list of questions with you, take notes when you are there, review them when you get home, and save them for future reference.

- Try always to have a family member or good friend with you when discussing your case with the doctor. People hear different things being said. It is important to have someone who is informed talk over the information with you.

- Do your homework. Ask your friends and family to help you search the library for any available articles on your specific illness. If a medical library is available to you, look for help there. So much new research is being done in so many places that you may find a clue to a treatment even your doctor hasn't heard of. Check with the nearest cancer center (there are toll-free phone lines available in many parts of the country; see chapter 23). Call your nearest American Cancer Society office; it will have a great deal of information and expertise on the illness.

- Expect some degree of depression. Cancer is a serious illness. Expect "down" days. Plan ways of coping with them. Call a friend. Take a walk down a favorite beach or pathway. Make a trip to a museum or wherever you feel happy.

- You need to do some thinking about whether quality or quantity of life—how good or how long—is more important to you. You may be faced with some decisions along the way where the answer to this question will determine which way to go.

- Don't be a martyr. Try to deal with your feelings honestly. Don't try to hide your illness and prognosis from your family and your friends. Try to face the facts openly. Accept and welcome the help of others. Only by tapping every resource will you be able to deal with your illness in an informed manner.

- Once you and your doctors have embarked on a course of treatment, your own unique style of coping will help to make you feel in control. You will be able to face your problems if you know what is being done to you, how it will be done, and what the prognosis is. You will undoubtedly find your optimism tempered with anxiety—and this is normal. You may be surprised that along the way you will experience a feeling of relief, or a feeling of calmness about what is happening, and even an increased zest for living. Many patients tell of a greater appreciation for the simple things in life once the initial decision on the course of treatment is made.

- Remember, your doctor will continue to work with you to control your disease. If the first treatment fails, there are others available that can be used.

- Go back over this chapter and check each of the areas where you will need further strengthening. Like any course of study, this will take practice and learning, but the more you learn, the better prepared you will be to make the right decisions for yourself.

Judging Your Own Attitude Toward Cancer

YOUR TRUE OR FALSE ANSWER		THE REAL ANSWER
_____	You will die if you have cancer.	False. Cancer, if discovered at an early stage, is curable in many instances.
_____	Smoking can cause lung cancer.	True. Heavy cigarette smokers get lung cancer 23 times more often than non-smokers.
_____	A lump in the breast means you have cancer.	False. Eighty percent of all lumps are not cancer.
_____	All cancers can be prevented.	False. However, preventive steps, such as not smoking or not being overexposed to the sun, have proved to reduce the chances of getting cancer.
_____	Cancer is contagious.	False.
_____	Cancer is hereditary.	False. However, the tendency toward breast and colon cancer, for example, seems to run in families.
_____	Cancer is more frequent in men and women over 35.	True. It is primarily a disease of middle age and old age—rare in children and young adults.

YOUR TRUE OR FALSE ANSWER		THE REAL ANSWER
_____	Cancer can develop in any part of the body.	True. All parts of the body are susceptible—the nervous system, bone, lymph, skin, etc.
_____	One-third of cancer patients are cured.	True. Of more than half a million newly diagnosed cancer cases each year, one-third are permanently cured, and many more lead normal lives for many years.
_____	The outlook for cancer therapy is hopeful.	True. The rate of cure is now one in three as compared to one in four in 1950.
_____	The doctor can tell how long you have to live.	False. Every case is different, and doctors' estimates on how long a patient will live are many times guesswork and often do a great disservice to the patient.
_____	There are no untreatable cancers.	True. There are always treatments that can be prescribed to make a patient more comfortable, although treatments are not always available to effect a cure.
_____	Putting off seeing a doctor can forfeit the possibility of a cure.	True. Of those who die each year, 100,000 will die needlessly because of late diagnosis and inadequate treatment.
_____	More people are having cancer diagnosed than ever before.	True. This is because more people are living to an age when cancer occurs more frequently, and diagnosis is better so more cases are being found.
_____	You should try to get a second or even a third opinion before having anything done.	True. A very wise idea, and any doctor who advises against another opinion is probably a doctor you shouldn't be using.

Suggested Reading

ROSENBAUM, ERNEST H., M.D. *Living with Cancer.* New York: Praeger. $4.95.

chapter 2

Deciding on Your Doctor and Hospital

Let's backtrack a bit and return to the basic question of who your doctor is at the moment. So much has been said and written about how to find a good doctor, yet so often in the cancer area the decision must be made on the spur of the moment. Most patients do not go through logical steps in making this important choice.

And once a doctor starts on a case, most people find it difficult to change, or even to bring up the subject of a second opinion. Remember, you are not alone in this problem. Most people find it difficult to challenge a doctor. On the other hand, most people even have a hard time changing hairdressers or standing up to their auto mechanics. It has only been in very recent times that people have felt they have the right to ask questions about their medical care.

Don't feel you are limited to the doctor you have right now. Use the checklist to help you determine if you are in partnership with the right doctor. This is one of the most important decisions you are going to make in handling your illness. (The right hospital is another important factor and will be discussed next.)

You might think that some of the questions that follow are irrelevant in your particular case—that they relate more to finding a good general doctor than an oncologist. But they are important for you to get an overall understanding of how the medical profession operates and will help you make some of those doctor decisions which will face you.

Judging Your Doctor

FILL IN HERE			SCORING		REASON FOR SCORE
+	−		+	−	

Kind of Practice

__	__	Multi-specialty group	5		Generally, a doctor who practices with a group which specializes in a variety of disciplines is better for your family doctor. Specialists who practice in a group or in a hospital are subject to constant review by peers.
__	__	Hospital-based office	5		
__	__	One-specialty group	5		
__	__	Loose association with others	2		
__	__	With partner	1		
__	__	Alone		1	

Hospital Affiliation

__	__	University or medical school hospital (part- or full-time staff member)	5		Same reasoning as above holds true here. You can be sure that a doctor who is a part- or full-time staff member at a university or medical school hospital or a larger community hospital has probably shown his merit and is respected by his colleagues. The doctor who practices in a small for-profit hospital might be just as qualified but should be more closely checked for other credentials.
__	__	On teaching staff of medical school	5		
__	__	Staff member, community hospital with 200 or more beds	4		
__	__	Staff member, community hospital with less than 200 beds	3		
__	__	Part owner, staff of small private hospital (proprietary hospital)	1		
__	__	No hospital affiliation (ask doctor for reason, then score either −1 or +1)	1	1	

FILL IN HERE	SCORING	REASON FOR SCORE
+ −	+ −	

Boards

__ __ Board-certified in his specialty and specialist in oncology   **10**

__ __ Board-certified and/or fellow of the board   **5**

__ __ Board-certified   **4**

__ __ Board-eligible   **3**

__ __ No longer eligible   **1**

The fact that a doctor has been certified in his specialty means that beyond training in his field he has subjected himself to the scrutiny of his peers in written and oral examinations. A fellowship is an extra flag of distinction. Oncology specialty means that the bulk of patients are cancer patients, but since this is a new specialty, many of the older and more experienced cancer doctors have not taken the boards in the field.

Manner

__ __ Explains procedures, asks and answers questions, keeps complete records, has laboratory tools in office or available nearby (x-ray, urine and blood-chemistry lab, etc.), takes full history at first visit   **5**

__ __ Difficult to communicate with, uses unfamiliar terms, doesn't seem able to communicate in plain language, forgets facts because doesn't take notes   **3**

Your own personal observations about how the doctor's skills measure up are an important part of the evaluation. Think back over his care of you before scoring this one.

FILL IN HERE	SCORING	REASON FOR SCORE
+ −	+ −	

___ ___ Seems interested but has never taken full history or given complete examination; lab tests done at different location   2

___ ___ Always in a hurry, doesn't care about problem, seems overly concerned about money   1

How Office Is Run

___ ___ Personable, warm, efficient office personnel; office looks cheerful, comfortable, neat; appointments kept on time or explanations given   5

The manner in which the doctor's office is run tells you a great deal about the doctor's own standards and probably reflects upon the way he conducts the professional side of his life. Taken alone, this part of the scoring is not as vital as the doctor's credentials, but added to the other material it stands as an important guideline to the kind of medical care you will receive.

___ ___ Clinical, impersonal atmosphere—both office and personnel; office always jammed; waiting the rule rather than the exception   3

___ ___ Concerned office staff— nurse seems more interested than doctor—but haphazardly run appointment schedule in attempt to keep everyone happy   2

___ ___ Messy, dingy office, inefficient personnel; record-keeping haphazard; over-emphasis on paying   1

FILL IN HERE			SCORING	REASON FOR SCORE
+	−		+ −	

Personality

___	___	Warm, concerned, listens, interested, willing to explain and answer questions	5	How well you relate to your doctor has a bearing on the kind of treatment you will get and how well you will respond. Therefore, it is important that he be someone for whom you have thorough respect and who sees you as a person as well as a patient.
___	___	Very professional but impersonal, cold and stiff	4	
___	___	Seems overly busy, average personality	3	
___	___	Doesn't relate well	1	

Other

___	___	Willing to make house calls or has 24-hour telephone accessibility to someone who knows you or has your records	5	These extra-point items are all pluses for a doctor since they give an indication of his compassion for his patients.
___	___	Willing to discuss fees	5	
___	___	Takes Medicare and Medicaid patients	5	

Do I have a family physician?

Today people commonly move from one area to another, and most of us do not have what is lovingly called a "family doctor." Ideally, your family doctor should be one who is either in general practice or in family practice or whose specialty is internal medicine (known as an internist or as a gastroenterologist or G.I. man). Your gynecologist/obstetrician and your pediatrician really should not be considered family doctors because of the nature of their specialties. Many younger doctors are turning to the specialty of family practice. This is a new or a renewed specialty which requires a three-year residency as well as a reexamination every three years to remain board-certified. Thus the new family practitioner is more highly trained than the old general practitioner.

How do I check out my doctor's credentials?

This is a relatively easy thing to do—and worth the half-hour it will take, especially when you consider that you will be spending hundreds of dollars for his expertise and putting your physical and psychological well-being in his hands. Go to the reference room at your local library and ask for a copy of either the Directory of Medical Specialists or the American Medical Directory. If possible, use the Directory of Medical Specialists, since it lists only those doctors who are "board-certified"—that is, those who have passed tests in their particular specialty, under the watchful eyes of their fellow doctors. The listings of doctors in the American Medical Directory, though it lists credentials, include any doctor who belongs to the American Medical Society, whether or not he has received board certification. If your library does not have either of these books, try calling your state or local department of health or medical society and ask them for the information.

What does board certification mean?

The specialty boards are private, voluntary, nonprofit, autonomous organizations founded to conduct examinations, issue certificates of qualifications, and improve and broaden opportunities for graduate education and training. Once a doctor finishes his required residency in his specialty, he becomes eligible to be certified by the board. This requires him to take a rigorous written and oral examination before other doctors who practice in his specialty. Many doctors are not "certified" on their first examinations by the board. Some boards require recertification after a specified number of years. An *F* after a doctor's name means he has been elected to a fellowship in the "college" of his specialty and is qualified to teach others. It is another step up the ladder and earns him an especially esteemed place among his colleagues.

Are there good doctors who are not board-certified?

Board certification and fellowships are designed to indicate a high level of competence, but there are many reasons why doctors who are equally competent may not be board-certified. In the field of cancer, especially, there are many doctors who treat only cancer patients, yet are not board-certified in oncology. This is because the boards in oncology are new and were not available to the older doctors when they started in practice. Many of the doctors in medical centers who are combining research with patient care never take boards. The main thing to remember is that if you are choosing a doctor without any personal recommendations from other physicians or health professionals, stick to those who are board-certified. You will have a guarantee from other physicians in his specialty that you have chosen a qualified person.

What is the difference between board-certified and board-eligible?

The physician who passes the examination of a given specialty is known as a diplomate of the board and is said to be board-certified. A physician who has completed a formal training program in the specialty but has either chosen not to take the exams or has not completed the exams is called board-eligible (newly trained doctors are board-eligible between the time they finish their residency and the time they take their boards and get the results). There are well-trained specialists who for good legitimate reasons are board-eligible, but these are exceptions. It is better to have passed the exams than not to have passed them.

Don't physicians have to be recertified periodically once they have passed their boards?

There are only two specialty societies at the present time which have taken definite steps to require periodic recertification—family practice and surgery. In general, most physicians are diligent in keeping up with the latest knowledge. However, there are obviously some doctors in practice who are not as up-to-date as others.

How do I use the medical directories to check out a doctor?

The book will tell you the year the doctor was born, the medical school he attended, the year he was licensed to practice, if and when he was certified in his specialty, both his primary and secondary specialties, and his type of practice. The Directory of

Medical Specialists has more detailed information as to where he trained, what societies he belongs to, his appointment to medical schools, and his hospital accreditations. Each book has its own method of coding, which is carefully explained in the foreword. (Bring your glasses or magnifying glass with you as the type is small and hard to read.) There is nothing mysterious or difficult about getting this information—it takes only a few minutes and it is important to you in getting the very best and most advanced treatment possible. Take the time to search it out.

The listings in both books are geographical, so this is a good time to find out and jot down the names and credentials of other specialists in your area—such as surgeons, anesthesiologists, gynecologists, urologists, etc. Each specialty in the Directory of Medical Specialists is listed separately by geographic areas. If no one in your town is listed, look for nearby towns and you'll surely find a suitable doctor.

What kinds of things are important to look for in analyzing the listings in the book?
There are several questions you should be asking yourself:

- Does he have a teaching appointment at a medical-school-affiliated hospital? This indicates that he is up-to-date and respected by his peers.
- What kind of hospital is he affiliated with? Is it a medical-school-affiliated hospital? Requirements for this sort of hospital are rigid and must be earned through teaching appointments.
- If he is a surgeon, does he have privileges at three or more hospitals? This sounds impressive but it takes so much of the doctor's time that you might be better served by someone who concentrates his efforts on one or two hospitals. The quality of the hospital he is associated with is more important than the number!
- How large is the hospital? If you don't live in an area with a university hospital center, the larger the hospital (200 beds or more) the more equipment and facilities it will have.
- Is it a privately owned (proprietary) hospital? If so, the doctors who practice there are usually part owners—and though that is not a reflection on their abilities, it can mean that standards are generally not as high as in community hospitals.

- What societies does the doctor belong to? He should belong to several, for these help keep him up-to-date on the latest information being developed by others in his specialty.

Does my doctor belong to a multi-specialty group?

This is important if you are looking for a family doctor but not as essential for a specialist. If you are looking for a family doctor find a group with a family practitioner, a pediatrician, an internist, a general surgeon, a gynecologist, and possibly a radiologist. Groups vary by size and category—but they offer the best overall coverage for a patient as well as the most convenient kind of setup, since all services can usually be provided within one building. Blood counts, electrocardiogram, urinalysis, and x-rays can all be done without having the patient run from one end of town to the other. You can find such a group by writing to the American Group Practice Association (P.O. Box 948, Alexandria, Va. 22313) for information on whether there is such a group near you.

Can any doctor be a specialist?

After earning his M.D. degree (four years of study after college) plus one year of internship, a physician can be licensed to practice if he can pass certain requirements. There are still a few states which do not even require an internship for a doctor to become eligible for licensing. Once licensed, a physician can call himself anything he wants. Even if a physician has no training beyond internship, he can call himself a psychiatrist or an internist, and he can legally perform operations as a surgeon. That is why it is important to determine whether or not the physician has had additional training, is board-certified, and is practicing in a legitimate hospital. The best way to do this is to check his credentials in the Directory of Medical Specialists.

If my doctor has no hospital affiliation does that mean he is not a good doctor?

Not necessarily, though that once was the case. Some perfectly good family doctors confine themselves to an office practice and when the patient needs hospitalization, they recommend the specialist they feel has the proper skills. If, however, the doctor was once affiliated with a hospital and no longer has that affiliation, make sure you ask some questions.

If the doctor is in solo practice, is that a good sign?

This really depends upon the area in which the doctor is practicing. Many doctors practice in rural areas and may have no choice but to be in solo practice. However, in general the doctor who works with other doctors is usually a better bet than one who works alone. Solo practice limits the exchange of ideas and cuts off the possibility of someone else evaluating the doctor's practices. Some solo doctors practice in the same building with other doctors and cover for each other. This is better than a doctor who is off by himself in an office with no contact with other medical professionals. (You should check what covering means—if the covering doctor does not have access to your medical records, he is very limited in how he can treat you in your doctor's absence.) Your doctor may be part of a group that consists of several other doctors who practice the same specialty, such as a group of internists, each with a different area of expertise. This gives them and you the advantage of other opinions on a specific case.

What are the major specialties?

The Directory of Medical Specialists lists some 22 specialties. Among those which pertain to what might be needed for cancer treatment are:

- *Dermatologists:* doctors who treat skin diseases and conditions, including skin cancer
- *Family practice:* doctors specializing in the continuing and total care of the family
- *Internists:* doctors who treat a wide range of medical problems. Subspecialists who are internists take an additional one or more years of "fellowship":
  - Endocrinology: diseases of organs which secrete hormones into the bloodstream, such as the pancreas, thyroid, etc.
  - Gastroenterology (GI): diseases of the GI tract (mouth to anus, including stomach, liver, pancreas, intestines)
  - Hematology: diseases of the blood and blood-making tissues
  - Infectious disease: difficult cases of infection
  - Nephrology: disease of the kidneys, the rest of the urinary system, and related disorders of metabolism

- Neurology: diseases of the nervous system (brain, spinal cord and nerves)
- Oncology: diseases of abnormal tissue growth (cancer)
- Pulmonary disease: disease of the lung

- *Otolaryngologists (ENT):* doctors who specialize in the ear, nose, and throat, air tubes to the lungs, and neck region
- *Pediatricians:* doctors who take care of children up to age 16. Subspecialties are similar to internists: pediatric cardiology, pediatric endocrinology, pediatric hematology
- *Psychiatrists:* medical doctors who treat emotional and mental disorders. Board-certified psychiatrists have three or more years of residency training after obtaining an M.D. (Clinical psychologists deal with nonclinical matters such as education and have no formal medical training. They obtain a Ph.D. instead of an M.D. but have post-M.D. training similar to that of the psychiatrist.)
- *Surgeons:* doctors who treat by cutting out or operating. Subspecialties which take four or more years of special training:
  - General surgery: operations within the abdominal cavity and chest cavity
  - Neurological surgery: operations involving the skull, brain
  - Obstetrics and gynecology: operations on the female reproductive organs, childbirth
  - Ophthalmology: operations of the eye and optical structures
  - Orthopedic surgery: surgical treatment of injury and diseases of bones and joints
  - Plastic surgery: operations involving skin grafts, facial injuries, and tendon and nerve repair
  - Proctology: study and treatment of colon and rectal conditions
  - Thoracic surgery: operations in area of chest, including lungs, heart, and blood vessels
  - Urology: treatment of the urinary system (kidneys, bladder, and prostate)
- *Pathologists:* doctors who study, grossly and microscopically, abnormal conditions of all tissues and interpret blood tests and tissue specimens to determine origin, nature, causes and development of disease

- *Radiologists:* diagnostic radiologists perform and interpret x-ray studies; therapeutic radiologists or radiation oncologists treat cancer with x-rays

Is it better to use a younger doctor or an older doctor?

It is generally thought that the younger doctor is probably more up-to-date and the older doctor has more experience. This may be true in private practice, but in the medical academic area, the older doctor is probably both more up-to-date and more experienced. Teaching in a medical school means he must stay up-to-date and be ready to explain to the students why he is using a particular procedure or treatment.

Are psychiatrists interested in treating cancer patients?

Generally, no. Cancer patients are not usually mentally ill. Sometimes, however, both the patient and other family members need to talk with someone. For some, a small amount of psychotherapy is needed. A psychologist (rather than a psychiatrist) or someone who has had training in social work may fill this role. Many times nurses, clergymen, friends, family members, or other patients can be of the most help. The main point is for persons to recognize that they are living through a stressful situation, and that they should accept and seek help from others.

What is an oncologist?

If you have cancer, "oncology" and "oncologist" are words you should be familiar with. The word "oncology" is from the Greek word *onkos,* meaning "bulk" or "mass," and relates to that part of medical science that treats tumors. It is only in the past five years that medical oncology has been listed as a subspecialty for internists in the Directory of Medical Specialists. The bulk of the practice of these physicians deals with cancer patients. You are indeed fortunate if you can arrange to have an internist who is a specialist in medical oncology as your doctor.

What is a surgical oncologist?

Although this is not listed as a specialty, some surgeons who are known in their professions as dealing primarily with cancer patients are referred to as surgical oncologists. Because they see many cancers, their treatment can be expected to be more up-to-date than that of a surgeon who deals with a broader spectrum of general cases. There are also surgeons who do diagnostic biopsies, laparotomies (operations to open the abdomen either to make an inspection of the contents or as a preliminary to further surgery), and splenectomies (removal of the spleen to see if it contains cancer cells). These specialists are important to cancer patients especially because of their expertise in diagnosing the problem.

What is a radiation oncologist?

A radiation oncologist is a doctor who specializes in treating the cancer patient with radiotherapy. Sometimes this doctor is called a therapeutic radiologist, radiation therapist, or radiotherapist. You will also hear the term "diagnostic radiologist." This is a specialist who performs and interprets x-rays used in diagnosing your illness.

What is a medical oncologist or a chemotherapist?

A medical oncologist is a doctor of internal medicine who specializes in the administration of a variety of drugs needed to treat specific cancers. He can also be referred to as a hematologist (one who specializes in blood diseases) or a chemotherapist (one who specializes in chemotherapeutic drugs). Chemotherapy is far too risky to be administered by general physicians without special training. It is important if you are living in a community that does not have an oncologist to make sure that your doctor has consulted with a cancer center, a medical school, or an oncologist to determine which drugs are best for your case, the dose of drug to be given, and the side effects to be expected. This field of medicine is very new and changes constantly. At the present time, the newest, most experimental chemotherapeutic drugs are available only at the large cancer centers or specialized hospitals. The use of chemotherapeutic drugs is a very specialized field. The drugs have many side effects and should be administered only by qualified personnel. In some areas, doctors, nurses, and pharmacists work as a team in this newly emerging field.

What is the difference between an anesthesiologist and an anesthetist?

An M.D. degree. An anesthetist is a person who administers

anesthetics. An anesthesiologist is an M.D. whose specialty is the administering of anesthesia. This specialty has become an extremely important one in the last 30 years as anesthesia has become more sophisticated and diversified. The anesthesiologist should be your choice to administer anesthesia during the operation. He will check your specific needs during the operation—oxygen requirements, heart action, blood pressure, pulse, and body functions. For any operation which requires the use of anesthesia, you should make certain that your anesthesia is administered under the supervision of a board-certified anesthesiologist.

What is the role of the nurse in cancer care?

You will find that the nurse is a very important part of the health team in cancer care. There is a growing number of nurses in the country who are specializing in the cancer field. Some of these nurses work in medical centers with the physicians who are doing investigational work in the fields of chemotherapy and radiation therapy. Some work in the offices of oncologists. Others are ostomy nurses or enterostomal therapists who take care of the needs of patients who have had operations in the gastrointestinal areas. Some nurses give chemotherapeutic drugs under the doctors' supervision. Others are involved with teaching patients how to take care of themselves after leaving the hospital. Many of them take time to evaluate how the patient and his family are coping with the illness. Whether your long-term care is in the hospital, the outpatient clinic of a hospital, or in a doctor's office, get to know the nurses who are involved with your care. They can be your best allies.

Should I discuss finances with my doctor?

Absolutely. Cancer is a very expensive illness, and you should know what kinds of costs will be involved. You should never be afraid to ask the doctor about costs, about his fees, what the laboratory tests will cost, how much the hospital bill will be, or what x-rays and drugs cost. The earlier you have this kind of discussion, the better off you will be. If the doctor does not know all the answers, he can direct you to someone else who will. If the doctor refuses to discuss costs with you, you should think about getting yourself another doctor.

Judging Your Hospital

Score	Type of Hospital	Scoring Guide	Reason for Score
_____	Comprehensive cancer center designated by National Cancer Institute (see Chapter 23)	50	If one of these facilities is nearby, by all means take advantage of it. Use its expertise for your care or have your case reviewed by the experts on the staff. This is where much of the newest work on cancer is taking place; consider yourself fortunate if one of these facilities is available to you.
_____	Clinical cancer center designated by National Cancer Institute (see Chapter 23)	40	
_____	Approved hospital cancer program sponsored by American College of Surgeons (check Chapter 23 for listings)	20	Accredited hospitals have voluntarily been surveyed by the College of Surgeons and have set up a multidisciplinary cancer committee and fulfilled additional requirements.
_____	Directly affiliated with medical school which uses hospital for internship and residency programs	20	Provide excellent care, generally, since medical schools attract some of the top doctors as faculty members and range of services is extremely broad.
_____	Teaching hospital, residency and internship training, medical-school affiliation, but hospital located away from medical school	15	Have good facilities, usually not as wide-ranging as in hospitals directly connected with medical school.
_____	Residency and/or internship program, without medical-school affiliation	10	These programs are a sign of better than adequate care and put these hospitals a step above those which simply are accredited.

SCORE	TYPE OF HOSPITAL	SCORING GUIDE	REASON FOR SCORE
_____	Accredited by Joint Commission on Accreditation for Hospitals, but without approved internship and/or residency programs	5	Accreditation is a minimum standard assuring adequate care.
_____	Not accredited	0	About one-quarter of hospitals in U.S. fall into this category. Unaccredited hospitals are not eligible for Medicaid payments.
_____	Government-supported (so-called public) hospital (VA, Public Health Service, county, city, or state)	0	Care in these varies from excellent to substandard. No score suggested.
_____	Proprietary or for-profit hospital, owned by individuals or stockholders, including doctors who practice there	0 or −10	Medical services frequently limited, although there are a few outstanding exceptions. If local reputation is excellent, do not score this category. Generally, however, this type of hospital is poorly equipped or has serious problems because of efforts to keep costs low and profits high. Score −10 if local reputation is unacceptable.

Number of Beds

SCORE	TYPE OF HOSPITAL	SCORING GUIDE	REASON FOR SCORE
_____	Over 500 beds	20	Larger hospitals generally offer more services. Of the more than 3,000 hospitals with fewer than 100 beds, only a handful are medical-school-affiliated, less than 1 percent offer residency programs. Be aware that there are a few outstanding exceptions in this category and score accordingly.
_____	100 to 500 beds	15	
_____	Under 100 beds	5	

SCORE	TYPE OF HOSPITAL	SCORING GUIDE	REASON FOR SCORE

Location of Hospital in Relation to Your Home

SCORE	TYPE OF HOSPITAL	SCORING GUIDE	REASON FOR SCORE
_____	Within 20 miles	25	Location is important. If your local hospital does not seem adequate to provide you with the services you will need, you should ask your doctor to refer you to a specialist who is affiliated with a hospital which is better suited to your needs. However, weigh carefully your own need for the emotional support of having visits from friends and relatives and the added burden of having to travel long distances for your care. Generally, you can arrange to be evaluated by one of the specialists, who can then advise your doctor how to treat your case. The specialist is important in making the diagnosis and planning the treatment. Your local doctor and hospital can usually carry out the treatment plan successfully.
_____	Within 100 miles	15	
_____	Within 200 miles	5	

General Hospital Services

SCORE	TYPE OF HOSPITAL	SCORING GUIDE	REASON FOR SCORE
_____	Postoperative recovery room	5	20 percent of our hospitals do not have a room where the patient is monitored by specially trained personnel during the crucial first hours following surgery.
_____	Intensive care unit	5	Referred to as the ICU, this facility is designed to give seriously ill patients carefully monitored attention 24 hours a day.

SCORE	TYPE OF HOSPITAL	SCORING GUIDE	REASON FOR SCORE
_____	Pathology lab	10	Importance of adequate pathology services cannot be overstressed in cancer diagnosis and care.
_____	Diagnostic laboratories	10	Well-equipped and well-staffed diagnostic facilities are an important factor in good patient care.
_____	Pharmacy	5	Well-trained personnel with up-to-date knowledge of drugs, side effects, etc. contribute to overall quality of hospital.
_____	Blood bank	5	Careful, accurate, and rapid service by specially trained personnel around the clock is a must for a well-equipped hospital.
_____	X-ray equipment, radiation therapy such as cobalt, linear accelerator, radium implants	5	A great deal of expensive machinery used in cancer diagnosis and treatment is available only at sophisticated treatment centers.
_____	Radioactive scanning equipment	5	Newer diagnostic equipment
_____	CT scanner	5	Newer diagnostic equipment
_____	Brain-wave equipment (EEG)	5	Highly specialized testing equipment
_____	Tumor registry, tumor committee	10	Indicates cancer is being treated regularly, statistics are kept on treatment, and group discussions held.

SCORE	TYPE OF HOSPITAL	SCORING GUIDE	REASON FOR SCORE
_____	Respiratory therapy	5	Requires trained personnel. Necessary in many basic treatments. Should be available on a 24-hour basis.
_____	Physical therapy	5	Sounds like peripheral service but is important aspect of rehabilitation.
_____	Social services	5	Necessary to provide help with financial aid, post-hospital care, housing, homemaker service, etc. A sign of a "caring" hospital attitude.
_____	Anesthesiologists	10	Use of anesthesiologists (M.D.s) in operating room, rather than anesthetists, is an important dimension of good hospital practice.
_____	Nursing staff	10	Numbers depend upon patients and beds. Some hospitals practice team nursing. Reputation for caring attitude and prompt attention will determine score.
_____	Physician staff	10	24-hour-a-day staffing is an absolute must.

This hospital scoring checklist is designed to allow you to check your hospital on its ability to deliver cancer care. It is not meant to be used to judge your hospital on its adequacy for emergency care, general surgery, etc.

Over 250—Excellent
Over 180—Very good
Over 130—Good
Over 100—Adequate
Under 100—Poor

Is it a good idea to go to a research or a teaching hospital?

Naturally, this is a personal decision, based on many factors. Certain demands are made on patients in these hospitals which might be disturbing to some and comforting to others. Physicians, nurses, psychologists, and social workers often interview patients. Members of the medical staff other than the patient's physician may drop by to examine the patient's condition. Of course, the patient always has the option of refusing to be examined by or treated by anyone other than his own doctor (except in emergencies where quick decisions are essential). Some people object to being treated by anyone except their own personal physician. If you feel this way, it is important for you to understand how these hospitals operate. However, the care in research and teaching hospitals is extremely attentive, the staff is very competent, and the patient can be assured that the latest and most up-to-date treatment is available.

If I go to a research or teaching hospital will I become a guinea pig for a cancer-research project?

Many people are frightened at the thought of being used in a research project without their consent. Rest assured that each research project must first be approved by the hospital's research committee (usually called the human investigations committee), which has very strict guidelines it follows in evaluating whether or not the project can be carried out at that hospital. Moreover, each patient participating in the research project must sign a consent form which explains both the potential value and the possible risks.

What questions should I ask before consenting to becoming a part of a research project?

Good questions to ask include:
- Is the project designed to benefit me or is it aimed at benefiting future patients?
- Is the project planned to include a control group—that is, a group which will receive no treatment or only the type of treatment that was previously used to give the researchers a basis for measuring the effectiveness of the new treatment?
- Am I likely to be part of the control rather than the treatment group?
- What are the aims of the project?

What is a comprehensive cancer center and what services do they offer?

There are 21 comprehensive cancer centers in the United States, so designated by the National Cancer Institute. They vary from centers which treat only cancer patients to centers in medical schools or in community hospitals. All of them were well known for their expertise either in cancer research or patient care or both before being designated as comprehensive cancer centers. The centers are devoted to the diagnosis and multidisciplinary treatment of cancer patients, to basic clinical and pharmacological research, and to the training of personnel in cancer diagnosis, treatment, and research. In addition, most have facilities for rehabilitation, social services, convalescent and intermediate care, home-care support, and patient follow-up. They are responsible for maintaining a cancer registry and for giving public information. They are specifically geared to treating cancer with the most up-to-date methods. The list of comprehensive cancer centers appears in Chapter 23.

Should I go to a comprehensive cancer center for diagnosis and treatment of cancer?

If one of the 21 centers is nearby, by all means take advantage of it. Use its expertise for your care or have your case reviewed by the experts on its staff. This is where much of the new work on cancer is taking place. However, if you are not close to a comprehensive center, you can ask your doctor to be evaluated by one of the specialists, who can then advise your doctor on your treatment. Sometimes, the doctor can make a telephone call and talk to someone who is treating your kind of cancer—this is especially important if you have a rare type of cancer which your doctor does not see very often. Remember that a qualified cancer specialist at a local hospital is usually up-to-date on the standard, proven treatment. You need to weigh carefully your own needs for having the emotional support of family and friends against the added burden of having to travel long distances for your cancer treatment and care.

What are clinical and nonclinical centers?

Clinical and nonclinical centers are medical centers which have support from the National Cancer Institute for programs to

investigate promising new methods of cancer treatment or for
nonclinical research programs. Some of the leading medical
centers in the country are clinical or nonclinical centers; clinical
centers treat patients and can offer many of the same services as
a comprehensive cancer center. A listing of these centers is in
Chapter 23.

What are cancer clinical cooperative groups?

These groups, under the sponsorship of the National Cancer
Institute, include more than 3,300 doctors at nearly 440 different
institutions throughout the country. Each clinical cooperative
group specializes in a particular type of cancer and conducts
controlled studies to determine the best possible treatment for
patients with those diseases. The approaches may include
chemotherapy, radiotherapy, immunotherapy, and surgery alone
or in various combinations. Presently about 28,000 patients are
receiving treatment as part of clinical cooperative groups. These
groups allow many patients from different parts of the country to
be given the same treatments so as to compare the new therapy
with standard methods.

**Who pays for the treatment given to patients in clinical
cooperative groups?**

Most costs of medical treatment in clinical cooperative groups are
borne by the patient, although medical insurance usually pays for
the doctor's visit. Sometimes the drugs are paid for by the
clinical cooperative group. Drugs not yet commercially available
and extra tests not required in usual treatment may be provided
free of charge. In some specialized treatments, all costs are paid
for. In Chapter 23 you will find the name of the chairman of each
clinical cooperative group and the phone number for contact.
The address listed is not an indication of where these groups are
located. It is simply the information center for the specific type
of study group. Your doctor or you may contact that person for
information on what clinical trials are available in your area. You
can get information about physicians located in your area by
calling the Cancer Information Service listed in Chapter 23.

**How is someone treated at the National Institutes of Health
Clinical Center?**

The National Cancer Institute conducts clinical research

programs at the National Institutes of Health Clinical Center in Bethesda, Md. This combined research laboratory and hospital is operated by the federal government as part of the National Institutes of Health just outside the District of Columbia. At full capacity it can accommodate about 500 carefully selected patients. It is not a diagnostic clinic and it does not accept patients with conditions doctors have been unable to diagnose. The clinical center provides nursing and medical care without charge for patients who have been diagnosed as having the particular kind or stage of cancer being studied in their clinical research programs. It is principally interested in long-term conditions, many of which have no specific treatment. Medical miracles are not to be expected. Patients at the clinical center may be required to be hospitalized for much longer periods of time than in a general hospital, but will be discharged when the study is finished.

The following steps should be followed by those interested in being admitted to the National Institutes of Health Clinical Center:

- Discuss the matter with your doctor. To determine if you can be considered, the doctor must call or write the Office of the Director, The Clinical Center, National Institutes of Health, Bethesda, MD 20205. (Telephone: 301-496-4114.) Your physician must furnish the center with a full medical report.
- The medical report is studied by medical scientists to determine whether your condition is of a kind presently under study at the clinical center. The clinical center will reply to your doctor, who, in turn, will notify you.
- If you are accepted, correspondence between the clinical center and the doctor, and sometimes with you, will settle details as to when and how you will be admitted. When you are discharged, a full report on the results of studies and on treatment given is sent to the referring doctor.

How can I tell a good from a bad hospital?

Some people judge a hospital by the food it serves. This is *not* a criterion for choosing a hospital. The checklist lists the services important for consideration. It will help you sort out the pros and cons of your local hospital. You'll be interested to know that there are about 7,000 hospitals in the United States. Of these, about 500 are medical-school-affiliated and another 1,500 have intern/residency teaching programs. Approximately 1,600 hospitals continue to lack minimum accreditation. In the middle is a group of average hospitals which offer care ranging from superior to substandard. However, in surveys done among hospital professionals, only about 25–50 hospitals in the country are categorized as superior.

Why is the care in some big-city public hospitals considered comparable to that in many nonprofit private hospitals?

It is mainly because many of the top medical students choose the big public hospitals for their internship and residency training. The students know that these hospitals tend to get the widest range of cases and that the interns and residents are given more responsibility than in private hospitals.

Why is a teaching hospital considered to be superior to a hospital which does not have an intern/residency program?

Simply because there are more professionals on the job—more doctors checking up on the competence of other doctors. You will be seen on regular daily "rounds" by your doctor and other interns and residents. Doctors who receive appointments to these hospitals are usually tops in their fields. Teaching hospitals attract the finest medical minds in the country. (However, some people are annoyed by being "poked at" by countless interns and residents. If you should find this to be the case, you have a perfect right to state that you wish to be seen only by your own doctor.)

Is size an important factor in considering a hospital?

In our listing, we have given greater weight to a hospital with 500 or more beds than we have to one with 100–500 beds or one with less than 100 beds. This is a general rule of thumb. There are some excellent small hospitals. There are some poor large hospitals. Size is not all—but the number of patients with serious illnesses seen by the staff is an important factor. In a larger hospital, in the course of a week a doctor will probably treat as many patients with a specific illness as the small-hospital doctor will see in a year. Hospital death rates have been estimated to be 40 percent higher in less-than-100-bed hospitals than in larger hospitals. The overall capabilities of a large hospital are greater than those of a small one. People sometimes complain that large hospitals are impersonal. This can be true—but it can also vary from department to department, from floor to floor, and from person to person.

What if the doctor sends me to a hospital I don't approve of?

You do have a right to go to the hospital of your choice—and that is why, in choosing a doctor, an important consideration is his hospital affiliation. Most doctors have admitting privileges at more than one hospital. Therefore, if you have a specific request for a hospital, be sure to discuss this with your doctor.

What kinds of nurses are involved with taking care of me in the hospital?

There are many changes taking place in the nursing profession, and the field is becoming more specialized. It may be useful to understand what the functions of the various nurses are. In most hospitals, particularly the larger ones, you will find, in order of authority:

- Director of nursing (responsible for the entire nursing staff)
- Nursing supervisor (in charge of major nursing areas)
- Head nurse (responsible for a particular floor)
- Floor nurses or staff nurses (handle specific nursing problems)
- Licensed practical nurses or LPNs (assist staff nurses with patient care)
- Nursing assistants (handle routine patient needs)
- Aides (handle routine patient needs)

The first four in the list are generally registered nurses (RNs) who have completed a nursing training program (sometimes they have a bachelor's or master's degree) and are licensed by the state to practice nursing. RNs have fundamental knowledge of most diseases and know how to observe and manage patients. They handle patient care which requires special knowledge such as giving out medication, adjusting medical devices (such as tubes, drains, respirators, etc.), changing intravenous bottles, giving injections, and recognizing problems which need a doctor's care. An RN is a skilled practitioner in nursing management and care and, in the cancer field especially, is a very important member of the health-care team.

What are the duties of the licensed practical nurse?

The licenced practical nurse (LPN) is usually a graduate of a one-year course. Although the LPN has some medical knowledge, she is usually not as expert as the RN. An LPN must take a state examination to practice nursing, but because her formal training is not as extensive, she cannot do all the things an RN can do. Normally, the LPN takes a patient's temperature, pulse rate, and respiration rate, delivers medication which the patient takes by mouth, and helps the patient with personal needs.

What are the jobs of the nursing aides and nursing assistants?

Nursing aides and nursing assistants are usually trained by the hospital to take care of very routine patient needs. They usually do not have medical education or training, and they are not licensed. Their tasks include feeding patients who need help, helping patients get out of bed to go to the bathroom, helping patients move on and off bedpans, giving patients baths, and generally assisting patients to feel comfortable.

Is it true that hospitals seem to "shut down" on weekends and holidays?

Most hospitals, like many other businesses, seem to operate with a skeleton staff on weekends and holidays—so if you have any choice, and are not facing an emergency situation, be aware that it is wise to try to avoid holidays. If you are being operated on, try to check into the hospital on a Monday or Tuesday so that your tests and your surgery can be done before the end of the week.

Do I have a right to see my hospital records?

Though many nurses and doctors are extremely secretive about hospital records, you do have a right to see yours. You may not be able to understand much of what is in it because it is written in medical shorthand. Usually a nurse or a doctor will be present so that you will not misunderstand or misinterpret the information.

Can I refuse to be examined by a medical student?

This is a right that is yours—but many a helpful diagnosis has been made by a medical student who was doing his job as painstakingly as only a novice will. Usually, it will be to your advantage to allow the services of the soon-to-be-doctor. Of course, if you are feeling very ill and find the poking and probing troublesome, you have a perfect right to refuse such an examination.

Am I obligated to sign consent forms?

Consent forms are necessary before the doctor can go ahead with any procedure that entails any element of risk—surgery, anesthesia, spinal taps, etc. However, do not sign a blank consent form. Do not let the doctor get away with an explanation that he is not certain what the surgical procedure will entail and so is asking you to sign a consent form to be filled in later. Your doctor has an obligation to inform you of the risks and consequences of any procedure and to state the specific procedure for which you are being asked to give your consent. (Specifications for surgery should include the specific area to be operated on and the specific procedure the surgeon expects to perform.) Do not sign any form unless *all* your questions have been addressed.

How can I guard against medication errors in the hospital?

You should ask and know what medications your doctor has prescribed for you, what they are designed to do, and what they look like. If you have any question at all about a medication, ask the nurse to check the order book to make certain the doctor's orders have been followed or to check back with the doctor in case he has made an error. Many a medical disaster has been averted by a patient who asks: "Is this a new pill?" Be alert to what medications you are taking and why they are being given.

Suggested Reading

LEVIN, ARTHUR, M.D. *Talk Back to Your Doctor.* Garden City, N.Y.: Doubleday. $7.95.

chapter 3

Understanding What Cancer Is

What is cancer?
Cancer is a group of diseases in which there is irregular growth of abnormal cells.

How do normal cells and abnormal cells differ?
Normal cells grow in an orderly, controlled pattern. As normal cells wear out and die, new ones are produced. Just enough new cells grow to replace the old ones. Abnormal cells grow in an uncontrolled pattern; they never stop reproducing themselves, and soon there are many more of them than of the healthy cells in the tissue surrounding them.

Do all normal cells look alike?
No. Each normal cell has a specialized structure designed to do a particular job in a particular organ. For example, those cells which form the skin tend to be flat. The class of cells which make up the nerves are long and slender. Within each class, all normal cells are quite uniform in size and almost identical in shape. Each class of cells presents different arrangements when they join each other. For instance, glandular cells form circles which build upon each other like the stones lining a well. Skin cells stretch out in sheetlike layers row on row like a brick wall. These joined cells form tissues which arrange themselves in orderly patterns to form organs such as the breast, stomach, kidney, and so on.

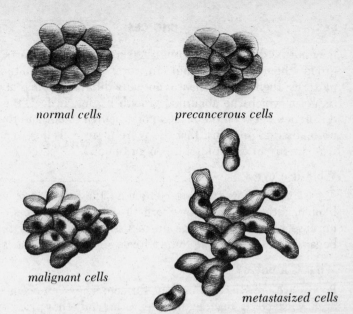

normal cells   precancerous cells

malignant cells

metastasized cells

How cancer grows

Are all growths or tumors cancer?

No. A tumor can be either benign (noncancerous) or malignant (cancerous). The word "tumor" itself is usually defined as "an abnormal mass of new tissue, the growth of which exceeds and is uncoordinated with that of normal tissue." The characteristic of a tumor is cell division—growth—that serves no useful purpose.

What is a benign tumor?

A benign tumor is a growth that is not cancerous. It has four main characteristics:

- It has limited growth potential and does not usually grow rapidly. It does not destroy normal cells while it is growing.
- It remains localized—that is, it does not metastasize (spread to other places).
- It usually does not produce any serious side effects, unless it is growing in a confined area such as the brain.
- It usually has an orderly and well-organized growth.

Are benign tumors dangerous?

Usually benign tumors do not endanger life, even though they are examples of abnormal growth. The cells in the benign tumor usually differ little from normal cells; in fact, as individuals they may not be distinguished from their normal counterparts. They group themselves together to form rather normal-looking patterns; their arrangement is not very different from that of the tissue in which the abnormal growth begins. In fact, the chief difference between the makeup of a benign tumor and that of a normal structure is just that there are more cells in a tumor.

A wart is an example of a benign tumor.

What is a cyst?

A cyst is a hollow swelling containing fluid. Cysts are usually benign, although cysts may form in cancerous tumors, either because the tumor is made up of tissue that secretes fluid or because the inside of the tumor breaks down and becomes fluid.

What is a polyp?

Polyps are growths in a mucous surface. They can occur in the nose, vocal cords, bladder, bowel, uterus, and other places where there is mucous membrane. Most polyps do not become malignant—but a small percentage are malignant from the start. Their removal is recommended by many doctors.

What do abnormal cells look like?

Abnormal or malignant cells vary in size and shape. They sometimes look almost like normal cells but most often are quite different-looking from the normal ones. The malignant cells do not organize themselves into normal patterns, although generally there is a tendency to reproduce the tissue in which they originate. For instance, skin-cancer cells tend to arrange themselves in the same sheetlike layers row on row as normal skin cells. But they do so imperfectly. Sometimes the cancer cells are so dissimilar from the normal structure that it is hard to identify the tissue from which the cancer started. The imperfection of the abnormal cell is the failure of the cancer cells to mature (or differentiate, as the physicians would say).

It has been said that cancer cells grow wild and uncontrolled. Is that true?

Not in the true sense of the terms. What the scientists are saying is that cancer cells are growing wild and uncontrolled in comparison with the normal cells around them. If a healthy normal cell is one that is slow-growing such as in the liver, then the cancerous liver cell is also slow-growing. There are also fast-growing and slow-growing tumors, which is why different tumors are treated with different kinds of drugs. The important fact is that the cancerous cells never stop reproducing and soon there are many more of them than of healthy cells in the tissue around them. Cancer cells do die but their death rate is lower than their birth rate.

Why are malignant or cancerous cells so dangerous?

Mainly because they deprive normal cells of nourishment and space. In most types of cancer, the cells build up into a mass of cells that compresses, invades, and destroys surrounding tissues. This mass is often called a growth, a tumor, or a neoplasm (new growth).

Do benign tumors become cancerous or malignant tumors?

In most cases they do not. The tumor that begins as a benign tumor usually remains a benign tumor. However, there are lesions that are considered precancerous, such as a thickening of the lining of the mouth. These should be taken care of before malignancy occurs.

What is a malignant tumor?

A malignant tumor is made up of cancer cells. This tumor also has four main characteristics:

- It divides and keeps dividing relentlessly; it reproduces in excess of the tissue's or organ's normal needs; it has a higher rate of cell growth than the normal tissues from which the cells came.
- It assumes, to a varying degree, a different appearance from the cells from which it came; the cells fail to maintain the boundaries of the normal tissues and organs; the cells resemble immature rather than mature tissues; they are without specific structure and function.
- It loses, to a varying degree, the ability to perform the functions of the tissues from which it came; the cells either stop that function, function differently, or function incompletely.
- It has uncontrolled movement; it is capable of breaking away and spreading throughout the body; the tumor tends to invade and destroy distant areas by spreading away from the

original site. This property varies from tumor to tumor.

Is it true that the more irregular the cells, the more malignant the cancer?

This is usually the case. As a general rule, the more abnormal (the doctors refer to it as undifferentiated) the cells look under the microscope, the more malignant the cancer. The greater the difference in their appearance from the normal cell, the more active the cancer is likely to be and the more uncontrollable its course. The term "differentiated" refers to malignant cells which resemble normal cells.

What is dysplasia?

Dysplasia refers to abnormal tissue development. It means that the cells or tissue are abnormal in their growth and organization for the location in which they are found. It does not mean necessarily that they are abnormal to the extent of being malignant, nor does it mean they have formed a tumor. Dysplasia occurs more often in tissues that "turn over" (or reproduce) frequently. Dysplasia may precede the development of some cancers by years or months. Not all dysplasia develops into cancer.

How many cells are in a cancerous tumor?

The number varies by the size of the tumor and the type of cell. First of all, you should understand that there is considerable variation in the size of cells making up the human body. The most numerous of the body cells are so small that it would take between 700 and 800 cells to cover the head of a pin. A 1-centimeter lump in the breast, which is a little larger than the size of a pea and is about the smallest lump which you can feel with your fingers, contains over a billion cells. This size tumor has undergone about 30 doublings since it first became an abnormal cell.

What is meant by doublings or by doubling time?

It is believed that cancer cells divide at a steady rate and the tumor steadily increases in size. One cell becomes two, two cells become four, four cells become eight. The body systematically continues the growth in this manner, with the number of cells doubling each time. The average length of time necessary for all the cells in a tumor to divide has been designated as the doubling time. With the passage of one doubling time, the number of cells in the mass is doubled and the weight of the mass is doubled. By the time a lump can be felt in the breast, for example, it has gone through at least 30 generations of doubling in size. The doubling time for breast cancer has been estimated to range from 6 to 540 days, depending upon the kind of cells and their rate of growth. That is why it is important that you see a doctor without delay as soon as you feel a lump.

Is cancer one disease?

No, cancer is believed to be not one disease, but many diseases. There are over 100 kinds of cancer, and each kind and site has its own distinguishing characteristics. Depending upon the location of the cancer in the body, the cause, symptoms, growth, kind of treatment, response to treatment, and possibility of cure are different. Cancer may behave very differently in different people. Generally, malignant tumors are divided into five main classifications, with many subdivisions in each group.

What are the five classifications of cancer?

The five classifications are:

- *Carcinomas:* These are the most common cancers. The tumors arise from tissues which cover a surface or line internal organs and passageways of the body (epithelial tissue). Skin, intestinal, uterine, and lung cancers are all carcinomas. There are several different kinds of carcinomas, including squamous cell, basal cell, transitional cell, and glandular epithelial.
- *Sarcomas:* These tumors arise in the connective tissue and muscles. They attack the bone, muscle, cartilage, and lymph system. Types of sarcoma include fibrosarcoma, liposarcoma, myosarcoma, chondrosarcoma, and osteosarcoma.
- *Myelomas:* These tumors arise in the plasma cells which are in the bone marrow. The plasma cells produce some of the protein that circulates in the blood.
- *Lymphomas:* These tumors arise in the cells of the lymph system. Lymph is a waterlike fluid that drains from all the tissues of the body through clusters of small glands called nodes. The nodes are the size and shape of lima beans and are

Major Classifications of Cancer

MEDICAL TERM	DEFINITION
Carcinoma	Originates from tissues that cover a surface or line a cavity of the body (epithelial tissue). This is the most common type of cancer.
Sarcoma	Originates from tissues which connect, support, or surround other tissues and organs. Can be either soft tissue or bone sarcomas.
Lymphoma	Originates in lymph system—the circulatory network of vessels, spaces, and nodes carrying lymph, the almost colorless fluid that bathes the body's cells.
Leukemia	Involves the blood-forming tissues and blood cells.
Myeloma	Originates in the bone marrow in the blood cells that manufacture antibodies.

Descriptions of behavior

Localized	Found only in the original or primary site; not spread to other parts of body.
Invasive	Cancer cells go beyond surface of tissues, invade tissues below but stay as one mass. A type of localized cancer.
Metastatic	Clumps of cells break off from original mass. Carried by lymphatic vessels or bloodstream to distant part of body. May also spread directly to another part of body.

found in many places in the body, such as the neck, the groin, the armpits, and the spleen. These glands swell up when bacteria or tumor cells drain into them or when the cells of which they are composed become malignant. The lymph system normally acts as a filter of impurities in the body. Hodgkin disease, for example, is a lymphoma.

• *Leukemia:* This is a cancer of the blood-forming tissues (bone marrow, lymph nodes, and spleen). It is characterized by the overproduction of white blood cells.

What does the doctor mean when he says I have a solid tumor?

A solid tumor means a tumor such as carcinoma and sarcoma which forms a mass of growth.

What is a disseminated tumor?

A disseminated tumor means a growth that is not confined to one area of the body; it has spread or has started to spread.

What is the meaning of the term "in situ"?

This is used to describe a noninvasive cancer. One of the most constant characteristics of cancer is the invasion of healthy tissues bordering the tumor. However, there appears to be a brief period before the invasion begins. Such growths are termed "in situ" and the results of removal are more positive than for cancers which have already begun to invade neighboring tissues. The term also applies to another group of tumors—usually found on surfaces—which have other characteristics of malignancy but in which normal cells may be completely replaced by tumor cells before there is evidence of invasion of surrounding tissues.

What is meant by the term "regression"?

Regression means that the tumor is getting smaller. This does not necessarily mean that the tumor has gone away, but if a tumor regresses far enough, it could eventually disappear altogether.

What is meant by the term "remission"?

Remission can be partial or complete. If it is complete, it means that all symptoms and signs of the disease are gone, although cancer cells usually remain in the body. The patient does not feel any of the former symptoms, and the doctors cannot find clinical signs of the tumor. A partial remission means that some of the signs and symptoms are gone.

Is a remission a cure?

A remission may or may not be a cure. Sometimes the disease can be in remission for anywhere from weeks to years, while undetected tumor cells in the body remain inactive. Eventually, though, they may begin to grow again until once more they produce symptoms.

Is cancer ever cured?

The term "cure" is used only after a patient's disease has been in remission for a long enough time to indicate that the cancer probably has been completely destroyed. Cure means that the treatment is successful and that all the cancer cells have been removed or destroyed. In terms of symptoms and test results, cure is almost the same as remission. For many kinds of cancer, five years of remission is considered a cure. This is because if cancer has spread to other areas it will usually become apparent and begin to cause problems within the five-year period. The length of remission necessary for cure differs for various kinds of cancer. In some kinds of skin cancer, for example, a person is considered cured as soon as the spot of cancer is removed. On the other hand, certain tumors are not considered cured until eight or ten years have passed.

What is meant by the term "high risk"?

Risks in medical terms are arrived at by looking at the various characteristics of a group of people and by comparing that to how often something occurs. Being at "high risk" means that your chances of getting the disease are somewhat greater than those of the general population, but it certainly does *not* mean you will get the disease.

What does the doctor mean when he says the cancer is localized?

When cancer is localized, it means that it is found only in the original or primary site; that it has not spread or metastasized to another part of the body.

What is invasive cancer?

Invasive cancer is when some of the cancer cells go beyond the surface of the tissues and "invade" the tissues around them. After invading, the cancer continues to grow, though for a time the cancer cells may remain as one mass. Sometimes the mass can be seen by the naked eye. As long as all the living cancer cells remain where the disease started, the cancer is still said to be localized.

Do all cancers spread the same way?

No. Cancer cells spread in several ways. Some cancers, like certain skin cancers, simply keep growing in the same location, becoming bigger and bigger until they invade normal neighboring tissue and destroy it. Other cancers keep growing in the original site but also spread, through the bloodstream and lymphatic system, to distant parts of the body.

What does the doctor mean when he says the cancer is about 2 centimeters in size?

Perhaps it will help if you can visualize the size of the cancer by comparing it with objects you know. For instance, a pea is slightly smaller than a centimeter; a marble or a dime is slightly larger than a centimeter. A cherry or a nickel would be about 2 centimeters. A ping-pong ball and a half dollar would be about 3 centimeters. A golf ball or a silver dollar would about equal 4 centimeters. A hen's egg would be about 5 centimeters, a baseball about 7 centimeters, and a grapefruit about 10 or 12 centimeters.

The doctor said my cancer has metastasized. What does that mean?

The process by which cancer spreads from where it began (that is, from the primary tumor) to distant parts of the body is called metastasis. Tiny clumps of cells break off from the tumor and are carried in the lymphatic vessels or the bloodstream to a distant part of the body. These "seeds" from the original cancer start growing in the new place. The new tumor is said to have metastasized to the new site, and such a tumor is often referred to as a metastatic tumor. The plural of "metastasis" is "metastases." Sometimes you will hear the word "mets," a shorthand term for "metastases."

Where does cancer usually spread to?

Different types of cancer have different tendencies to spread to certain organs. Breast cancer, for instance, generally spreads or metastasizes from the breast (primary site) to four places in the body: liver, bone, lung, and brain. More rarely, it can spread to the spinal cord, to distant lymph nodes, and to other places such as the face, lips, urological and genital areas, and alimentary tract. The identification of metastases is the most decisive factor in the choice of treatment and the success of the treatment.

When a tumor metastasizes or spreads, is it called by the organ to which it has spread?

No. If the original tumor is in the breast and it has spread to the bone, it is not then bone cancer. It is breast cancer in the bones. The type of cancer cells found in the bones will be the same type as the cancer cells found in the breast. These cells will grow, reproduce, and behave according to the pattern of metastatic breast cancer (breast cancer which has spread into other areas) and not like bone cancer. Because of this fact, metastatic cancer of any kind is generally treated in the way the original cancer responds best. In other words, cancer that starts in the breast and spreads to the bones is not treated the same way that cancer which starts in the bones would be treated, but is treated like breast cancer.

We hear so much about cancer these days—is it a new disease?

No. Cancer is more than a million years old. Evidence of cancer has been found in skeletons of prehistoric animals and in Etruscan, Peruvian, and Egyptian mummies. The reason you hear more about it today is that it is a general disease of older people, and as people live longer (since we have cured many of the ailments which used to cause people to die younger), more people are getting cancer.

At what age do persons usually get cancer?

Cancer is predominantly a disease of middle and old age. In the United States, 66 percent of cancer in men and 63 percent of cancer in women is diagnosed at age 55 or over. Persons at about the age of 70 account for a higher number of cases than any other age group. Overall, in new cases of cancer, men and women account for about the same number.

Don't young children sometimes get cancer?

Cancer is quite rare in children and in young adults. However, for children under 15, cancer is the second leading cause of death, accounting for 1 out of 28 deaths. Leukemia is the most common form of childhood cancer, followed by tumors of the central nervous system.

What does the word "oncology" mean?

"Oncology" is from the Greek word *onkos*, meaning "bulk" or "mass," and refers to the study and treatment of a large variety of tumors. The doctors who specialize in cancer treatment are called oncologists. There are surgical oncologists, medical oncologists, radiation oncologists, pediatric oncologists, and gynecological oncologists.

Does cancer run in families?

Cancer is a common disease, and some "clustering" of cases in families will occur by chance alone. However, there is some limited information which suggests that there is some increased family risk of developing cancer of the same site for cancers of the female breast, stomach, large intestine, endometrium, prostate, lung, and possibly ovary. It is known, for example, that a woman whose mother and/or sisters have had breast cancer is at a risk approximately two times higher than average. Brain tumors and sarcomas also seem to occur more frequently than expected in brothers and sisters of children with these tumors. When an identical twin has childhood leukemia, the probability that the other twin will develop the disease within two years of the date of diagnosis of the first twin is about one in five, far greater than the rate for the general population. A rare cancer of the eye, bilateral retinoblastoma, also seems to run in families. The chances that a patient cured of this kind of cancer will have a child with it are high. Scientists still do not know whether family clustering of cancer cases is due to inherited characteristics or to other factors, such as diet or occupation, which may continue unchanged from one generation to the next.

Is a cancer patient likely to develop a second cancer?

Persons with cancers of the skin, mouth, colon, and rectum run an increased risk of a second cancer in the same organ. Patients with cancers of the breast, ovary, and, perhaps, lung run a slightly higher risk of developing the disease in the paired organ. There is some evidence that tumors of certain different sites often occur together. Such combinations include colon and breast, colon and endometrium, uterine cervix and rectum, and combinations of sites in the female reproductive organs, digestive tract, and respiratory system.

Is there a cancer "smell"?

Not as such. There are some open wounds which do have an odor, whether the person has cancer or some other disease. It is important, if the patient has such a wound, to change the dressing often and to dispose of the dressing when it is changed.

Can you "catch" cancer?

There is no indication that cancer can be considered contagious in the popular sense of the word. You should not be afraid that you will "catch" cancer. There is no evidence to suggest that living in the same household with a cancer patient over a long period of time, sharing his or her possessions, kissing, or having intercourse with a cancer patient will increase your chances of getting cancer.

Are there any basic warning signs of cancer?

There are seven basic symptoms of cancer as emphasized by the American Cancer Society:

- Unusual bleeding or discharge
- A lump that does not go away
- A sore that does not heal within two weeks
- Change in bowel or bladder habits
- Persistent hoarseness or cough
- Indigestion or difficulty in swallowing
- Change in a wart or mole

Any of these symptoms signal you to see a doctor. They might mean you have cancer, but in most cases the doctor will find you do not. The most important thing is that the symptoms should be checked out by a doctor, for only a doctor can make a definite diagnosis.

Can I have cancer without any of these symptoms?

It is possible. But the symptoms seem so trivial to most people that they may be ignored. For example, coughs are so common that we do not get alarmed when we have one. Usually you can tell yourself that you have been smoking too much or blame your sinuses or say that everybody is coughing at the office. However, coughing can also be the first visible sign of lung cancer. Irregular vaginal bleeding can be due to a whole list of causes, which can lull you into not bothering to see a doctor. But irregular vaginal bleeding can also be the first sign of cancer of the uterus. What all this means is that any suspicious symptom that persists longer than expected should be investigated by a qualified physician.

What does "staging" mean?

Staging is the process doctors go through to tell how much cancer there is in the body and where it is located. It is necessary for the doctor to have this information to plan your treatment. Staging is also a way for doctors to communicate with each other about your specific case.

Why is staging needed?

The doctor needs to understand the amount of cancer in your body in order to give you the right treatment for your specific kind. The treatment for breast cancer at one stage of the disease, for example, is different from what it is at another stage. Your doctor also needs to anticipate the course your disease is likely to take. Staging also makes it possible to compare the results of the different treatments being used by different physicians in different parts of this country and around the world.

What is the doctor looking for when he stages cancer?

The doctor wants to know basic information about the original (primary) tumor—what size and type it is, where it is in the body, whether or not it has spread to other areas around the original site, and whether or not it has spread to other parts of the body away from the original site.

Are the answers to these questions important?

The answers to these preliminary questions are vital. Tumors must be staged at the beginning of the diagnosis to the fullest extent possible in order to give you the most effective treatment. For example, if the doctor finds that the cancer which began in your lung has already spread to other parts of your body, he may decide to treat you with chemotherapy and radiation rather than surgery, since an operation might offer little or no chance of cure for you and could seriously weaken your system.

How does the doctor decide on the stage of the disease?

There are four types of evidence used for classifying the extent of disease at different sites and at different time periods:

- *Clinical-diagnostic staging:* This is determining how much cancer there is by what the doctor can see and feel by any means other than looking at cells under the microscope. This includes examination of the tumor by x-rays and tests.
- *Surgical-evaluative staging:* This term is used to describe the extent of the disease as known after a major surgical exploration or biopsy or both.
- *Postsurgical treatment—pathologic staging:* This is determining the stage of the disease by examining the tumor directly, looking at cells under the microscope.

- *Retreatment staging:* This is determining the extent of the disease when additional or new treatments are being given for the same disease.

What do the letters "TNM" stand for in the TNM classification system?

Cancer is sometimes classified by the letters TNM.

T, plus the numbers 1 through 4, stands for the primary tumor. This is used to describe the size and/or level of invasion. The higher the number, the larger the size of the tumor and/or the depth or amount of involvement in the local area of the tumor. TX means the tumor cannot be assessed. TO means there is no evidence of primary tumor. TIS means carcinoma in situ.

N, plus the numbers 1 through 4, indicates whether or not there is evidence that the tumor has spread to the regional lymph nodes, the size of the nodes involved, and the number of nodes involved. NX means the regional lymph nodes cannot be assessed clinically. NO means regional lymph nodes are not demonstrably abnormal.

M, with a zero or plus sign, indicates the absence or presence of distant metastases (cancer which has spread to other parts of the body). A letter is sometimes added to the M to show the other areas involved. P, for instance, would indicate "pulmonary"—that the cancer has spread to the lungs. MX means the metastasis is not assessed. MO means there are no known distant metastases.

Do these letters and numbers mean the same thing for every kind of cancer?

Each tumor type has its own classification system. Some sites of cancer do not as yet have an agreed-upon classification and staging. Some types of cancer, such as lymphomas, use a different system from the one just described.

A T1 in lung cancer and in breast cancer means about the same, although a T1 breast tumor is less than or equal to 2 centimeters in size and a T1 lung tumor is less than or equal to 3 centimeters in size. Also the treatment for the two types of cancer would be different. The variation depends upon what the doctors know about each kind of tumor, how it spreads, what treatments are most effective at each stage, and what the prognosis is.

What does it mean when the doctor says I have Stage I disease?

This means your disease is curable in the highest degree. Staging numbers were originally used by doctors to indicate how far the disease had advanced—Stage I being the most curable, Stage IV the least curable. Staging is still used to define cancers, but more refined designations include the T, N, and M categories. Many hundreds of doctors and many national and international committees are working at trying to standardize cancer language so it can be interpreted accurately by all doctors.

What are examples of how to interpret the letter designations?

Here are a few examples of how to interpret a series of letters when you see them on your reports or when they are used as a reference by the doctor.

- *Stage I, T1, NO, MO.* This would tell you that clinical examination reveals a mass or tumor limited to the organ where it appears. The tumor is operable, with only local involvement. There is no nodal spread or signs of metastases.
- *Stage II, T2, N1, MO:* This indicates that there is evidence of local spread into surrounding tissue. The tumor is operable, but because of its location and size, there is uncertainty as to completeness of removal. There is evidence that there is spread to the lymph nodes but no signs of metastases.

Most parts of the body which are commonly affected by cancer have their own sets of designations, although some sites have not yet been classified by the medical profession. The T classifications are designed to pinpoint the size and location by individual area. The N (node) and M (metastases) designations follow a fairly standard pattern. Unfortunately, because many new advances in diagnosis have been made in the past few years, many of the classifications are in the process of evolving and new, changing criteria are being used. The material in this book, both in this chapter and where it appears in other parts of the book dealing with specific parts of the body, is meant to act as a guide to you in better understanding your disease. You can ask your doctor for further explanations, if the information is not detailed enough.

chapter 4

Diagnostic Tests

Questions You Should Ask Your Doctor When He Orders Tests

- What is the test for?
- What will the procedure be like?
- What will you learn from the test?
- Why is it important for me to have the test?
- Will I need to be hospitalized for the test? For how long?
- Can it be done on an outpatient basis instead? Why not?
- How much will the test cost?
- What risks are there in doing the testing?
- When will we get the results of the test?
- What decisions will I have to make if the test is positive?

Questions You Need to Ask Yourself When You Get Your Diagnosis and Before You Make Appointments for Surgery or Other Treatment

- Is this the doctor I want to handle my case?
- Am I comfortable with him?
- Is he someone who understands how I feel and is sensitive to my needs?
- Do I have enough information about my case to make a judgment?
- Who do I want with me when I receive my diagnosis?
- Should I have a second opinion?

- Should I go to a large medical center for more diagnostic work or for my treatment?
- Which hospital will I go to for my surgery and treatment?
- Have I had the appropriate tests to see if the cancer has spread before surgery is done?

Questions to Think About When You Are Facing a Diagnosis of Cancer

QUESTION	REMARKS
Do I want to know exactly what plans the doctor has for my treatment and what alternative treatments there might be for my type of cancer?	Many people want to participate in the decisions about the treatment of their illness. Knowledge about the treatment plan is important to you if you want to be a part of the decision of how and where you will receive treatment.
Do I want to ask the doctor for a second pathologist to do an independent report?	The pathology report is the basis on which all future decisions will be made. You should think about talking with your doctor about how the pathology report was done, whether he has talked with the pathologist, whether or not there is any question or doubt about the diagnosis. If there is, ask to have the pathology checked by the laboratory of a large hospital or medical center.
Do I want to know specifically what kind of cancer I have and the stage it is in?	Some people do. They like to have all the facts so they can do research at the medical library to find out what treatments are being offered. Others do not. However, if you have a rare type of cancer, you should know it, because you need to decide whether you want to go to one of the cancer centers or medical schools that are specializing in your type of disease for consultation or treatment. Or you should at least ask your doctor to have a phone consultation with a physician doing research in the area.
Do I want my doctor to consult with the nearest cancer center or cooperative group about my case? Do I want to make some phone calls myself?	There are clinical cooperative groups across the country specializing in treating particular types of cancer. Controlled studies are being conducted to determine the best possible treatments. Your doctor needs the latest information to give you the best possible treatment.

QUESTION	REMARKS
Do I want to go to a cancer center or medical school for my treatment?	You need to weigh this decision most carefully. The cancer centers and other hospitals specializing in cancer treatment have on their staffs doctors who are especially trained in the various cancer disciplines. In the course of a week, they will probably be treating more patients with your illness than many local doctors see in a year. On the other hand, the practical question of geography and your emotional energy will have to be considered.

What are the kinds of tests used to help detect cancer?

The tests used to detect cancer depend upon the kind of cancer and the degree to which it has spread. They fall into the following categories:

- Clinical history and physical examination, routine blood, urine, heart exams, chest x-ray
- X-ray examinations
- Optical instruments (endoscopy)
- Examination of sloughed-off cells (cytology)
- Radioactive scans
- Ultrasound
- CT scans (also called CAT or ACTA scans)
- Biopsies

Do doctors do too many diagnostic tests?

Sometimes, but in the area of cancer, it seems that the problem is that too *few* diagnostic tests are done before operating rather than too many. Laboratory tests are a vital part of any diagnostic workup, but especially so in the treatment of cancer. It is of major importance for the doctor to determine if the cancer has spread to other areas from the primary site of the growth. If it has already spread from the primary site, in many cases an operation may not be advisable. Instead chemotherapy or radiation treatment may be used. The treatment for cancer which has spread, therefore, is different from the treatment for cancer which is located only in the primary site. A good, thorough workup is vital before any surgery at all is done for cancer.

Are the risks great in waiting to do the surgery while spending time to do the diagnostic tests?

There is very little conclusive evidence to show that there is harm in delaying a short time (such as two weeks) while you are having the diagnostic tests. Of course, occasionally rapid treatment is necessary for some specific problems of cancer patients. There is, of course, harm in delaying seeing the doctor if you have suspicious symptoms such as a lump in your breast or blood in your stool.

What are some of the things the doctor should tell me about the tests he is going to do or going to order?

The doctor should tell you what the test is for, what the procedure will be like, what he feels he will learn from the test, why it is important for your symptoms, what the risk of the test is, whether you need to be hospitalized, how much it will cost to do the test, and when you can get the results. If the doctor does not offer this information, ask for it.

What kind of risks are there in the tests done for cancer?

The risks depend upon the test and on the condition of the person on whom the test is being done. Certainly the more simple ones, such as blood counts, involve little or no risk. X-rays which involve small amounts of radiation are low-risk tests. However, some of the x-rays, as well as some of the procedures, do involve quite a bit of risk. Risks are discussed in this chapter, along with the procedures. You should ask the doctor to discuss the risk versus the benefit of the tests he recommends. Generally in the area of cancer, the benefits of the tests are worth the risks.

What is the best place to go for laboratory tests?

In general, the most reliable laboratories are in the hospitals. However, there are many independent labs (independent of doctors' offices or hospitals) which also do an excellent job. Many small independent laboratories do so few of some tests that the results may be questionable. The results are only as accurate as the person or laboratory doing them.

Is it all right for me to ask for information about testing, test results, and other procedures?

It certainly is. You are entitled to all information that the doctor has about your case.

How long does it take to establish a diagnosis?

Ask your doctor about the time it will take. This will depend upon several factors—and the slightest delay will seem like an eternity because you will be living with the fear of the unknown. A full evaluation can take from several days to several weeks—or may even have to be postponed because a decision cannot be made for any of a number of reasons. Don't be in a rush for that final diagnosis. Allow time for as many diagnostic procedures, additional consultations, and reviews as you can. This is the point in your treatment that is most important to you—because what happens at this point sets the stage for determining much of the future course of your disease.

It is at this point that you must evaluate the following:

- Is this the doctor I want to handle my case?
- Do I have enough information about my case to make a judgment?
- Am I comfortable with him?
- Is he someone who understands how I feel and is sensitive to my needs?
- Whom do I want with me when I receive my diagnosis?
- Should I have a second opinion?
- Should I go to one of the large medical centers for more complete diagnosis and treatment?
- What hospital will I go to for my surgery and treatment?

Won't my doctor be offended if I ask for another opinion?

If he is, you should find yourself another doctor. The important thing to remember is that most doctors *welcome* a second opinion. Because the public has held doctors in reverence for so long, many people think that the doctor will be upset if they ask for a second opinion. But *a second opinion does not mean you are questioning your doctor's competence.* If you have cancer, a decision about how you proceed with treatment is probably the most important decision you will make in your life. You need the best advice you can get before proceeding with a course of treatment. You don't hesitate to check out various makes and models of cars when you are making a decision about buying one. Certainly you should not hesitate to check out all the possible angles when making a decision about your health.

Can I do this tactfully?

Yes. Often it is easier if you ask your husband, wife, sister, or whoever usually accompanies you to help you with this. He or she can simply explain to your doctor that before going any further you would like to have a confirming opinion. This is *not* an unusual or unreasonable request. It is a very *necessary* step for you to take. The doctor may explain that the x-rays and tests are conclusive as far as he is concerned. Don't let that put you off and agree to go along with his treatment. A second opinion will strengthen his conclusions and set your mind at ease.

Who will recommend a specialist to me?

Usually, this is something that your primary doctor will do. Sometimes he will give you more than one name. You should ask about the specialist's credentials, such as:

- Why do you recommend this particular doctor?
- Is he a specialist in the operation (or field)? How often does he perform this particular operation (or service)?
- Is he board-certified?
- Is he on the staff of an accredited hospital?

There are some competent doctors who are not board-certified, but your doctor should be able to tell you why he has chosen the specific specialists he is recommending.

What do I tell the doctor who is doing the consulting?

When you call, explain that you have already had a diagnosis and are coming to him for a consultation. Don't make the mistake of trying to let him think you haven't been to another doctor. Using him on a consulting basis means that you will get a straight answer, since he has nothing to gain from recommending one treatment over another.

How do I go about finding the right doctor for a second opinion?

- You can ask your own doctor to suggest the name of someone to see for a second opinion.

- You can make the appointment yourself or you can ask the doctor to make the appointment for you.
- You should always discuss your plans for consultation with your doctor. He has your original x-rays and tests, which the other doctor will need in his deliberation. If your doctor is uncooperative, then you have other decisions to make about continuing your relationship with him.
- You can call the nearest cancer center (many of them have a toll-free 800 number) and ask for names of doctors who will give second opinions. If there isn't one close to you, you can call the toll-free number of the National Cancer Institute (see Chapter 23).
- You can call your nearest medical school and ask for suggestions.
- You can call the nearest unit of the American Cancer Society or state or local medical society.
- You can check the Directory of Medical Specialists at your library and call the specialist directly.
- You can check the Directory of Medical Specialists, get the names of two or three top-notch doctors in the area, and ask your doctor to suggest which one he thinks you should see.

Is a medical school's outpatient clinic a good place to go for a second opinion?

Yes. This is probably one of the best places to turn for a second opinion. Physicians who practice there are on the faculty of the medical school and are usually using the latest methods of treatment. Because most outpatient clinics are divided into specialties, this is where some of the top specialists in the country are practicing. You can contact the clinic by calling the medical school and explaining that you are interested in contacting a doctor at the clinic who specializes in the area of your specific problem. Don't be afraid to explain that you want to get a second opinion and what your experience has been to date. Each clinic, of course, has its own setup—but most have appointment secretaries who are very knowledgeable about the clinic and the doctors in their service and will be most helpful in making arrangements for a consultation.

What will such a consultation cost?

You will be amazed to find that some of the finest physicians in the country charge no more—and sometimes much less—than doctors with far less experience and expertise. Fees may range from $25 to $100. Part of the reason is that medical-school-faculty clinic physicians are often salaried and their fees return to the medical school.

Does such a consultation mean I have to go to that institution for my treatment?

No, you have free choice in this matter—and the decision should be yours. Sometimes people shy away from getting expert advice from doctors at a large medical center because they feel this will mean that they will have to return to the medical center for their treatments. However, this is not the case. Many medical and cancer centers diagnose and recommend treatment for patients to be followed by doctors in local communities. If the medical center is a long distance from your home and you do not want to be bothered with the expense and inconvenience of returning there each time you need treatment, you can take advantage of a consultation and continue to be treated at your local hospital by your own doctor—but with the added experience and continuing advice of the specialist at the medical center.

Who pays for a second opinion?

Some insurance companies now pay for second opinions. Even if your particular insurance company does not, the cost should be less than for the first consultation, because all of the test results and x-rays are available to the second doctor.

What if the second opinion differs from the first doctor's advice?

Second opinions can sometimes be confusing. If the first doctor recommends a course of treatment different from the second, you are left more confused than when you started. You have three alternatives in this case: Ask the two doctors to discuss the case to see if they can resolve the conflict, ask for a third opinion and accept the majority decision (two out of three), or follow your own instincts about what is best for you.

What is the difference between a referral and a consultation?

If your doctor decides that your illness requires the attention of a specialist, he will recommend the names of one or several specialists for you to see. This is called a referral and differs from a consultation. A referral means that once you see the specialist you become his patient. For a consultation, a consultant is called in to advise you and your doctor but does not take over responsibility for treating you.

If I am unhappy with my doctor, should I ask him for a referral or a consultation?

When you are satisfied with your doctor but want to get a second opinion because you want confirmation of a diagnosis, you should ask for a consultation. However, if you are really unhappy with your doctor and the kind of treatment he has been giving you and if you really feel that someone else should be handling your case, what you want is not a consultation but a referral. Ask your doctor to refer you to the top specialist in the area dealing with your condition. Many times, this is a step that may be difficult for the patient to take and can be more easily handled by a family member or a friend. The important thing to remember is not to waste time trying to be patient about the treatment being received when in your own mind you know that things are not going as well as they should. Be bold and ask the doctor for a referral.

Can I take advantage of a comprehensive cancer center or research center while using my own local hospital?

Yes, you can, and it is wise to do so. You can make an appointment to be seen by the specialists at the cancer center or research center for a consultation. Most of the comprehensive cancer centers maintain a "hotline" service; your doctor can call for information on getting a consultation with a doctor on the staff to discuss a case, or you can call for information. As stated before, these centers are designed for treatment of cancer patients and most have the most up-to-date cancer information available.

What do I do if I want a second opinion and I am already hospitalized?

It is a little more difficult to arrange unless your doctor is agreeable to your having it. Explain to your doctor that before you go ahead with any treatment you would like to have another consultation. If there is a specialist on the hospital staff who is qualified, arranging a consultation will be easier than if the specialist is located at another hospital. However, don't allow difficulties to deter you from seeking a consultation that will give you further insight into what alternatives are open to you. Even when you are hospitalized, it is still your right to demand that your doctor find another physician—even one from another hospital—to give you an independent opinion. Some hospitals have patient advocate services which can be helpful in this kind of situation.

Is it a good idea to get a second opinion on a pathology report?

The kind of treatment you will get and the outlook for your future are often based on the pathology report. Pathologists are human—and pathology is not an exact science. The diagnosis of cancer sometimes requires more than just the examination of a very thin slice of tissue through a series of lenses which magnify the tissues several hundred times. Question the pathology report. Ask your doctor whether he has consulted personally with the pathologist. Many doctors do this as a routine matter. If the doctor has not already done so, indicate that you would like the opinion of a second pathologist to confirm the first report. In most large hospitals where several pathologists are employed, consultations are routine, assuring the patient that the report is the consensus of a number of trained pathologists.

How are clinical histories taken?

First, the physician or a trained medical assistant takes a family history, exploring the kinds of illnesses and diseases you have had, whether or not there has been a history of cancer in your family, and the kinds of medication or radiation administered to your mother during pregnancy and to yourself during your lifetime. He asks questions about your body's organs and any suspicious symptoms you may have noticed. You may be asked about your work area, whether or not you are exposed to carcinogens such as asbestos or vinyl chloride, and your smoking habits.

If I have no cancer symptoms and I go to a doctor for a complete cancer-detecting physical, what should that physical consist of?

There is certainly not full agreement on what a comprehensive cancer-detecting physical should consist of. Here are some of the items a complete checkup for detecting hidden cancer could involve:

- Complete medical and family history
- Complete blood count
- Complete urinalysis
- Digital rectal exam
- Proctosigmoidoscopy for persons over 40
- Pelvic exam and Pap test for women
- Chest x-ray
- Manual examination of the abdomen, thyroid gland
- Examination of the prostate gland in men and breasts in women (mammography if called for)
- Check of all skin areas
- Mouth check using a mirror to see into throat and larynx
- Eye exam with a lighted instrument
- Test for occult blood in the stool

Why does the doctor always order basic blood and urine tests?

These simple tests, sometimes called CBC (complete blood count), SMA 12 (serum factors), and UA (urine analysis), give the doctor a great deal of basic information about your general health problems. They can usually be done in the doctor's office.

What does the complete blood count consist of?

The technician takes whole blood from your vein as well as a blood smear from your finger and uses it to check the hemoglobin, white blood cell count, and complete red and white cells in the blood and the platelets. The hematocrit test requires that the blood be spun in a centrifuge and measures (usually on an automatic counting machine with computer printout) the volume of red cells as a percent of the total volume. This test can help detect if anemia is present, though it cannot identify the type of anemia. The hemoglobin test measures the number of grams of red cell pigment in 100 cubic centimeters of blood. A low count is a sign of some type of anemia. The white cell count (listed as WBC) shows the number of white cells per cubic millimeter of blood. Usually if this count is elevated it points to infection.

The microscopic examination and count of the blood smear

helps to determine the type of infection, type of anemia, or blood-clotting conditions. The technician examines the smear to determine the proportions of various types and numbers of white cells (called differential), the size and shape of red cells, and the number of platelets present.

What does the urinalysis tell the doctor?

The degree of concentration of the urine (weight of urine relative to plain water), called specific gravity (SG), indicates urinary obstruction with kidney damage if the count is low or dehydration if the count is high. Using a simple plastic strip with a series of chemically sensitive patches, the doctor or his nurse or technician can also check the amount of acidity, protein, sugar, and ketones in the urine—to diagnose acidosis or alkalosis, kidney damage, diabetes, etc. The microscopic examination of centrifuged urine called the urine sediment exam checks for red cells, white cells, kidney cells, crystals, and microorganisms in the urine which might indicate kidney damage, urinary-tract infection, or gout.

Are blood tests used for detecting cancer?

At the present time there is no one blood test which conclusively tells if cancer is present, either for the initial diagnosis of cancer or for monitoring disease recurrence. The tests now available are not sufficiently accurate—they may be negative when no cancer is present and also when it is known that the person has cancer. Sometimes they are positive when cancer is not present. Therefore they are currently being used only along with other cancer detection exams. There are several studies now being conducted to determine whether or not there might be some blood tests which can be used to tell if cancer is present.

Is the CEA (carcinoembryonic antigen) test now being used?

The CEA test detects changes in the body that often accompany cancers. This test is now being used but only in combination with other established procedures for both diagnosing and managing cancer. Although it may be useful as an early indication of recurrence in some patients previously treated for cancer, alone it is not a conclusive test either for initial diagnosis or for monitoring disease recurrence.

What is the hemocult test?

The hemocult test, also called the occult stool test or the guaiac test, detects blood in the stool not visible to the naked eye. Usually the doctor will tell you to eat a diet containing a lot of roughage and no meat for four days. Starting on the second day of the diet, two samples are taken from each of the next three stools passed. Each sample is smeared on a labeled slide. The slides are impregnated with guaiac, a resin which when mixed with blood and treated with hydrogen peroxide turns a deep-blue color. The slides are analyzed for human blood in the stool, which might be an indication of a precancerous or cancerous condition. Though the reliability of this test is still being evaluated, it is used as a supplement to other rectal examinations and may someday be used as a widespread screening device for colon cancer.

What routine is followed in doing an ECG (EKG) exam?

The electrocardiogram is an electrical record of the performance of the heart. When the heart muscle contracts and relaxes, changes are produced which can be picked up from the skin surface by electrodes applied to the various parts of the body. This test is part of most routine physical examinations when a patient is past 40, and is a part of most routine hospital examinations. The electrodes—round, cold metal discs—are smeared with a jellylike substance to heighten conductivity. They are attached to the wrists and ankles. Another disc is used by the operator to move in a series of prescribed positions on the chest. The wires or "leads" record the vertical peaks and horizontal lines made as the heartbeat travels from an upper chamber to the lower chamber of the heart. An inked stylus traces the pattern on graphed paper affixed to a drum that rolls through the electrocardiograph machine. From this tracing, the doctor has a graphic record of the patient's heartbeat.

What is a lumbar puncture?

A lumbar puncture is a diagnostic procedure usually performed under local anesthesia in which a thin needle is inserted in the space between the two lower vertebrae of the spine to remove fluid that normally is in this area. Lumbar punctures (also called spinal taps) are used in cancer, for instance, to diagnose leukemia in the central nervous system. This examination indicates the pressure within the spinal fluid system and can show evidence of tumor, infection, or inflammation in the central nervous system.

When are x-rays used in diagnosis?

X-rays are an important part of the diagnostic workup. X-rays are used to detect and diagnose many forms of cancer, including cancer of the lung, digestive tract, and breast. They are also used to determine whether the cancer has spread to places such as the lung or the bone. Properly taken and read, x-rays are one of the doctor's most valuable diagnostic tools.

What are the main kinds of x-rays?

There are two major types of diagnostic x-rays: plain films and contrast films.

What are plain films?

These are the regular, standard x-rays you have always known. They are ordinary films of various parts of the body. A chest x-ray is an example of a plain film. For a tumor to be seen on a standard x-ray it must be big enough and it must be more dense than the surrounding normal tissues. Tumors are not always detectable on an x-ray.

What are contrast films?

A contrast film is used when some foreign substance is put into the body to contrast with normal body tissues. For example, a chemical dye or air or a radioactive material may be introduced into the body to allow some organ to be outlined on the x-ray. A barium-enema x-ray is an example of a contrast film.

What is meant by air-contrast x-rays?

This is when air is introduced into a selected part of the body. It is used to outline soft-tissue structures within the body. Since air does not absorb x-rays like the surrounding tissues, it provides a contrast on the film. Depending on the test, the air may be inhaled, swallowed, injected, or obtained from carbonated beverages. For example, a deep breath held during a chest x-ray fills the lungs with air. X-rays pass through the air readily so the tissues surrounding the lungs will show up, and any areas where the lungs do not readily fill up with air will be cloudy on the x-rays.

What are the names of some of the different kinds of contrast-film tests using dye?

There are many of them, and their names normally correspond with the part of the body being tested:

- *Barium enema (BE)* outlines the colon (intestines) and rectum. Barium is given rectally by enema.
- *Barium swallow* outlines the upper digestive tract including the pharynx and esophagus. Barium is swallowed.
- *Bronchogram* outlines the bronchial tree. Dye is injected into the lung bronchi (air passages). High-risk procedure.
- *Cerebral angiogram* outlines the blood vessels in the neck and brain. Dye is injected into carotid and/or vertebral arteries in the neck. Also called an arteriogram. High-risk procedure.
- *Coronary angiogram* outlines the heart chambers, valves, and surrounding arteries in the veins. Dye is injected into the chambers of the heart. Also called an arteriogram. High-risk procedure.
- *Cholecystogram* outlines the biliary tract (gallbladder and bile ducts). Contrast medium is given as pills twelve hours before x-rays are taken.
- *Cystogram* outlines urinary bladder (cystourethogram outlines bladder and urethra). Dye is placed in bladder by means of urinary catheter.
- *GI series* outlines the stomach, duodenum, and remainder of the small intestine. The contrast medium is swallowed.
- *Hysterogram* outlines inside of uterus and the fallopian tubes (hysterosalpingogram outlines uterus and oviducts). Dye is injected through a vaginal catheter into uterus.
- *Intravenous pyelogram (IVP)* outlines the urinary tract (kidneys, ureters and bladder). Dye is injected into the arm vein.
- *Lienography* outlines the spleen. Dye is injected.
- *Lymphangiogram* outlines the lymph nodes. Dye is injected into involved lymph system—usually used for patients with Hodgkin disease, lymphomas, or testicular cancer.
- *Myelogram* outlines the spinal cord and adjacent structures. Dye is injected by needle into the fluid surrounding the spinal cord.
- *Pneumoencephalogram (PEG)* outlines the chambers and

surface of the brain. Air is injected and rises into the brain. High-risk procedure.

- *Pulmonary angiogram* outlines blood vessels (arteries and veins) in the lungs. Dye is injected into the pulmonary arteries as they leave the heart. High-risk procedure.
- *Venogram* outlines the venous system of the body. Dye is injected into vein.

Why are some of the contrast films noted as high-risk procedures?

Most of the contrast films involve little risk. The high-risk procedures are those in which a stroke might be induced, nerve damage may be caused, or other complications may happen when the dye is being introduced into the body. Those which involve more risk include the bronchogram, cerebral angiogram, coronary angiogram or arteriogram, pneumoencephalogram, and pulmonary angiogram. These tests demand skilled personnel. Also some people are allergic to the dye, particularly that of the intravenous pyelogram (IVP).

Why is lymphangiography important in the diagnosis of cancer?

Lymphangiography is important to cancer diagnosis because one of the ways that cancer spreads is through the lymph nodes. Lymphangiography can be useful in the diagnosis and staging of persons with Hodgkin disease and lymphomas and sometimes for other cancers. It is a procedure which is done in an outpatient setting or in a hospital. A blue dye is injected into the small lymph vessel after a cut is made in the big toe. The lymph system in the abdomen can then be looked at by means of x-rays. Since the lymph glands are very small, it usually takes two to three hours for the dye to reach the lymph nodes. Lymphangiography is used to localize and determine the extent of the tumors. The surgeon can use it as a guide to finding specific lymph nodes and showing the size of the tumor. The radiotherapist uses it to evaluate how a person is responding to therapy. Since the dye stays in the system some three to four months, progress usually can be followed through x-rays without repeating the procedure.

Do some of the parts of the body absorb more x-ray beams than others?

If you put a part of the human body in front of a beam of x-rays some of the rays will pass through while others will be absorbed and scattered inside the body. The bone, for example, which is more dense, will absorb x-rays more readily than surrounding tissues. It is the shadows of these denser parts of the body which show up on the developed film or screen.

What kinds of contrast media are used for x-rays?

X-rays are absorbed by dense substances such as barium or iodine. These contrast media can be swallowed, injected into the bloodstream, or inserted with a plastic tube or catheter. Sometimes dye and air are both used in contrast films. For example, often both barium and air are used for gastrointestinal examinations.

What kind of physician should read diagnostic x-rays?

Diagnostic x-rays should be interpreted by doctors who are board-certified (or board-eligible) radiologists.

What kind of background does a radiologist have?

A board-certified radiologist (certification is by the American Board of Radiology) must be a graduate of an approved medical school, have four years of postgraduate training in the department of radiology and must include training in pathology, nuclear radiology and therapeutic radiology, and have successfully completed written and oral examinations administered by the board.

What is the difference between a diagnostic radiologist and a therapeutic radiologist?

A diagnostic radiologist performs and interprets x-rays used in diagnosing illness. A therapeutic radiologist (also sometimes called a radiation therapist, a radiotherapist, or a radiation oncologist) specializes in treating cancer with radiotherapy. The American Board of Radiology gives separate certification to these two specialties.

How do I know where to go for my diagnostic x-rays?

This is a subject you should discuss with your physician. Ask questions. If you can, have your x-rays done in the outpatient department of a medical school hospital or by a private board-certified radiologist.

What questions should I ask before I have x-rays?

There are several things you should ask about:
- Are the x-rays clearly necessary for diagnosis?
- Are there any x-rays which I have had taken recently which might be used instead of taking new ones?
- What is the approximate dose of x-ray?
- What do you think you will find out from the x-rays?
- What dosage is the particular machine giving?
- When was the machine last inspected?
- What kind of shielding will be used during the procedure?

Is there really a difference between machines in one office and another?

Yes, there is definitely a difference. You should know that both the quality of the x-ray equipment and the quality of the technician or doctor doing the x-ray make a difference in whether or not you receive a low or high dose of radiation. The expertise of the operator also makes a difference in how good the x-ray will be. Another variable is in who reads the x-ray after it is taken.

What kind of training do x-ray technicians have to have?

There are few states which require that radiology technicians be properly trained and certified. The 1970 X-ray Exposure Study conducted by the Public Health Service shows that those x-rays supervised by radiologists in private offices involved less exposure than those supervised by non-radiologists in private offices. However, many states have been working with the FDA's Bureau of Radiological Health on radiation-control regulations and on training programs for personnel.

Are the machines inspected regularly?

There are presently no U.S. government inspection requirements. Although some states do have requirements, in many states the equipment is not inspected every year. Many machines, particularly those in doctors' offices, go uninspected for long periods of time. There should be a certificate posted near the machine. Look at it to see when the last inspection was performed. If more than a few years ago, go elsewhere.

When should x-rays be considered a necessity?

As noted earlier, x-rays are an important part of the diagnostic workup and when properly taken and read they are one of the doctor's most valuable tools. However, the benefits of the x-ray must be weighed against the risks. A qualified professional is a better judge of when x-rays are needed than you are. You, however, need to know the right questions to ask so that you can assure yourself you are in the hands of a skilled and competent practitioner.

What is the major risk of diagnostic x-rays?

The amount of radiation which x-rays deliver to your body is the biggest risk. It is believed that the risks of x-ray dosage are linear—that is, the more dosage a person receives during a lifetime, the greater his or her chance of developing cancer or another abnormality.

Who can tell me what the approximate dosage should be for the various tests?

Your doctor should be able to give you approximate dosages so that you can ask the technician where you are having the test done what dosage his machine is giving. For example, a standard chest x-ray involves about 5-10 millirem (.005-.010 rem or rad); a mammogram should be under 1 rem or rad.

Do the x-rays belong to me?

There is quite a bit of controversy over this issue. However, you have a right to ask that the x-rays taken in one place be sent to another doctor or hospital of your choice. Some doctors and hospitals will give them to you directly, others will insist on mailing them to the other physician or hospital. It might be a good idea to explain that you are concerned about x-ray overexposure.

What is a fluoroscope?

This is a kind of x-ray in which a special machine (the fluoroscope) takes a continuous x-ray so that the doctor can see the movement of internal organs. A fluorescent screen, coated with a special substance, is mounted in front of an x-ray tube. The x-ray shadow is cast on the screen. The fluoroscopic image can be amplified and displayed on a television screen. Fluoroscopy can show the expansion of the lung or a barium liquid passing through a patient's esophagus to his stomach. Fluoroscopic techniques sometimes provide important information which cannot be provided in any other way.

How much radiation exposure do you get from a fluoroscope?

Fluoroscopes take longer to perform and often expose you to more radiation than do the conventional x-ray exams recorded on film. There are new machines which give better images with less exposure, particularly those which amplify the light from the fluoroscopic screen and then provide a brighter image on a TV monitor, but the exposure is still higher than for a standard x-ray film. Make sure this procedure is done only by a board-certified radiologist and only when necessary.

Will the doctors use x-rays taken by someone else?

Some doctors will not use them because they are not aware they are available, they don't want to be bothered asking for them, or they don't trust the manner in which they were taken. There may be good reason for having x-rays retaken, such as if the first set is on poor-quality film. But you should make sure that your x-rays are being redone for good reasons and not just because the doctor or hospital does not want to share them. You should keep a record of your own x-ray history so that you can tell the doctor what has already been done, especially on high-dose film such as gallbladder or GI series. More and more doctors are accepting x-rays taken by others.

How is the dose of radiation measured?

You will hear the terms "rad" or "rem" used in describing the dose of radiation. "Rad" stands for *r*adiation *a*bsorbed *d*ose. A rem is equivalent to a rad. The terms apply to all types of radiation and take into account the energy actually imparted to the tissue. (Sometimes the terms "millirads" and "millirems" are used to describe the dosage.) The effects of diagnostic x-rays on the body depend in a complex way on a number of factors, such as the distribution of energies of x-ray photon in the beam, the total intensity or quality of radiation, the distance between the x-ray tube and the individual being x-rayed, the type and location of tissues and organs in the main beam, and the age and sex of the person being examined. The unit of exposure is the roentgen, named after Wilhelm Roentgen, who discovered x-rays in 1895. However, most radiologists now measure the absorbed dose, which is the amount of energy dumped by incident radiation into a gram of material. The dose absorbed by a gram of skin or muscle can be much less than that of a gram of bone placed in the same x-ray beam. This is because the heavy atoms of calcium in the bone absorb x-rays more easily than lighter elements abundant in tissue. X-rays pass through tissue more easily and don't leave as much energy behind.

What is skin dose?

This refers to the dose of radiation immediately on the surface of the skin. The outer layers of material absorb x-rays readily and thus, particularly with older machines, the exposure inside a body will be less than the exposure at the skin. The absorbed dose in the outer layers of skin is often referred to as the skin dose, while x-ray energy deposited in a gram of bone, tissues, or an organ at a certain location inside the body is referred to as the depth dose at that location.

What x-rays give relatively high overall radiation doses?

Several examinations are of special concern because they involve relatively high overall radiation doses. They include examinations of the breasts, gastrointestinal system (upper and lower), thoracic spine (middle and dorsal), lumbosacral spine (lower), lumbar spine, cervical spine, gallbladder, kidney, ureter, bladder, skull, pelvis and hip or upper thigh, and fluoroscopic procedure.

What other things should I watch for when having x-rays taken?

A good operator will measure carefully the thickness of the part of your body which is to be exposed and consult a technique chart to set the tube current, voltage, and exposure time for each type of x-ray. If the operator hurries, there is more likelihood that a poor exposure will require additional x-rays. You must be careful not to move, since blurred images mean additional x-rays. The operator must also carefully align the beam, using the minimum beam-size possibilities.

When are lead shields used?

Shielding can help reduce the amount of scattered radiation absorbed, especially by reproductive organs. There are several kinds of shields such as lead aprons, lead-lined panels, scrotal cups, flexible lead-lined drape cloths, and shadow shields. If they are not offered to you, ask about them before being x-rayed. Newer machines have built-in shields to avoid scattering.

What kind of x-ray is a mammogram?

A mammogram is a soft-tissue x-ray of the breast. It is but one of several techniques used in diagnosis of breast cancer. The mammogram and the other techniques used in diagnosing breast cancer—xeroradiography, thermography, graphic stress telether-mometry—are discussed in Chapter 11.

What is endoscopy?

Endoscopy is the examination through optical instruments of the interior of the body. There are many different kinds of instruments designed to perform this examination on different parts of the body. Several new tools use fiberoptics for this procedure—tiny flexible fibers that carry a powerful light and a telescope which allows the doctor to peer inside the body. These instruments allow the diagnosis of various kinds of cancer without performing a major operation. Sometimes they are used in combination with other tests, such as x-rays, to confirm the diagnosis.

What are some of these endoscopic instruments called?

You can identify these instruments because they end in the suffix "scope"—cystoscope, hysteroscope, colposcope, laparoscope, bronchoscope, proctosigmoidoscope, esophagogastroduodeno-scope, etc.

Why are these instruments important in diagnosing cancer?

For many years, these procedures have offered a fairly simple method of detecting malignancies, precancerous growths, and non-cancer-related diseases without the necessity for major exploratory surgery. This means you can return to work, be free from postoperative complications, and save money. The doctor can see the exact location of tumors and cytology can be done without a major operation. Since the introduction of fiberoptic equipment in the 1970s, new areas of the body can be examined without surgery.

What is a cystoscopy?

A cystoscopy exam allows the doctor to inspect the lining of the urinary bladder for the presence of diverticulum, fistula, stones, or tumors in the bladder. The bladder is first enlarged by filling it with air or water. A cystoscope—a thin, hollow tube with a light at the end of it—is inserted through the urethra. The doctor can then actually look at the walls of the bladder. Cystoscopic brushes can be passed along to the tract to obtain cells for microscopic examination. Small tumors can sometimes be removed through the hollow tube. This test is usually done if you have repeated urinary tract infections or if you have bleeding associated with urination.

When is a hysteroscope used?

A hysteroscope can determine the presence of fibroid and endometrial tumors as well as helping to find lost IUDs or treat cases of infertility. The hysteroscope looks somewhat like a skin diver's spear gun with an eyepiece and a trigger that controls a flexible tip that provides a full view inside the uterus. The instrument is inserted through the vagina and threaded through the cervix into the uterus to view the uterine cavity and entrance to the fallopian tubes.

What is a colposcope examination and how is it done?

The colposcope is basically a microscope on a stand which gives a lighted, magnified view of the vulva, vagina, and cervix—an area which previously could not be seen without major surgery. It allows the doctor to look through a microscopic eyepiece into the area. No part of the instrument is inserted into the vagina. Further details about colposcopy are covered in Chapter 16.

Is the laparoscope used as a diagnostic tool?

Yes, the laparoscope is used to examine a woman's reproductive system for diagnosing disease as well as in performing a quick, relatively painless operation for sterilization. With the laparoscope, the doctor can inspect the uterus, the ovaries, the fallopian tubes, and even the appendix if the other organs are moved aside. He can sometimes use it to differentiate fibroid from ovarian cancers and various other pelvic problems by looking inside the abdominal cavity. A small slit is made in the abdominal cavity near the navel. This procedure is usually done under general anesthesia in the hospital. Normally you can leave the hospital the same day. Sometimes the laparoscope is used for detecting liver lesions, either alone or in conjunction with an ultrasonic probe.

When is a bronchoscope used?

A bronchoscope is a slender, tubular instrument that slides down the throat into the larger breathing passages. Its light at the far end allows the doctor to look directly into your bronchi. The doctor normally sprays anesthetic into the throat and bronchial tubes so that they are numb. Since it is inserted into only one bronchus at a time, you should have no trouble breathing normally during a bronchoscopy. The fiberoptic bronchoscope is a more flexible instrument which allows viewing of less accessible parts of the respiratory tract to locate early lesions.

What is a proctosigmoidoscope?

This is a lighted instrument that can be inserted to a maximum of 10 inches into the colon. It can be used for viewing the lower interior portion of the colon. Two-thirds of all cancers of the colon and rectum are accessible to detection by this means.

What is a colonoscope?

The colonoscope allows the doctor to examine the entire length of the colon. It is used to detect cancers which sometimes are not seen in x-ray studies. It is a highly flexible, four-directional instrument, no thicker than a finger, that can be maneuvered through the curves and around the bends of the colon. It gives off brilliant rays of light and gives the doctor an excellent view of any damage or abnormality in the tissue. The colonoscope permits tiny tissue samples or biopsies to be taken. Since the delicate walls of the colon can be penetrated by this instrument, it requires a skilled physician to perform this test. Often it is used in conjunction with a fluoroscope to help the doctor follow the course of the tube. It is usually performed under light anesthesia on an outpatient basis.

If the doctor sees polyps (cherrylike growths on the intestinal wall) he can sometimes remove them entirely, safely, and easily through working channels in the colonoscope which allow a variety of instruments to be inserted.

What are esophagoscopy, gastroscopy, and duodenoscopy?

These three procedures use flexible fiberoptic instruments to examine several parts of the gastrointestinal tract. A doctor can look at the esophagus (esophagoscopy), see problems in the stomach (gastroscopy) or in the pancreas (duodenoscopy). These instruments permit photography, biopsy, and collection of cytological materials. Several different models of instruments are available of varying lengths. They have working channels through which various tools can be inserted, and they have controls for air, water and suction. Some anesthesia is used, especially in the area of the throat, to allow painless swallowing of the tube.

What kind of doctor should do these examinations?

Several of the new instruments require doctors who are qualified, trained specialists to perform the tests and to understand what is being seen by these tools. They can be dangerous in the hands of untrained practitioners. In most cases the average general practitioner has not had enough experience. Make sure a trained proctologist, internist, or surgeon will be doing your tests.

What is involved in a barium enema with air-contrast examination?

This method uses a contrast medium to visualize the lower bowel. By carefully x-raying the colon, small and large lesions overlooked by other tests (such as palpation, proctosigmoidoscopy, or colonoscopy) may be seen. Sometimes if a barium-enema exam is negative, but suspicious signs and symptoms continue, the exam is repeated.

What is cytology?

Cytology is that branch of medicine which deals with the formation, structure, and function of cells. When it is mentioned in the area of diagnosis for cancer, it is sometimes called exfoliative cytology and refers to the technique of examining cells which have been normally shed or which are scraped from living tissue. The cells, which cannot be seen by the naked eye, are examined under the microscope, usually by a pathologist or a technician trained to know whether the cells look normal or not.

What kinds of tests are cytological exams?

There are several:
- Pap test to detect cervical cancer
- Vaginal pool aspiration or endometrial aspiration to detect uterine cancer
- Sputum tests to detect lung cancer
- Urine-sediment tests to detect cancer of the urinary tract, especially bladder
- Scrapings from the mouth to detect oral cancer
- Cell samples from the esophagus, stomach, pancreas, or duodenum
- Fluid tests from areas such as breasts, spinal cord, thyroid, prostate
- Bone-marrow tests

How are cytological exams performed?

A little fluid taken from the organ—either from cells which have been sloughed off, cells which have been scraped off, or body fluid which has been taken by needle—is spread on a glass slide. The fluid is stained with dyes and examined through a microscope. When cancer cells are present in the fluid, they can usually be spotted. The cytological exam of cells is based on the fact that cells on the surface of an organ are constantly being shed and falling off. In some places, these cells, both malignant and benign, can be scooped up in the normal fluid secretions. There are structural differences between the cancer cells and benign cells which can be seen under the microscope. The smear technique was first used in the Pap test. Today the new fiberoptic instruments make it possible to obtain smears from less accessible organs such as the stomach and the pancreas.

Can a final diagnosis of cancer be made with a smear test?

Most smear tests are used for screening to detect abnormal cells. Most doctors do not feel that the smear can be used to provide the final diagnosis of cancer. The smear consists only of individual scattered cells, sometimes clusters of them. A smear diagnosis gives strong evidence of the presence of cancer, but biopsy is still held to be essential for a final decision.

What are the advantages of the smear method?

There are several. Some smears, such as used in the Pap test, can be done easily and cheaply for testing large groups for cancer. Some smears, such as in the Pap test and the lung sputum test, can detect the presence of cancer before any signs or symptoms appear. And in hard-to-reach areas such as the stomach, exfoliate cytology smears can provide evidence of the presence of cancer without performing an operation.

Does the Pap test detect any cancers other than cervical?

The Pap test is approximately 97 percent successful in detecting cervical cancer; the cervix is the opening to the uterus and is where most cancers involving the uterus and female genitals begin. However, the Pap test will show only about 50 percent of cancers of the uterine lining (endometrium), and is of little or no value in picking up cancers of the ovary.

What are radioactive scans?

Radioactive or nuclear scans are tests in which the patient is given a weak radioactive substance—called a radioactive isotope—by injection into the bloodstream. The material is taken up by the body. A machine, which looks like an x-ray machine, moves over the area being tested and draws a series of pictures.

How can the doctor tell if cancer is present?

Deposits of cancer may show up as areas of either increased radioactivity or decreased radioactivity, depending upon the organ being studied, the type of radioactive substance used, and the kind of scan being done.

What kinds of substances are used in nuclear scans?

The kind of isotope used depends upon the part of the body which is being studied. Certain isotopes accumulate in certain body organs. In the area of cancer detection, technitium 99m is sometimes used for brain, liver, spleen, bone, and thyroid scans. Radioactive iodine can be used for thyroid scans and for liver and renal function studies. Gallium is capable of showing rapidly dividing cells. New substances are constantly being tested and reviewed.

Where are radioactive scans done?

These tests must be done in special laboratories by doctors and technicians who are trained in handling radioisotopes. Other conditions can, at times, look similar to cancer on the scans, so it takes a skilled practitioner to interpret them. Nuclear scans have been commonly used for detecting tumors since the early 1950s, and initially the tests were an offshoot of radiology. Now many hospitals have departments of nuclear medicine and it is a rapidly growing field in its own right. There is an American Board of Nuclear Medicine which certifies physicians in this field.

Who performs radioactive scans?

A skilled physician who has had special training after completing medical school—including several years of intensive postgraduate training to qualify as an expert in diagnosis with extensive technical knowledge of the machinery used, the chemistry of radioactive compounds, and nuclear physics and radiation safety—is responsible for nuclear scans. The American Board of Nuclear Medicine certifies doctors in this field. A nuclear medicine technologist assists the doctor, positions you, and operates the equipment during the examination. The technician has had special training and experience in nuclear medicine technology.

Are nuclear scans different from x-rays?

Yes, they are. X-rays involve passing radiation through your body from an external source (an x-ray tube) and recording the image on a film (radiograph) which the radiologist can examine. In a scan, the radioactive substance is introduced into your body, usually through an injection in your vein. The machine translates the substance into spots of light that expose the film, which is developed and called a scan. By observing how and where the radioactive compounds go in your body, the doctor can detect changes in your body's processes.

What kinds of machines are used?

There are two main types. A "scanner" moves back and forth in straight lines, and as it moves it records images of the radiation given out. The other machine, called a "camera," records the radiation without the machine moving. It is larger than the scanner. The areas where the radioactivity is concentrated are seen as dots on the film. Places where there is high activity have more dots than those where there is low activity.

Is there any discomfort or danger to radioactive scans?

The scans involve little discomfort. The danger involved depends upon the part of the body. Some of the radiation given off by the tracer substance can be absorbed. However, the radioactive substance is weak, so the risks associated with nuclear scans are similar to those associated with diagnostic x-rays.

When are radioactive scans done?

It depends upon the kind of cancer suspected and the stage of the disease. Scans can be used to detect the primary source of cancer. They can also be used to estimate the progress of the treatment. Scans are also part of what is known as a metastatic workup—that is, checking the body for distant cancer. A metastatic workup is usually used before treatment is begun if there is a diagnosis of cancer or if a very high suspicion of cancer is present. Metastatic workups are part of the "clinical staging system" which determines the person's state of cancer at the time it is diagnosed.

What kinds of scans are done for a metastatic workup?

Again it depends upon the kind of cancer and knowledge of where that cancer is likely to spread. A metastatic workup can include bone scans, liver scans, and brain scans along with a battery of other tests.

How are bone scans done?

The liquid which has been "tagged" with the mildly radioactive substance is injected into a vein and carried by the bloodstream to the bones. Cancerous areas in the bone will usually pick up more of the radioactive material than normal bone, so these show up as "hot spots" on the films taken of the area. Most of the liquid injected into the body for the bone scan disappears within a few hours. The liquid is excreted from the body within 48 hours after the test is done.

Are bone scans difficult to interpret?

Yes, because injured bone, arthritis, infection, and certain other abnormal conditions may show up as hot spots on the bone scans.

Do bone scans show different things than routine x-rays?

Yes, bone scans can detect cancerous areas in some cases earlier than x-rays. They are more sensitive. Bone scans are also better than x-rays in following the disease; they can show progress or regression. Routine x-rays have some drawbacks. Approximately 50 percent of the bone tissues must be destroyed by cancer in a given area before it will show up on an x-ray. On the other hand, x-rays also have some advantages: they are quick, easily obtained, involve no discomfort and little risk, and are relatively accurate.

Do brain scans also show hot spots?

The picture that appears as a result of a scan depends on the person's individual situation, because each kind of lesion in each particular organ creates its own variation in the isotope's pattern. In a brain scan the picture is of the blood pools carrying the isotope around. The isotope accumulates within a lesion to form a hot spot. Regions that are only lightly represented on the scan of a normal brain usually show up much more darkly when they contain a lesion.

What are liver scans?

A substance is injected in a vein and goes through the entire bloodstream. Because of the size of the particle injected, it is trapped by the normal cells in the liver and spleen (the major organs in the body which will trap that particular size particle) and accumulate enough of it to give an image. If there is a lesion, it is seen as a "cold spot" because the abnormal liver cells aren't performing their normal trapping function. Liver scans are used to evaluate liver size, shape, and position and to detect the presence of lesions in the liver. Liver scans are usually routinely recommended before major tumor operations in many sites.

When is a thyroid scan done?

A thyroid scan is done if a tumor is suspected after the doctor has examined the thyroid area with his hands. A small amount of radioactive material is swallowed or injected. A cold spot (showing decreased concentration of the radioisotope) makes the physician suspicious of cancer, although a great percentage of cold spots can also prove to be benign. A hot spot of great activity is usually a sign of a benign growth. Thyroid scan is used in determining the size, position, and function of the thyroid gland and to detect metastases of thyroid cancer. Sometimes two thyroid scan readings are taken—usually at 2 and 24 hours after administration of the radioactive material.

Would having a radioactive scan be a problem for a pregnant woman?

You certainly should tell the doctor in the nuclear-medicine department that you are pregnant. The radioactive material can be carried to your baby through your circulation system. The amount of radiation is small, but you and the doctor should discuss the problem and the alternatives together. Be sure you tell the doctor if you are pregnant or think you are pregnant.

What is a gallium scan?

A gallium scan is used to determine if the cancer has spread to more than one area of the body because it is capable of showing rapidly dividing cells. One of the main uses of this test is in detecting lymph-node involvement in lymphoma or other tumor masses.

How much do radioactive scans cost?

Radioactive scans cost from less than $75 for some organs to $125 or more for complete bone scans.

What is ultrasound?

It is one of the new methods used to locate and measure solid tumors in the body. Ultrasound, or sonar, was used extensively during World War II for tracking submarines. Today it is used to clean teeth, age alcohol, and prospect for oil. It has been adapted for medical application and is a common technique for watching the heart in motion and for examining unborn babies.

How does ultrasound scanning work?

It works just like sonar. If a destroyer captain wants to locate a submarine, he sends bursts of sound through the water around him and waits for some of them to bounce off his target. By analyzing these echoes, he can tell where the submarine is and how large it is. An ultrasound technician, or sonographer, uses exactly the same principle.

How is ultrasound scanning done?

The technician presses a microphone-like probe across the patient's skin. This probe is called a transducer. The probe sends out sound waves at 1 million to 10 million cycles per second. When the probe picks up an echo, a dot registers on the screen (called an oscilloscope screen). The probe sends out sound waves 0.1 percent of the time it is on and listens 99.9 percent.

How can ultrasound tell a solid tumor from one that is not solid?

As the technician moves the probe across the skin surface, a composite picture emerges on the screen showing what's inside the body. A solid tumor looks solid on the screen because echoes are returning from all the particles inside it. But a cyst filled with fluid looks hollow, because fluid doesn't reflect ultrasound waves. The technician can make a permanent record of the picture with a special camera attached to the oscilloscope.

Can ultrasound tell the difference between a malignant tumor and a benign one?

No. Ultrasound can confirm that the mass is a tumor. It outlines it and shows the extent of it. But an ultrasound machine that by itself can distinguish a malignant tumor from a benign one has yet to be invented. A doctor, by looking at the shape and consistency shown by ultrasound and combining it with the clinical history of the patient, can say that a tumor is "highly suspicious" of being cancerous.

Is ultrasound like an x-ray?

No. Ultrasound has no radiation. It uses high-frequency sound waves to scan the body—sound waves that are far beyond the range of human hearing. The range of human hearing is about 20 to 20,000 cycles per second. The probe used in ultrasound scanning sends out sound waves at 1 million to 100 million cycles per second. The vibrations from these sound waves are reflected off body tissue and transformed into electrical signals that show up on a screen as a two-dimensional image.

Does the patient have to make any special preparation when going to get an ultrasound scan?

No. You will be put on an examining table. Your skin in the area to be scanned will be covered with mineral oil in order to eliminate most of the air gaps that block sound transmission. You need no anesthesia and you will feel no pain. The ultrasound scan itself takes only a few minutes to perform, especially if it is being done only on one small area of your body.

What are the advantages of ultrasound scanning?

With ultrasound, you have no radiation exposure. You need no incisions or injections. You do not have to swallow any substances. There is no discomfort. Ultrasound can be used many times on the same patient without risky side effects, even to pregnant women. Studies to date have revealed no known biological damage to humans from diagnostic exposure to ultrasound waves, although it is a form of energy being transmitted through tissues.

Is ultrasound new?

The procedure has been around for 20 or 25 years. In the past it was used mainly for obstetrical tests. Since 1970, there has been a dramatic change in its use in the United States. Now ultrasound is being used for the whole pelvis, and about two-thirds of the scans now being done are in the abdominal area. It is a field which is changing very quickly, with new technology being introduced constantly. However, there is only a small number of doctors who know how to use and interpret the tests accurately.

Is ultrasound being used in other areas besides diagnosis?

Yes. Ultrasound experts can measure a tumor's progress during therapy—whether it is getting smaller as a result of chemotherapy or radiation treatments. It can be used to tell the doctor whether or not the treatment is working. It is thought to be a good monitoring device because it can be used often, since there is no radiation involved. Ultrasound is used to help the doctor more accurately aim radiation during treatment. It is also used as a guide for operations.

What kinds of tumors are being diagnosed with ultrasound?

Ultrasound scanning has proved to be helpful in diagnosing tumors of the stomach, pancreas, kidney, uterus, and ovaries. It has helped detect tumors of the eye and thyroid gland. In the thyroid area, it acts as a complementary test, mainly to get the size of the lesion. It can actually differentiate between fluid or solid tumors in about 98 percent of the cases.

How is ultrasound used in the gynecological area?

This is where the use of ultrasound began. It can be used in the urinary area. In the ovarian area, it can detect whether the tumor is cystic, partly cystic and partly solid, or all solid.

How is it used in liver and pancreas areas?

Ultrasound is useful in scanning the pancreas, especially in thin patients. In the liver, ultrasound scans are often used when a patient is jaundiced—since it can help to differentiate between normal consistency and pancreatitis. However, it cannot tell the difference between pancreatitis and cancer of the pancreas. Small tumors of the pancreas can be discovered by ultrasound.

Is ultrasound used in detecting breast cancer?

At the present time, investigation is being done in this area. It may be that it will be useful for lumpy breasts or for high-risk younger patients. Another area of future use could be for follow-up purposes—doing a baseline mammogram and following it up with ultrasound.

Is ultrasound useful in the chest area?

No, ultrasound has not been found to be useful in this area.

Is ultrasound used for detecting cancer of the kidney?

Ultrasound can be used for a more definitive diagnosis after IVP (intravenous pyelogram) testing is done. It can help differentiate between solid and cystic kidney masses.

Do ultrasonic scans give different information than standard x-rays?

Although ultrasonic scans can be used as a substitute for x-rays for certain kinds of examinations, they yield different types of information, so often both ultrasonic scans and x-rays are ordered. They are complementary tests. The boundaries between different types of soft tissue can be highlighted with ultrasonics and the characteristics of blood flow can be studied, for example. However, for viewing structures such as bones, x-rays are presently preferable.

Where can I have ultrasound scans done?

Ultrasound is presently available in the larger cities and in medical centers. It is more readily available than some of the other new diagnostic machines, such as CT scanners. However, ultrasound is much more dependent upon the operator for good results than is a tool such as the CT scanner. There must be a qualified expert available to interpret the results of the test.

Can ultrasound be done on an outpatient basis?

Yes, it can. However, in many of the major centers which have the scanning equipment, inpatients take preference over the outpatients for use of the machine.

How much does an ultrasound scan cost?

It depends upon the extent of the scan. Presently, average costs for a one-organ scan run from $75 to $125.

What is a CT scan?

"CT" stands for "computerized tomography." A new way of looking inside the human body, it uses pencil-like x-ray beams to scan the section of the body being studied. It combines the speed of a computer with the sensitivity of the x-ray detectors. Sometimes you will hear the terms "tomographic scanner," "ACTA scanner" ("ACTA" stands for "automatic computerized transverse axial scanner"), or "CAT" ("computerized axial tomography"). They all mean the same thing. We have used the term CT scan to refer to this procedure in this book.

How does the CT scanner work?

The CT takes a three-dimensional look inside the body. The scanner has an arm which directs the beam through the body as it rotates around you. The x-rays pass through the body and are detected by an electronic device. About 160 scans are made in one position; then the detectors are rotated and the 160 scans are repeated.

What does the computer do?

As the beam moves around the body in the same plane, a minicomputer analyzes how much of the x-rays are absorbed as they pass through the various internal organs and structures. Up to eight slices 1 centimeter apart may be taken at any one time. Each target area in the slice has between 100 and 200 x-ray beams going through it. The approximately 100,000 bits of information are fed into a computer that performs a billion calculations to convert the data into an image. The image can be seen on a TV screen or in printed form.

How does the CT scan differ from the standard x-ray?

X-ray machines send a broad x-ray beam over a large area. CT scanners direct a pencil-point-thin line of electromagnetic energy through a narrow cross-section or slice of the body. Ordinary x-rays take a "flat" view, superimposing organs in the front of the body on organs in the back, giving a two-dimensional picture. CTs give a three-dimensional picture. CTs also give better pictures of soft tissues than do x-rays.

What is ECAT?

ECAT stands for "emission computerized axial tomograph." It is a cousin of the CT. Patients swallow radioactive material. The charged particles (positrons) given off from deep inside the body are recorded on the ECAT scanner, giving the doctor a picture taken from the inside of whatever organ is under study. It is very expensive machinery and there are very few presently available.

Is it uncomfortable to have a CT scan?

There should be little discomfort. The total time needed to complete a series of scans making up a complete examination is about an hour. Sometimes contrast material is used. If it is needed, an intravenous needle is put in your vein and the solution passed through it.

Can I move during the CT scan?

No. It is very important that you not move during the examination. If you do, the examination may need to be repeated.

Do I need any special preparation?

Ordinarily not. If your head is being scanned, however, an elasticized stocking cap will be put over your scalp to assist the technician in positioning your head for the examination. Tape will also be used to ensure proper positioning. You will be asked to remove all jewelry, ornaments, dentures, and other similar objects in the head and neck area so that they will not interfere with the scanning examination. If the scan is of your chest, stomach, pelvic area, arms, or legs, you will be given a gown to wear.

Who will do the actual scan?

The technician will prepare you and position you for the examination, and will be operating the equipment. The diagnostic radiologist will view and interpret the scanning information. The report of the examination will be given to your doctor by the radiologist.

Has the CT scan taken the place of other tests?

The hospitals with CT scanners have reduced the number of pneumoencephalograms and angiograms significantly. Both are conventional brain x-rays using contrast media, and both are high-risk procedures because of the injection of contrast medium. A CT scan is not considered a high-risk procedure.

How much radiation do you get from a CT scanner?

Some radiologists claim that the thin x-ray beams expose patients to less radiation than a conventional x-ray examination. They do not expose the patient to *more* radiation than the conventional x-ray. And the scan avoids the risks associated with the injections of contrast dyes needed in some of the conventional procedures.

How long does it take to do a CT scan?

It depends upon the question the doctor wants to have answered by the scan. A single scan takes anywhere from a few seconds to a couple of minutes, depending upon the type of scanner and the extent of the examination. A full body exam could take from 15 minutes to an hour, depending upon the questions to be answered. The CT scan can be done on an outpatient basis, with a minimum amount of discomfort.

What are CT scanners used for?

Originally, CT scanning was used only to see brain abnormalities. Today it is a tool which can be used for cancers such as those of the lung, bladder, prostate, liver, and pancreas. It is used to spot tumors, detect organ disorders and abnormal structures, follow blood vessels, spot blocked ducts, differentiate between normal and abnormal tissues, and see blood clots. It can detect small differences in the physical characteristics of tissues. It can tell the difference between white matter and gray matter and between blood and water. It can be used by radiologists in making out treatment plans because it can provide detailed information about the absorption of radiation by a particular tumor. Some scanners now take the scans in color, but these are not usually used for routine diagnosis since the black-and-white image at this time gives more detail.

What is the average cost of a CT scan?

That depends upon the test being done. The average cost to the patient of a CT scan is about $275. Many health plans do not pay for CT scans.

Are the CT scanners and ultrasound ever used for one patient?

Sometimes. For example, for heavier persons, the ultrasound scan is usually performed first. If it does not give the information the physician is looking for, then a CT scan is performed. It is usually done in this order because since the ultrasound scan gives out no radiation, it is felt to be a safer test for the patient.

Which should be used first—CT scan, ultrasound, or nuclear devices?

There is still no consensus on which scan may be best for a particular symptom, disease, or area of the body. The techniques for the tests are quite new, and the fields are changing almost monthly. At the present time, for example, kidney lesions seem to be seen more clearly with the CT scanner and ovarian and uterine tumors seem to be better detected with ultrasound scans. Many doctors themselves are unsure which diagnostic tool should be used first. As the uses of the machines evolve, the first choice of testing for the particular machine changes. The main problem is that if all three are used as complementary techniques, tests could easily cost over $1,000. You need to be sure that your doctor is up-to-date and communicating with the various specialties.

Types of Biopsies

TYPE	PROCEDURE
Needle or aspiration biopsy	Fluid or tissue is removed by suction through a pointed needle.
Endoscopic biopsy	Fluid or tissue is obtained by using long instruments, usually with a needle or knife; the optical instrument allows the doctor to see into the body cavity.
Incisional biopsy	Part of the tumor is cut out to be looked at microscopically by the doctor.
Punch biopsy	Specimen is removed by means of a punch.
Total biopsy or excisional biopsy	The entire tumor is removed for examination under the microscope.

What is a biopsy?

A biopsy is the procedure in which a piece of tissue is obtained and examined under the microscope to determine whether cancer or other disease is present. This microscopic examination of the biopsy specimen is accepted by doctors in determining the nature of tumor with complete accuracy. Therefore, whenever possible a doctor insists on obtaining a sample of every tumor that could be cancer before treatment is attempted. The biopsy provides the most reliable basis for a diagnosis of cancer.

Who determines if the biopsy cells are cancerous?

The biopsy is "read" by a pathologist—a physician who specializes in the study of normal and diseased body tissues.

What kind of training does a pathologist have?

In order to be certified by the American Board of Pathology, the person must be a licensed doctor of medicine or osteopathy and have four years of training in both clinical and anatomic pathology or three years of training in either specialty or eight years of practical experience under circumstances acceptable to the board. The doctor must also successfully complete the examinations administered by the board. The pathologist is a vital member of the health-care team, especially in the field of cancer.

Are all pathologists skilled in diagnosing cancer from slides?

As in all other specialties, the skill and the competence of pathologists vary. A decision regarding whether cancer is the disease in the tissue being examined depends on the interpretation the individual pathologist makes of the cellular structure of the biopsy. Frequently, tissue or slides are sent to experts of larger institutions for consultation, especially by pathologists practicing alone in small communities. If your diagnosis of cancer is based on the single pathological report of a single pathologist in a small community, be sure to ask that the slides or tissues be sent to other pathologists for confirmation. As important is the relationship between the patient's doctor and the pathologist. They need to be talking with each other and working together as a team.

How can the pathologist tell if cells are benign?

When a piece of tissue is taken from the body and examined microscopically, the normal cells have an orderly appearance. They possess the distinctive features of the organ from which they came. The cells from the thyroid gland, for example, are very different from those of the lymph nodes. Normal cells from different organs carry genetic "messages" that determine their structure and function.

What does the pathologist look for when he reads the biopsy?

The pathologist does many things. First he looks to see whether the specimen is malignant or benign. If it is malignant, he tries to identify the specific type of cancer cells present in the tumor and attempts to determine just how fast they reproduce themselves. With special stains and fixes, he can tell much from the tissue samples. He looks to see if the blood vessels or lymph channels have been invaded. With some kinds of tumors, he may test for hormone dependency. The pathologist gives the other doctors information which will allow them to determine the proper course of treatment.

How important is the pathologist in a cancer diagnosis?

The pathologist is the key to the entire diagnosis, since a diagnosis is nothing more or less than a carefully considered opinion. It is important first of all that there be adequate and properly prepared biopsy material, since no diagnosis is better than the evidence that it came from. Sometimes, it is found that the kind of specimen presented to the pathologist is inadequate for a true diagnosis to be made or the cellular structure is difficult to identify. Further, like everyone else, the pathologist is just one individual with the same burdens and problems as we all have. He may be swamped with work and may not have the time to do an adequate job of preparation in, or reflection upon, the report he makes. His relationship with the physician in charge of the patient may be poor. All these factors have a bearing on the kind of pathological study and report that is done on your biopsy—and underlines the need for a second pathological opinion. As was noted earlier, in large hospitals and medical centers where there is more than one pathologist, second opinions on biopsies are often routinely done.

What are the different kinds of biopsies?

There are three general techniques for getting the tissue for a biopsy: incisional, excisional, and needle.

What is an incisional biopsy?

In an incisional biopsy, a part of the tumor is cut out and looked at microscopically. This method is usually favored if the suspicious mass is a large one. The object is to get as large a sample as possible, cutting down on the chances of getting a false reading from a bit of tissue that is not representative of the whole.

What is an excisional biopsy?

In an excisional biopsy, the tumor is removed totally. This method is decided on when the tissue has been identified as cancerous, when strong suspicion exists that part of it may be or become cancerous, or when the tumor is small. Many skin tumors, for example, are totally removed before the biopsy is performed.

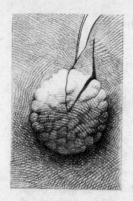
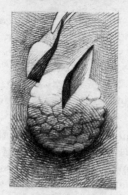
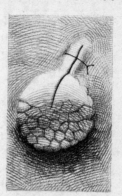

Incisional biopsy

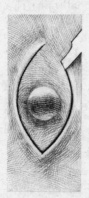
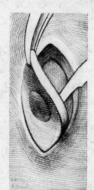
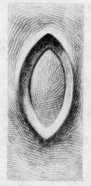
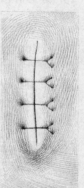

Excisional biopsy

What is a needle or aspiration biopsy?

In a needle biopsy, a needle is used to extract either fluid or tissue for a biopsy. In the United States, the usual needle biopsy is performed by inserting a fine needle into the lump to draw out fluid or tissue juice. A smear of this fluid is then examined for cancer cells. This method is also called an aspiration biopsy. In some places in the country, thin-needle aspiration is being used by urologists to take tissue samples to detect prostate cancer and by other physicians to detect breast cancer.

What is a wide-bore needle biopsy?

It uses a wide-bore needle to extract tissue. It is being used sometimes for liver and bone marrow samples. It is a method used extensively in the Scandinavian countries and in Great Britain. A tiny cutting instrument is inserted through the needle to obtain a tissue sample of the tumor and its immediate surroundings.

What are the advantages and disadvantages of the needle biopsy?

The advantages of the needle biopsy are that generally it can be performed in the doctor's office and requires only local anesthesia. It is a simpler and less expensive way to get the biopsy done. The big disadvantage, especially of the thin-needle biopsy, is that it is easy to get the needle in the wrong place and miss the tumor completely, especially if the growth is a small one. The wide-bore needle biopsy is more reliable.

How does the physician decide which kind of biopsy to perform?

There are no set rules. The size of the lesion, the location of it, and the suspected diagnosis affect the doctor's decision on the type of biopsy to perform.

I keep hearing the term "frozen section." What kind of biopsy is that?

The frozen section can be done with either an excisional biopsy or an incisional biopsy. It refers to the procedure of preparing the tissue for the pathologist to read. There are two ways to prepare the tissue—via the frozen section, which is a quick procedure taking 15 to 20 minutes, or via a permanent section, which takes several days. The frozen section is a quick-reference method of determining whether or not cancer is present. The permanent section is a more accurate method.

When is a frozen-section biopsy used?

The frozen section is performed while the patient is in the operating room. It is used when the surgeon has a suspicious mass which cannot be reached to obtain tissue by means other than an operation. The patient is prepared for the major surgery; the tissue is obtained and the surgeon does not proceed with the operation until the report is relayed to him from the pathologist.

How is the frozen section done?

The surgeon sends the section of tissue he has cut to the pathology laboratory. The tissue is cut and a "touch-prep" slide is made by touching a slide against the tissue so it makes an imprint. Solutions are added to another slice of tissue (about three-sixteenths of an inch thick), which is put into a machine (cryostat) for fast freezing. In about three minutes it is frozen and cut into thin slices. The cut sections are placed on slides and dipped in wood alcohol for about ten seconds. These slides and the touch-prep slide are stained. The frozen-section slides are used to look quickly at the structure of the tissue and the touch-prep slide is used to look at the cellular structure. The two types of slides should agree.

How does the permanent section differ from the frozen section?

The permanent-section biopsy takes considerably longer than a frozen-section biopsy. In this process, the tissue is put through a time-consuming multistage procedure that is highly complicated and that gives a high-quality slide. The tissue is put through a series of solutions to take out the water and fatty substances from it. It is then saturated with warm liquid paraffin. When it has cooled and hardened, the tissue in paraffin is sliced into thin slices. The slices are placed on slides and stained so that the tissue can be studied under the microscope. Proper staining, which brings out cell formations and their nuclei, requires exact timing.

Why is there so much controversy about the frozen section versus the permanent section?

The controversy between these two types of biopsies comes mainly in the area of breast cancer, and whether the patient will have a one-step or a two-step operation. The permanent section, done on an outpatient basis, allows for a complete workup and for alternative treatments.

How is the permanent section done on an outpatient basis?

The permanent section on an outpatient basis is being performed in some of the major medical centers around the country. The patient is told not to eat or drink after midnight, checks into the hospital in the morning, and receives a premedication injection for relaxation and a small amount of local anesthetic in the area to be biopsied. The lump or suspicious tissue is excised, and the wound sutured closed. The patient returns home after a few hours and the pathologist returns a complete report within three or four days.

What are the disadvantages of the frozen section?

In the frozen technique, there can be some distortion of cells because of the freezing process, shrinking in alcohol, and the fact that the stain is a rapidly performed one. The technical appearance of the tissue may not be of the highest quality. The tissue can be wrinkled, torn, and fractured by the cutting processes of the frozen section. The pathologist thus must make the decision based on examination of tissue that may be distorted by the way it has been processed. He must be able to understand which of the changes he sees are processing distortions and which changes are due to the actual abnormalities of the tissue.

Are there any advantages to a frozen section?

There is still considerable controversy about this. It depends upon the kind of cancer and the extent of it. If it is in an area where a permanent section *cannot* be done under local anesthetic, then the frozen biopsy eliminates a second operation. If general anesthesia must be administered to do the permanent section, then a frozen biopsy is called for because no anesthetic agent is perfect and each anesthetic entails a risk. In the area of breast cancer, however, since permanent sections can be done under local anesthetic and the risk of general anesthesia is not involved, it is usually to the patient's advantage to have a permanent section.

What are the advantages of a permanent section?

The advantages of this method are many. The tissue is first fixed in formaldehyde for from three to twelve hours. The fix is better, the tissue shrinkage is more uniform, and the whole process is slower and therefore it reduces tearing of the tissue and distortion of its structure. The tissue cuts thinner in this manner. The method of fixation allows tissue to take up the stain better than the frozen section. The pathologist has the whole tissue block available for cutting samples at a later date. The definition and character of a single cell is much clearer and more precise than in a frozen section. The pathologist usually has better tissue to work with, and therefore you are assured of a more technically correct diagnosis.

Is a second opinion ever called for on a biopsy?

If the diagnosis is malignant, some surgeons send the slides to another pathologist, without including the conclusions of the first, for a second, uninfluenced decision. It is not possible to do this with a frozen section, only with a permanent section. You, as a patient, can request that the slides be sent to a consulting pathologist at another medical center for a second opinion.

Have there been advances in the kinds of microscopes being used by the pathologists?

The electron microscope, which is being used at several medical centers, sorts out tumor cells by exposing fine structures visible only at magnifications at least ten times as high as a light microscope provides. It gives information which the standard microscope cannot give and permits the pathologist to tell the difference between primary and metastatic tumors and often to identify where in the body the cancer began.

What is bone-marrow aspiration? What is bone-marrow biopsy?

These are two similar tests. The biopsy needs a whole piece of the marrow. For both tests, the doctor, using novocaine, inserts a long, hollow needle through the skin and other tissues into the bone marrow—the soft, spongy center of the bone which produces blood cells. A small specimen of the marrow is then removed by suction. The specimen is examined under the microscope for the presence of cancer cells. For a bone-marrow biopsy, the doctor pushes the needle in further until there is a piece of whole marrow in it.

When will the doctor usually order a bone-marrow study?

Usually bone-marrow studies are ordered if some abnormality shows up in the complete blood count or peripheral smear. It is a routine test for suspicion of leukemia or to check if cancer has spread to the bone marrow. The presence of abnormal blood cells is frequently an early sign of tumor-cell invasion of the bone marrow.

What is a metastatic workup?

A metastatic workup is done to see if cancer has spread to other parts of the body. It usually consists of bone and liver scans; sometimes brain and lung scans are added.

Why would the doctor order a bone scan if my cancer is in the breast?

This is a routine check, so don't let it frighten you. It is done because metastasis to the bone is common with breast cancer.

What does the doctor determine from the liver-scan test?

These tests are valuable in alerting the doctor to the presence of liver involvement, although they are not truly diagnostic. The intravenous injection of radioactive material helps to accurately outline liver size, shape, and position and to detect the presence of abnormalities that alter the structure of the liver.

What specific tests does the doctor do to find out whether or not the cancer has metastasized?

For the most common sites to which cancer spreads, the general diagnostic techniques and treatment are:

- *Lung:* This is the most common site for cancer of other organs to spread. X-rays, tomograms, bronchial brushings, scans, fiberoptic bronchoscopy, and biopsies are used in diagnosing lung metastases; chemotherapy and sometimes surgery are used for treatment.
- *Bone:* Metastases to the bone from cancers which start in other organs are more common than is primary bone cancer. Diagnosis is done by x-ray, bone scans, and gallium scans. Radiation, chemotherapy, and hormonal therapy are used for treatment.
- *Liver:* Metastases to the liver from cancers which begin in other organs are more common than is liver cancer itself. Ultrasound and liver scans are used to diagnose it. Radiation and chemotherapy can be used for treatment, depending upon the primary site of the cancer.

- *Brain:* Brain metastases are detected by physical examination and then usually confirmed by brain or CT scan. The treatment is usually radiotherapy or corticosteroids.

Am I wise in not wanting to know the extent of my disease?

It is certainly your privilege to specifically tell your doctor that you not be informed if your diagnosis is bad. However, knowledge of what is happening to you really is more valuable than not knowing.

Should I ask my doctor to explain my case to me?

If you are interested enough to be reading this book, you probably are interested enough in the progress of your own case to want to know the details. The fact is that the better you understand what is happening to you and what the alternatives are, the more likely you are to help in making the right decisions about your own care. The doctor has both a right and a duty to give the patient reasonable knowledge about his condition.

chapter 5

Treatment

Cancer can be treated in several different ways, depending upon the kind and the extent of the tumor. Among them are:
- *Surgery:* removal of the tumor by cutting
- *Radiation:* the use of x-ray or radium
- *Chemotherapy:* the use of drugs and hormones
- *Immunotherapy:* the use of the body's immune system
- *New, experimental or investigational treatments*

Questions to Ask About Treatment

- What treatments are available?
- What treatment do you recommend?
- Is this treatment necessary for me?
- Are there any other alternatives? What are they?
- Why do you think this treatment is preferable?
- What do you expect the results to be?
- How safe is the procedure?
- What are the side effects of the treatment and what can be done to relieve them?
- Can I be put on a program that doesn't interfere with my work schedule?
- How will we determine how well the treatment is working?

Types of Treatment

TREATMENT	DEFINITION	WHEN USED
Surgery	Removal of tumor by cutting	Most often used if tumor is small, if it is limited to a single area of the body, and if cancer has not spread to other parts of the body. It is the most frequently used method.
Radiation	Use of x-ray or radium	For those cancers extremely sensitive to radiation; used as cure attempt when cancer is localized; can be used to control growth; often combined with surgery (before or after); used to cure or palliate in 50-60 percent of all cancer cases.
Chemotherapy and hormone therapy	Use of drugs and hormones	Used after surgery or radiation as "adjuvant" or preventive treatment. Used when cancer is in body system rather than localized in one spot. Used to control growth and for palliation. Often combined with surgery and radiation.
Immunotherapy	Use of body's immune system	Newer, experimental treatment; stimulates or enhances body's own response.

- When can I call you to ask further questions—can I leave a list with the nurse or do you have hours when I can call and talk with you directly?
- Do I have a type of cancer which would be better treated at a specialized center?

Are there any general rules as to when the various treatments are used?

There are some general rules, but you must understand that the treatment will vary depending upon the kind of cancer, the extent of the disease, and how the person reacts to the treatment being given.

Are the kinds of treatment ever combined?

Yes. Often several types of treatments are given to the same patient in hopes of achieving better results than with one type of treatment alone.

How is my specific treatment decided?

Your doctor will consider many factors in determining the treatment for your cancer. Among them are:

- What kind of cancer you have and its pattern of growth and spread
- Aggressiveness of the cancer
- Predictability of the spread of cancer
- The sensitivity of your cancer to specific drugs or other modes of therapy
- Morbidity and mortality of the treatment procedure
- Cure rate of the treatment procedure
- The areas of your body affected by your cancer
- Your physical state

Can I withdraw from a type of treatment once I have started the treatment?

This depends upon you and your doctor. Your doctor should explain in detail the pros and cons of your recommended treatment as well as alternative forms of therapy which might be available to you. Of course the final decision is yours, but you should understand you may be losing valuable time which can never be regained.

How can I get treatment with the newer experimental or investigational drugs?

Information on treatment with newer experimental or investigational drugs approved by the National Cancer Institute is included in Chapter 8.

How can the doctor measure the effectiveness of the various kinds of treatment on the tumor?

Different patients have different responses to treatment. The doctor uses physical exams, x-rays, scans, and various laboratory tests to measure each patient's tumor's response to therapy.

What if the treatment chosen for me does not work?

With the exception of a few cancers, there are many alternative treatment programs which can be used. One may result in controlling the disease even after another has failed to adequately control it.

Why are there so many different kinds of treatment?

Since no two cancers are truly alike and since people respond differently to treatments, patients with seemingly identical diseases may receive different treatments. Each type of cancer has its own way of growing and spreading. Therapy must be tailored to each individual cancer, to its size and location in the body, and to the physical condition of the patient.

What is meant by a curative form of treatment?

A curative treatment is one that is being used to cure the disease.

What is meant by adjuvant forms of treatment?

An adjuvant treatment is one that is being used in addition to a primary form of treatment.

What is meant by palliative treatment?

A palliative treatment is one that is intended to improve the condition of the patient. It may be to reduce pain, to eliminate the worst symptoms, to prevent complications, or to give a psychological uplift.

What is meant by treatment of choice?

The treatment of choice is usually the main kind of treatment of that stage of the illness. In many types of cancer, surgery is the treatment of choice with radiation or chemotherapy used as adjuvant treatments.

What is the most frequently used treatment for cancer?

Surgery is still the most frequently used method of treating cancer, both alone and in conjunction with other methods of therapy, although chemotherapy and radiation are increasingly used today. Surgical resection—the taking out of a portion of an organ or other body structure—was the treatment of choice in 55 percent of all cancer cases in the years 1955–64, according to the National Cancer Institute.

Why has there been a change away from using surgery alone for the treatment of some cancer?

There seems to be an increasing realization that cancer in many instances is a systemic disease—a disease of the body system rather than localized in one spot. Therefore, the use of surgery alone or radiation alone, two forms of treatment which are successful in treating tumors which are confined to one spot, are not adequate when the tumor has spread. In some kinds of cancers, although surgery might remove all visible signs of cancers, based on patients whose disease has recurred, it is thought that micrometastases (small colonies of cancer cells which cannot be detected by any known means) have escaped from the original tumor site and are looking for a home elsewhere in the body. Today there is more work being done in using surgery, radiation, chemotherapy, and immunotherapy to assist one another in a systemic attack against the disease.

Are the different kinds of treatment given one at a time or all together?

It depends upon many factors, including the tumor and the extent of the disease. Sometimes, they are given in sequence. Other times, two or more treatment modes are intermixed. Sometimes, radiation therapy is given first, after which surgery is used. For other kinds of tumors, surgery is the first kind of treatment used.

What is meant by "informed consent"?

Informed consent is a legal standard which defines how much a patient must know about the potential benefits and risks of therapy before being able to agree to undergo it knowledgeably with legal responsibility for the result. The question of informed consent is a very controversial and complex one, particularly if one is talking about surgery or other treatment procedures which carry some risks. Basically, you have the legal right to know everything you want to know about a treatment that is being proposed for you. In experimental or investigational treatment, you will be asked to sign a paper which explains the pros and cons of the treatments before they are performed. In most cancer treatment, however, it is up to you to ask about the major risks involved versus the benefits to be expected.

What is meant by the term "prognosis"?

Your prognosis is an estimate of what the outcome of your disease will be. The doctor bases his prognosis on your general physical condition plus his accumulated information about the disease and its treatment.

What is meant by the term "quality of survival"?

This term is often used when talking about cancer treatment. It means how good the life is that you will be leading. Some people feel that they would rather live a shorter period of time than undergo disfiguring operations or long periods of painful treatment. Influencing the quality of survival are such things as general health, the ability to function normally, pain, the patient's personal attitude, economic status, and physical condition. Each of these items needs to be examined as you assess the treatment for the illness.

chapter 6

Surgery

General Types of Surgery

TYPE	DESCRIPTION	WHEN USED
Specific	Local removal of tumor	When tumor appears to be localized and there is hope of taking out all of cancerous tissue
Radical	Removal of tumor and adjacent tissues or organs affected by cancer cells as well as lymph glands	When surgeon believes this is necessary because of possibility of regional or local spread
Preventive	Removal of growth not presently malignant	If surgeon feels growth might become malignant if left untreated. Used for precancerous conditions such as polyps in colon and moles on skin.
Palliative	Treatment of complications incidental to the disease	To relieve pain; to try to stem spread of disease; to give patient several more years of useful life
Electrosurgery	Use of high-frequency current	For some cancers of skin, mouth, rectum

General Types of Surgery (continued)

Type	Description	When Used
Chemosurgery	Use of chemotherapy drugs on tumor before or instead of surgery	Primarily for skin cancers and melanomas of eyelid
Cryosurgery	Destruction of tumors by freezing	Best for tumors easily seen or felt; usually head and neck and skin cancer
Laser Surgery	Use of laser beam	Experimental

Questions to Ask Your Surgeon Before Operation

- Why do you want to do the surgery?
- Exactly what will you do? Please explain it to me in simple terms.
- How long will I have to stay in the hospital?
- What are the chances for cure with the surgery?
- What other kinds of treatment can you use instead of doing the surgery? Are there any less extensive, less deforming, less painful operations than the one you are suggesting?
- What are the risks of having the surgery?
- What are the risks in the other kinds of treatment?
- What is the risk of death or serious disability?
- Do you feel the benefits outweigh the risks? Why?
- What are the consequences of postponing the surgery?
- What happens if I don't have the surgery?
- How much will the operation cost?
- How long will I be in the hospital?
- How long will the recovery period be?
- How disfiguring will the operation be?
- How disabling will the operation be? Temporarily? Permanently?
- Will I have drains, catheters, intravenous lines, transfusions?
- What are the possible aftereffects?
- How many times have you performed this operation?
- Whom do you recommend I see for a second opinion?
- Can the diagnostic tests be done on an outpatient basis?

Questions to Ask the Anesthesiologist

- What kind of medication will I be given before I go up to the operating room?
- Who will be administering the medication and anesthesia?
- How will they be given to me?
- Are you an anesthesiologist or an anesthetist?
- Will my allergies be a problem?
- What kind of anesthetic are you going to give me?
- What are the side effects?
- What are the risks?
- How long will the operation take?
- How long will it take before I regain consciousness?
- Will I go to a recovery room after the operation?
- What are the fees for your service?
- If you do not want to be fully unconscious during surgery, are elderly, or have lung problems ask: Is general anesthesia absolutely necessary?

Questions to Ask When You Are in the Hospital

- What will be happening to me tomorrow?
- Why is this blood test/x-ray being taken?
- What will this test determine?
- What will this drug accomplish?
- What drugs have you prescribed for me to take and for what purpose?
- This pill/medicine is different from the one I have been taking. Will you please check to make sure it is prescribed for me?
- Do I have to stay in bed?
- Am I allowed to walk to the end of the hall?

Questions to Ask Your Doctor Before Leaving the Hospital

- How long will I have to take it easy after I leave the hospital?
- Will I be a bed patient at home? How long?
- Will I need help at home?
- Will I be able to take care of myself?
- When will I be able to engage in normal activities? (Ask specific questions based on your case: When can I drive a car?

When can I play tennis? When can I resume sexual activities?)
- Will I have to have some special regimen?
- What symptoms, if any, should I report to you? (If you are under the care of several doctors, ask which doctor you should report to if you have questions or problems, and how you can reach the doctor at night.)
- What symptoms should I ignore?
- When can I safely go back to work?
- What medications should I continue to take?
- What exercises will I be permitted to do?

When does surgery offer the best chance of cure for cancer?

If surgery alone is being used, it offers the best chance for cure if the disease is still confined to one site and if the tumor can be fully removed by the surgeon's tools.

Do surgeons remove more than the cancer they can see?

Surgeons usually try to remove the visible cancer tissue plus some of the surrounding tissue, even if it seems normal. This is in case nearby tissue is hiding cancer cells that could later lead to the recurrence of the cancer.

Is surgery safer now than it was some years ago?

Cancer surgery, as well as surgery in general, is safer now than it was 20 or 30 years ago because of many advances in the areas of anesthesia, antibiotics to control infection, and transfusions to build up the patient's blood supply. All surgery has some risk to it. The complications of surgery are often related to the anesthesia. The problem is to weigh the benefits against the risks.

What is specific surgery?

That is when a tumor appears to be localized and there is hope of taking out all of the tissues which are cancerous.

What is radical surgery?

Radical surgery involves removal not only of the tumor but also of adjacent tissues or organs that may have been invaded by the cancer cells; in addition, lymph nodes in the vicinity of the tumor may be removed for staging the cancer to determine prognosis and treatment.

What is preventive surgery?

Preventive surgery is when a surgeon takes out growths which are not presently malignant but might become so if left untreated. These may be precancerous growths. They can be, for example, polyps in the colon, cysts in the breast, or moles on the skin.

What kinds of palliative surgery are performed on cancer patients?

Palliative surgery is sometimes necessary to treat complications incidental to cancer, such as abscesses which are a result of the tumor. The surgeon may sever nerves to relieve pain. Sometimes in patients with advanced breast cancer, the surgeon may remove hormone-producing glands such as ovaries, adrenal glands, or pituitary glands.

What is electrosurgery?

Electrosurgery uses the cutting and coagulating effects of high-frequency current. This is applied by needle, blade, or disk electrodes. It is used as a treatment for some cancers of the skin, mouth, and rectum.

What is chemosurgery?

Chemosurgery is treatment with a chemotherapy drug before or instead of removing the tumor by surgery. The doctor coats the tumor with zinc chloride fixative paste; this paste destroys the upper layer of the tumor. The remaining tumor is then removed by surgery layer by layer until microscopic examination shows that all tumor cells have been eliminated. It is used primarily in the treatment of skin cancers and melanomas of the eyelid. Chemosurgery is gaining wider acceptance; it allows the surgeon to completely remove all cancer cells with a minimum destruction of normal cells.

What is cryosurgery?

Cryosurgery destroys tumors by freezing them with liquid nitrogen. The liquid nitrogen is applied to the tumor through a probe. Instead of a scalpel, the cryosurgeon uses a hollow metal probe that contains liquid nitrogen which is circulating constantly at a temperature of about −196° Centigrade (−320°

Fahrenheit). The tip of the probe is inserted into the tumor or applied to its surface until the tumor has frozen solidly enough to kill the cancer cells. Sometimes liquid nitrogen is sprayed on the tumor surface to freeze the cancer cells.

Does cryosurgery take place in an operating room?

Yes. You are usually taken to an operating room and local or general anesthesia is used just as it is in other surgery. When cryosurgery begins, the cold metal probe is applied to the tumor until it turns into a ball of ice. The temperature of the tissue around the outside of the tumor is measured by insertion of needle thermocouples—a kind of miniature thermometer. The surgeon takes regular readings from the thermocouples to determine just when the tumor has been cooled to the desired temperature.

Is the tissue then allowed to thaw?

When the tissue temperature drops below -30° Centigrade, the probe containing the circulating liquid nitrogen is taken out. The frozen tissue is then allowed to thaw slowly, because the process of thawing helps kill tumor tissue. Usually this process of freezing and thawing is repeated twice or three times at the same operation to make sure the tumor is destroyed. Within four to five days after the surgery, the treated area begins to slough off, as the body rids itself of the dead cells. This leaves a sore which eventually heals.

When is cryosurgery used?

Cryosurgery works best for tumors that are easily seen and felt. It is sometimes used to treat tumors of the head and neck and certain skin cancers. Recent reports show that it may eventually prove useful in the treatment of other forms of cancer such as cancer of the pancreas and localized bone tumors.

What should I know before agreeing to an operation?

Check the list at the beginning of the chapter of questions to ask the doctor before an operation is performed. The doctor should describe the operation in terms you can understand. He should be willing to answer your questions. You should ask what other types of treatment might be used instead of an operation. You should ask the kinds of risks involved in each of the treatments. You should talk with your doctor about getting a second opinion on the treatment. Remember, once the operation has been performed, you cannot change that decision. Check your understanding of what the doctor has told you about your condition and the treatment of it before you leave the office; repeat to him what he has told you so you are sure you understand correctly.

What if the doctor won't take the time to explain what the surgery is all about?

If you think that his explanation is not satisfactory, you should tell him. If the doctor tries to pass it off—"Don't worry about it, I'll take care of you"—and won't answer your questions, you should seriously consider switching to another doctor, especially if you are the type of person who wants to share in the decision-making. Before you agree to any operation you should know what is wrong with you and how the doctor arrived at his diagnosis. The surgeon should be able to tell you what benefits you might gain from surgery and what risks you will face. Be wary if the doctor is not willing to talk about these items.

What if I think of questions after I've left the office?

This happens to almost everybody. The best thing is to have a list of questions you want to ask before you go into the surgeon's office. Bring paper and pencil with you so you can write down the answers. Bring another person in with you so that you have moral and mental support. If you have more questions when you get home, write them down and bring them to your next appointment. Or call the surgeon and arrange a time to discuss them with him.

Does it make any difference what day of the week I go into the hospital for surgery?

You usually do not have a choice, but normally go when there is an empty bed. But there are a few general rules that you should be aware of. It is better not to go into the hospital before a weekend or a holiday. It is best if your surgery is done during the week, rather than just before a weekend, when the hospital may not be as fully staffed. It is better to go into the hospital, if possible, at the beginning of a full work week.

Is it unusual to have drains, catheters, intravenous lines and transfusions when you return to your room after an operation?

Doctors often forget how shocking it can be to a patient and his family to discover that a tube has been connected to his nose to drain his stomach while another has been placed in his chest to drain air, that intravenous feedings are underway, and a catheter is in place to collect urine. Ask your doctor which of these procedures you should expect. Most of them are routine for many operations and if you are prepared for them, and have prepared your family, no one will be alarmed but will accept them for the routine procedures they are.

What kinds of things should I know in order to make an "informed choice" about the surgery?

There are several things you should know if you want to make an informed decision. Among them are:

- The likelihood of being cured, repaired or made better by the operation
- The risk of death or serious disability from the operation or from its complications
- The benefit and the risks of *not* having the operation
- The alternative kinds of treatment which are available
- How disabling and disfiguring the operation is going to be

Are there some operations which are considered overdone?

There was a study done in 1973 in which the surgery done at a large medical-school-affiliated hospital was compared with that done at a smaller unaffiliated suburban hospital. That study showed there were some operations performed much more often at the suburban hospital than at the medical-school-affiliated one. Among the overdone operations that had a relationship to cancer were D&C, hysterectomy, thyroidectomy, and radical mastectomy. In addition, overall, there were generally more operations performed at the suburban hospital than at the medical-school-affiliated hospital. Another study showed that these same operations were also performed more often in the United States as a whole than in either England or Wales.

What can a person do to make sure the operation being performed is necessary?

One of the best ways to make sure that your operation is necessary is to obtain the opinion of at least two surgeons before you agree to an operation. It is also best to choose someone other than a surgeon as your primary-care physician.

Is surgery dangerous?

Yes, all surgery has some risk to it. How much risk is involved depends upon many factors: the kind of operation being performed, the physical condition of the patient, the skill of the surgeon and his team performing the operation (especially the skill of the anesthesiologist), and the caliber of the hospital and its facilities. Again, however, the problem is to weigh the benefits against the risks. It is certainly a subject you should discuss with the surgeon before going ahead with the operation.

What determines whether the doctor will operate or whether another type of treatment will be used?

There are several items which the doctor considers before the decision to operate is made. Among them are:

- Is the person in good enough physical condition to survive the operation?
- Is the operation worth the risk in terms of choice of cure?
- What cell type is the cancer?
- Is there any indication that the cancer may have spread outside the primary site?
- Is it technically feasible to remove the primary tumor and a reasonable margin of surrounding healthy tissue?
- Can similar results be obtained from a different kind of treatment?

What determines how radical the surgery will be?

Different kinds of cancer have different tendencies to spread. The surgeon must understand the history of the kind of cancer he is operating on, the growth rate, and how the tumor spreads. He takes into consideration whether or not the lymph nodes are involved and whether there is any indication that the cancer has spread to other parts of the body. The physical condition of the patient is also a determining factor. The surgeon will remove as much of the organ involved as is reasonable along with a generous margin of apparently normal adjacent tissues and often the neighboring lymph nodes.

What does the surgeon look for during the operation?

The surgeon gathers as much information as is possible about the cancer before the operation. But in some cases, all the questions cannot be answered before the doctor actually looks at and examines the diseased area.

How can the doctor determine if the tissue is malignant during an operation?

If the type of cancer and the degree of malignancy are not definitely known before the operation, the doctor cuts out a piece of the tumor and sends it to the pathologist for a "frozen-section" biopsy at the beginning of the operation. When the test results come back from the laboratory—it usually takes 15 to 20 minutes—the surgeon will then decide whether or not to continue with the operation to remove the tumor.

What if the doctor finds that the tumor has spread too far to remove it?

The doctor's decision in that case will depend upon the kind of operation being done, the condition of the patient, and the history of the disease. In lung surgery, for example, if the tumor has spread too far for the doctor to remove all of it, he will usually leave the lung alone and close the incision. Radiation or chemotherapy will then be used. In other kinds of cancer, the doctor may remove all he can of the tumor and then treat the patient with radiation or chemotherapy.

Are there some types of cancers which respond better to surgery?

The general rule is that the smaller the tumor, and the more differentiated or mature the tumor, the better chance it has to be cured by surgery.

What kind of evaluation should be done before the operation?

There are several things which should be done before any operation for cancer is performed. All the necessary testing should be done so that the diagnosis is as certain as it can be before the operation. More problems result from going ahead with an uncertain diagnosis than from the delay for more review and consultation. This does not mean, however, that you should shop around to try to find a doctor who will tell you that you do not have the disease. Also, the surgeon should consult with the other specialists who might be carrying on further treatment after the operation has been completed.

Is there a special kind of surgeon who works with cancer patients?

There are doctors known as oncological surgeons and gynecological oncologists who specialize in treating cancer patients, although these are not board-certified specialties. Before you have an operation, you should know whether or not your doctor has had special training in cancer treatment, and you should find out about his experience in treating your particular kind of cancer. There are no easy guidelines, but one or two cases of treatment of a particular kind of cancer a year does not qualify as extensive experience. Each cancer has its own special history of how it grows and where it spreads. The choice of a surgeon is a very critical part of cancer treatment. It is very important that the doctor know how your cancer might spread so that the proper operation can be done.

What is the American Board of Surgery?

The American Board of Surgery was established in 1937 by a group of prominent American surgeons, mostly college professors of surgery. Rigorous testing, written and oral, is administered to those who qualify with full training in approved surgical residencies. The board certification is a high point in the surgeon's career, proving to his fellow surgeons and to others that he has the judgment and ability to be a specialist in surgery. While it is true that some excellent surgeons are not board-certified, those who are not should be carefully checked before you allow them to operate on you. Although the board certification is not an absolute guarantee that the surgeon is a competent one, it is one of the criteria by which you can judge a surgeon.

What does F.A.C.S. mean?

The initials F.A.C.S. mean that the surgeon is a Fellow of the American College of Surgeons, a criterion to be used in evaluating the competence of the doctor. The American College of Surgeons, though it at present requires qualification for membership similar to that of the American Board of Surgery, does not demand rigorous testing before a candidate is admitted as a Fellow. Most first-class surgeons are members of the American College of Surgeons as well as being diplomates of the American Board of Surgery, and they operate in accredited hospitals. Either of these professional recognitions is indication that the surgeon is well trained and has proved to other surgeons that he is qualified in his area of specialization.

What kinds of qualifications does a doctor need to be a general surgeon?

To be certified as a surgeon by the American Board of Surgery, the person must be a licensed doctor of medicine, have had a minimum of four years of residency training in general surgery, and have successfully completed a written and an oral examination given by the board. Specialized surgeons must take additional years of training to be qualified.

Do all surgeons have to pass boards of the American Board of Surgery?

No. You should know that a doctor can be a surgeon without having passed the boards. It is worth checking to see what kind of qualifications the doctor has before you agree to let him operate on you.

What is a thoracic surgeon?

A thoracic surgeon is a highly specialized doctor. He operates on patients with problems in organs in the chest area. In the cancer field, this includes lungs and the esophagus. To be certified by the American Board of Thoracic Surgery, a doctor must have been certified by the American Board of Surgery, have had two additional years of training in thoracic surgery, and have successfully completed the written and oral examinations given by the board.

What are the qualifications of a plastic surgeon?

To be certified by the American Board of Plastic Surgery, the person must be a licensed doctor of medicine, have three years of training in general surgery or prior certification by any one of several surgical specialty boards, have had a minimum of two additional years of training in plastic surgery, and have successfully completed the written and oral exams given by the board.

What is a proctologist?

Doctors certified by the American Board of Colon and Rectal Surgery are often called proctologists. A proctologist is especially qualified to examine and perform operations of the colon and rectal area. To be certified by the board, a person must be a licensed doctor of medicine, have had four years of training in general surgery, and have had one year of training in colon and rectal surgery. The doctor could substitute three years of general surgical practice and two years of colon-rectal surgical training or certification by the American Board of Surgery if he plans to limit his practice to colon and rectal surgery and has demonstrated special competence in that field.

What is a neurosurgeon?

A neurosurgeon is concerned with the diagnosis and treatment of diseases of the nervous system (brain, spinal cord, and nerves) and its surrounding structures. To be certified by the American Board of Neurological Surgery, he must be a licensed doctor of medicine, have had one year of training in general surgery, four years of training in neurological surgery, and two years of independent practice of neurological surgery, and have successfully completed examinations given by the board.

What is the difference between a neurologist and a neurosurgeon?

The neurologist has many skills in common with the neurosurgeon but is not qualified to perform operations. Your internist will probably refer you to a neurologist if you have a problem of the nervous system. If you need an operation, the neurologist will send you to a neurosurgeon. The neurologist, certified by the American Board of Psychiatry and Neurology, must be a licensed doctor of medicine, have had three years of specialized training in neurology, have had two additional years of satisfactory experience in neurology, and have successfully completed the written and oral examinations. A neurological surgeon must be qualified as a surgeon, plus having completed four years in neurological surgery.

Is a gynecologist also a surgeon?

The gynecologist is trained to deal with problems related to the female genital system. He is also a surgeon with the skills necessary to correct diseases of the ovaries, fallopian tubes, uterus, and vagina. Many gynecologists also perform breast operations. Some gynecologists who specialize in cancer treatment are known as gynecologic oncologists. To be certified by the American Board of Obstetrics and Gynecology, the person must be a licensed doctor of medicine, have had three years of residency in obstetrics and gynecology, have successfully completed the written examination of the board, have had at least twelve months of independent practice, and have successfully completed an oral examination given by the board.

Does an ophthalmologist perform surgery?

The ophthalmologist treats the diseases of the eye and surrounding structures and has had extensive training and experience in the complex and delicate surgical treatment of eye diseases. To be certified by the American Board of Ophthalmology, the person must be a licensed doctor of medicine, have had three years of residency and basic science courses in ophthalmology, have had one year of independent practice or research, and have successfully completed the written and oral examinations given by the board.

What is an orthopedic surgeon?

The orthopedic surgeon is a specialist in the diagnosis and treatment of diseases of the bones, joints, tendons, and muscles. In the cancer area, he treats a great variety of bone tumors. To be certified by the American Board of Orthopedic Surgery, the person must be a licensed doctor of medicine, have had four years of general surgery, two years in the orthopedic area, and have successfully completed an examination given by the board.

There are orthopedic surgeons in the larger medical centers who have special interest in cancer. If you have bone cancer, check to see if the specialist you are going to is treating a majority of cancer cases in his practice.

What kind of doctor is an otolaryngologist?

An otolaryngologist specializes in the diseases of the ear, nose, throat, and larynx. Sometimes this doctor is called an ENT specialist. He is qualified to examine and perform surgery on these organs. To be certified by the American Board of Otolaryngology, the person must be a licensed doctor of medicine, have had one year of residency in general surgery, have had three years of residency in otolaryngology, and have successfully completed oral and written examinations administered by the board. Again, some ENT specialists are primarily involved with cancer cases.

Does a urologist perform surgery?

The urologist is a specialist in the diseases which affect the kidneys, ureters, urethra, bladder, prostate gland, and male sex organs. He is an expert in both the diagnosis of the disease and in surgical treatment in the area. To be certified by the American Board of Urology the person must be a licensed doctor of medicine, have had two years of post-medical training, have had three additional years of training in urologic surgery and eighteen months of independent practice, and have successfully completed the written and oral examination given by the board.

Are there some suggestions you have for choosing a surgeon? How can I be sure I have a competent person?

You probably have more influence over the choice of your surgeon than of your primary physician. Check out the surgeon's credentials and check out the hospital where he will operate to make sure you are getting "one of the best." (See Chapter 2.)

Remember these basic points:

- It is best to have a surgeon who is board-certified and a Fellow of the American College of Surgeons. Although this professional accreditation is just a guide, it tells you the doctor is well trained and has proved to other surgeons that he is qualified in his area of specialization.

- It is best to choose a doctor who has performed the operation many times. Although this does not prove he is competent, as a general rule the more experienced the surgeon, the more competent he is.
- It is best to be in a hospital which has an approved cancer program sponsored by the American College of Surgeons or is part of a comprehensive cancer center or is directly affiliated with a medical school. At the very least, the hospital should be accredited by the Joint Commission on Accreditation for Hospitals (JCAH) or the American Osteopathic Association.
- It is best to choose a surgeon who is willing to answer your questions and to give you the time and attention you feel you need. Check your understanding of what the doctor has told you about the operation by repeating it to him in your own words.
- It is best, if you wish, for you to know the risks of the surgery. Ask the doctor to tell you the risks based on your particular physical condition added to the statistical evidence (both national and local) compiled over the years for the particular operation you will have. You should also ask what the risks are if you do *not* have the surgery.
- It is best to have a surgeon who knows and can work with your general practitioner or internist. Remember it is the surgeon who will most probably be in charge of your care while you are in the hospital.
- It is best to choose a surgeon who is part of a group or who is hospital-based, since this will probably offer you the best total care both before and after the surgery.
- If you are getting a second opinion, it is best to get it outside of the particular group practice where your primary physician is located, or where the first surgeon is located.
- It is best to get a second opinion before having the surgery done.

Are there different kinds of anesthesia used in operations?

Anesthesia primarily means the loss of feeling, particularly the senses of touch and pain. You will either have a general anesthesia or anesthesia applied to a specific part of your body. Among the terms you might hear are:
- General anesthesia

- Regional anesthesia
- Topical anesthesia
- Inhalation anesthesia
- Intravenous anesthesia
- Spinal anesthesia
- Epidural anesthesia

Is general anesthesia dangerous?

Anesthesia is necessary for surgery. In most cases, general anesthesia must be given, so you will be asleep during the operation. In some cases, local or regional anesthesia can be used. In general, the surgery is less risky if local anesthesia is used. If you are aged or have a history of lung problems, you may want to ask your doctor and the anesthesiologist to explore whether general anesthesia is absolutely necessary.

When is general anesthesia used?

The doctors use this term when referring to any anesthesia which puts you to sleep so treatment can be done on any part of the body. The anesthesia may be light, such as for a superficial procedure upon the skin. You may be given a deep anesthesia so that operations upon the heart, lungs, or abdomen can be carried out. The anesthesiologist aims at producing a sleep of just enough depth to permit safe surgery.

What is regional anesthesia?

Needles can be put in various parts of the body and anesthesia such as novocaine can be injected to block or temporarily deaden those nerves supplying particular parts. That means that an arm, hand, neck, or side of the face alone, for example, can be anesthetized so that the operation can be performed. The advantage of regional anesthesia is that your heart, lungs, blood pressure, and general condition are unaffected because only specific nerves are blocked. This means many poor-risk patients can be operated on who could not withstand a spinal or general anesthesia.

What is topical anesthesia?

An anesthetic is sprayed or painted onto a mucous membrane surface (a lubricating layer lining an internal surface or an organ).

Topical anesthesia is usually used for eye, nose, and throat procedures. Sometimes it is followed by injections of novocaine or similar local anesthetics. It is also commonly used when tubes are being put into the trachea (windpipe) or esophagus (food passage).

What is inhalation anesthesia?

This is a common type of general anesthesia. You inhale an anesthetic gas which is pleasant to breathe. Many gases are used for this purpose, such as ether and nitrous oxide (laughing gas), in combination with oxygen. The gases go from the lungs into the bloodstream to the brain, where they induce anesthesia. Inhalation anesthesia is administered through a mask which is connected by rubber tubes to a breathing bag and then to the anesthesia machine and gas tanks.

What is intravenous anesthesia?

This type of anesthesia is injected directly into your bloodstream through a vein. Usually sodium pentothal is the drug used. You will go to sleep almost at once. Sometimes an intravenous anesthesia is given to you before you get inhalation anesthesia. After the initial needle injection into the vein of the arm or foot, a solution containing the medication is allowed to drip into the bloodstream at a controlled rate of speed.

How is spinal anesthesia given?

A long, thin needle is put into the fluid surrounding your spinal cord and the drug is injected. This drug, actually a local anesthetic, blocks pain impulses in the spinal cord. You will have no feeling in your legs and pelvis. It is the kind of anesthesia often used during childbirth.

Are there different kinds of spinal anesthesia?

Spinal anesthesias are called by different names depending on where they are being injected. A high spinal anesthesia is used when organs in the mid- or upper stomach area are being operated on. A low spinal anesthesia is used when the rectum or genital organs in the lower area are the site of the operation. A saddle block is a form of spinal anesthesia used when the rectum or genital organs are being operated on. Spinal anesthesia completely anesthesizes that part of the body served by the nerves at the site of the injection into the spinal canal. Thus you can be awake and alert and your abdomen and lower extremities can be insensitive to pain.

What are epidural and caudal anesthesia?

These are similar to spinal anesthesia except that the drug is injected into the area outside the spinal canal rather than within it. It has some advantages, especially in protecting patients against the post-spinal headaches they sometimes get with spinal anesthesia. Its big disadvantage is that it needs a skilled operator to give it and it is not as complete an anesthetic as is the spinal.

What is meant by a nerve block?

Anesthesia can be given around the boundary of an area to make a nerve block. For example, lack of feeling around your hand can be caused by putting in a local anesthetic around the nerve in your elbow—the doctor has "blocked off" the sensory nerves some distance away from the actual site of the operation. It is a regional anesthetic.

Are different kinds of painkillers ever used in combination?

The anesthesiologist has many kinds of painkillers to choose from, such as sedatives, muscle relaxants, analgesics, narcotics, and gases. Sometimes one or two are used; at other times as many as six or more might be needed. Some are pills, others must be injected. Some can be given through a face mask or by putting a tube into the windpipe. The anesthesiologist combines various painkillers and uses one drug to reinforce another so that in total a lesser amount is needed. This keeps undesirable reactions to a minimum.

Will I be awake during spinal or local anesthesia?

You can be. Or if you wish, intravenous drugs can be given to you to put you to sleep during such anesthesia.

Who gives the anesthesia?

Anesthesia should be given either by an anesthesiologist or under the direction of an anesthesiologist. An anesthesiologist is a doctor specializing in anesthesia—the physician who can choose the most appropriate type of anesthesia to be used—and during surgery is responsible for maintaining all the body's vital functions.

What is an anesthetist?

Anesthetists are non-physicians, usually specially trained nurses who give anesthesia under the direction of a doctor. A hospital's department of anesthesiology, besides being responsible for the administration of anesthesia during surgery, usually sets the standards for the way in which the operating room and the recovery room are run.

Does the anesthesiologist work only in the operating room?

No, he works in the recovery room as well. It is the responsibility of the anesthesiologist to alleviate pain, relieve anxieties before the operation, increase the safety in the operating room, provide the best conditions for the surgeon during the actual operation, and help assure complete and comfortable recovery afterward. Anesthesiologists have made it possible to operate on patients who not long ago would have been considered poor surgical risks because they were too young, too old, or too feeble.

What will the anesthesiologist do during the operation?

He will be present during the operation and after it, monitoring your condition. He will watch your blood pressure, pulse rate, temperature, and the electrocardiographic recording of the action of your heart. He can administer glucose, plasma, whole blood, and various other drugs as needed.

What are the qualifications of a board-certified anesthesiologist?

If the anesthesiologist is certified by the American Board of Anesthesiology, he is a licensed doctor who has completed at least two years of specialized training in anesthesiology plus one year in other medical training, and has passed qualifying tests. If he is listed as a Fellow of the American College of Anesthesiologists, his proficiency has been certified by the college's board of governors after qualifying tests.

Can I decide what kind of anesthesia I would like?

The decision on the kind of anesthesia to be used should be made by your anesthesiologist and surgeon. However, you can discuss any feelings and desires you have, and if you do not want a particular kind of anesthesia, you should discuss that with the doctors. If you wish to be asleep instead of awake during the surgery (even though you will not experience any pain) you should talk to the doctor about that.

How does the anesthesiologist decide what kind of anesthesia to use?

It depends upon the kind of operation, what the surgeon needs during the procedure, and the physical needs of the patient.

How long can a person stay under anesthesia?

It varies depending upon the kind of drugs used and the condition of the patient. Surgeons are not under the same pressure to hurry through operations as they once were, mainly because of advances in methods of anesthesia and better monitoring of patients during surgery.

Will I meet the anesthesiologist?

In some hospitals, the anesthesiologist comes to your room the evening before your surgery. He will try to ease any anxiety you feel, explain what will happen, and answer your questions. He will also ask you some questions, such as whether you have any allergies, whether you are sensitive to any drugs, and whether you have any illnesses other than the one for which you are being operated on. He might ask you whether you have ever had anesthesia before and whether you had ill effects from it. He will want to know about any past history of liver or kidney disease, since these organs eliminate certain anesthetic agents from the body. He needs to know what medications you are taking because anesthetics could cause dangerous reactions when combined with a number of other drugs, particularly tranquilizers, antidepressants, sedatives, and drugs used to lower blood pressure. The anesthesiologist will get some of this information from your medical history and other available medical records as well as by consulting with your surgeon.

Are there any special questions I should ask him if he comes to visit me before the operation?

You might want to know things such as the drugs he is planning to use, what discomfort, if any, you will have, when you will go to sleep, and when you will wake up consciously. If you have a special request—such as wanting to be asleep during a "minor" procedure that is ordinarily performed with a local anesthetic, or not wanting a spinal anesthetic—be sure to talk with him about it. The anesthesiologist will often do what you want if it is medically sound. Be sure you tell the anesthesiologist about all your allergies, whether they are drug-related or not.

How do I know that the doctor will not start the operation when I can still feel pain?

One of the jobs of the anesthesiologist is to make sure that you can feel no pain. He will conduct tests to make sure that before any surgery begins, you cannot feel the pain.

Will I have any medication the night before the operation?

It depends. The doctor might order tablets or injections the night before your surgery to make sure you have a good night's rest. If you are a heavy smoker or drinker, the doctor may tell you to stop for several days before the operation because these could cause complications with the anesthesia both during and after the operation.

Is anesthesia painful?

Not with today's procedures. Probably an hour or so before the operation, you will be given something to make you drowsy and relaxed. You may also be given medication (such as stropine or scopolamine) to dry up mucous and salivary-gland secretions, which will help in the anesthesia. The anesthesia will be given in the operating room. Anesthesia, even types which were once painful, is now an almost painless procedure.

How will the anesthesia be injected into me?

After you reach surgery, the anesthesiologist will probably insert an intravenous (IV) needle into you so that any drugs which need to be used during the operation can easily be injected. If you are to be asleep during the operation, a drug will be injected and within seconds you will be sleeping. If a mask is to be used or an endotracheal tube is to be inserted, this will be done after you are asleep so you will not be aware of it. Sometimes you will be given a short-acting muscle relaxant to make it easier to pass a tube.

Will the IV needle be used for drugs other than the anesthetic?

It depends upon the operation. If you need additional drugs, these can easily be put in through the intravenous needle. The needle is joined to a length of flexible tubing attached to a bottle hanging over the operating table. The drops of whatever drug are needed, when released into the tube, will go immediately into the bloodstream.

What kinds of tests are done before the operation?

In cancer-related operations, many tests are performed to make as complete a diagnosis as possible. These tests are described in Chapter 4 and also in the chapters which discuss the particular kinds of cancer. There are some general tests which are performed for all operations. Included in these are:

- Blood sample to test for hemoglobin (oxygen-carrying pigment of blood) to discover anemia; count of red and white blood cells; sometimes a routine test for syphilis
- Blood-type test if surgeon feels there is the slightest chance of need for blood transfusion
- Urine analysis for presence of sugar, blood, pus cells, crystals and other materials

Is it important for me to know what blood type I am?

You should know your blood type, especially if it is a rare one. Ask your doctor and carry this information with you. If you do not know, blood types are quickly and easily determined in a laboratory by a simple slide or tube test.

What are the blood types?

Most people in the United States have either O Positive blood or A Positive blood. The frequency of the various blood types varies geographically and by racial or ethnic groups. In the United States whites are more likely than blacks to have type A blood, and blacks are more likely to have type B blood. Both races have about the same frequency of type O and type AB. This table shows the overall blood-type frequencies in the United States:

BLOOD TYPE	RH FACTOR	PERCENT OF THE POPULATION
O	Positive	39
A	Positive	35
B	Positive	9
O	Negative	6
A	Negative	5
AB	Positive	4
B	Negative	1.5
AB	Negative	0.5

Are there special procedures which are done the night before the operation?

There are several procedures which may be done.

- *Shaving:* Since the skin and hair hide organisms which can cause infections, a wide area is usually shaved and cleansed before the operation. Usually a nurse or orderly will shave and clean with antiseptic an area larger than the proposed incision; skin preparation may start as much as 24 hours before the operation.

- *Enema:* Because there may be temporary interference with normal functioning of the intestines after some kinds of surgery and the bowels may not move for several days, an enema may be given the night before the operation to clear out the bowel.

- *Fasting:* You will usually not be allowed to eat or drink for about 12 hours before the operation so that it can be done on an empty stomach. You will probably be told to have a light evening meal and then nothing by mouth after midnight the night before surgery.

- *Sedatives:* Usually you will be given a sleeping pill so that you will have a good night's sleep before the operation. An hour or two before you go to the operation room an injection is usually given so that you will be in a calm, semiconscious state.

- *Stomach tubes:* If you are having an operation in the stomach area, a rubber tube is usually inserted through the nose into the stomach so that the stomach and bowels will be empty and free of fluids and gas. Sometimes this is done the night before or in the morning. It is usually left in place throughout the operation.

- *Urinary catheter:* For some operations, especially those in the pelvic and bladder area, a rubber catheter is inserted so that the bladder will be empty. This may be done in your room or in the operating room.
- *Blood transfusions:* Depending upon the operation and your own condition, you may receive a transfusion of blood before the operation. In many cases, blood is given before, during, and/or after the operation. Sometimes plasma is given instead of whole blood.

Are intravenous feedings usually a part of surgery?

The bottle of clear fluid is usually a part of both the preoperative (before the operation) and postoperative (after the operation) procedures. Doctors have found that surgery is much safer when carried out on patients with normal blood chemistry. Various substances such as water, salt, sugar, protein, potassium, calcium, and vitamins can be given to the patient via the intravenous route, through the veins of the arms and legs, to substitute for the solid food which you cannot have until normal digestive processes are reestablished. (You will hear the term "IV," which is the shorthand for "intravenous.") It is not unusual for intravenous treatments to be continued for the first four or five days after a serious procedure has been performed.

What is meant by being "prepped" for an operation?

To ensure a perfectly sterile operation, several steps are taken. Usually a wide area around where the incision is to be made is shaved. The area is first washed with a mixture of iodine and soap and all body hair is removed. The entire abdomen, genital area, and upper legs are often shaved for an abdominal procedure. For a brain operation, the head is shaved.

Why is a catheter needed for a surgical operation?

A catheter, a narrow tube which is inserted through the urethra to the bladder, is sometimes used during surgery to drain off urine. It is usually put in place before you are brought up to surgery. Thanks to modern materials, the flexibility of the catheter now permits it to be inserted with little or no discomfort.

What does the doctor mean when he says he'll write a "stat order"?

The medical profession uses the term "stat" fairly frequently and in several contexts. The word comes from the Latin *statim*, meaning "immediate" or "rush." A stat order is simply a request for fast service.

Who is usually in the operating room during the surgery?

Several people help with any operation, no matter how minor. The team, depending upon the extent of the operation, may be composed of:

- Surgeon
- One to three assistant surgeons, depending on the position, nature, complexity or technical peculiarities (even some minor procedures need more than one hand).
- Anesthesiologist or anesthetist
- Chief operating room nurse who is the overall supervisor
- Nurse in charge of surgical supply
- Scrub or suture nurse who handles instruments
- Circulating or chase nurse who gets additional supplies and is responsible for the sponge counts (sponges are layered gauze pads used to blot blood so the surgeon can see)
- Additional persons, as needed, such as a cardiologist during a heart operation

How are stomach tubes inserted?

With the head tipped back, a thin tube is inserted in the nostril and pushed up and backward. You then swallow and the tube slides smoothly into the throat and to the stomach. Sometimes some kind of anesthetic is given when the tube is inserted. The tube is usually left in place throughout the operation and sometimes for a number of days after it to help suction off fluid and gas.

Does the length of time I spend in the operating room indicate the seriousness of the operation?

It depends upon the individual case. There are several items which can make your time in the operating room longer but have no bearing on your own operation. For instance:

- The patients are sent for, some time in advance of the actual operation.

- The anesthesiologist can make additional preparations that last 30 minutes or even an hour.
- The surgeon can take longer than he expected on the operation before yours, thus starting on your operation later than scheduled.
- You could spend more time than anticipated in the recovery room.

Your family and friends should never judge the length or seriousness of an operation by the amount of time you spend in the operating room.

Will I need to go into the recovery room after my operation?

Yes, it is the usual procedure so that you can be watched and checked by a medical team until you awaken. The recovery room has equipment for monitoring your heart action and respirators for assisting you to breathe if you need them. You can get intravenous fluids and blood in the recovery room. Normally the recovery room is run by a physician anesthesiologist so that you can be monitored when you wake up from the anesthesia. Respiration therapists will probably help you cough and inflate your lungs as soon as you wake up. You may spend several hours or even days in the recovery room.

What if I have my operation late in the day—will I still go to the recovery room?

It depends upon the hospital. Some will take you to the intensive-care unit rather than the recovery room if you are on the afternoon surgical schedule because in some hospitals the night-patient load in recovery rooms doesn't warrant maintaining a staff through the night.

How long will it take for the anesthesia to wear off after the operation?

Once the operation is finished, it can take anywhere from minutes to hours before you wake up. It depends upon the kind of anesthesia you are given and the dose. If you have had local, regional or spinal anesthesia, it will wear off within one to three hours after the operation.

Will things seem hazy as I come out of the anesthesia?

Sometimes they do. Voices may seem to be coming from a long

way off. You may not hear them distinctly. People may seem to be moving differently from the way you think they should. Vision, hearing, and sense of balance can all be affected by anesthesia and it takes time for it to wear off.

Will I be able to get painkilling drugs after the operation if I need them?

You may experience some pain as you become fully conscious. There are many painkilling drugs which can be used with perfect safety. The doctor will be trying to balance your immediate comfort with your recovery. Some of the drugs tend to slow up vital functions. Since it is important after an operation that your vital functions get back to normal as quickly as possible, you may be asked to put up with some pain to speed your recovery. But if you are feeling a substantial degree of pain, be sure that your nurse and your doctor know about it. Try to keep your reports as factual as possible.

What are the general procedures that are followed after an operation?

It depends upon your doctor, the hospital, the operation performed, and your own physical condition. You will usually spend some time in the recovery room. Then, some of the following common procedures will probably be followed:

- *Bedrest:* You will most probably spend some time lying flat in bed. After your recovery from the anesthesia, you will be encouraged to change your position and move your legs often. This is to stimulate your circulation and make you breathe deeply so you will not get blood clots or pneumonia.
- *Getting out of bed:* Usually you will be made to get out of bed and walk a little the day after the operation with most major types of surgery, although sometimes it will be a few days or even a week or longer. Again, it depends upon many factors. Getting out of bed as soon as possible speeds your recovery and minimizes complications of the operation.
- *Eating and drinking:* Unless you have had surgery of the stomach or intestinal tract, you usually will be given sips of water or tea within a few hours after your operation and will be allowed a bland diet the next day. Stomach and intestinal-tract patients usually don't eat or drink for 48–72 hours.

- *Gas or urinary problems:* If you are having trouble with stomach gas, you will be encouraged to move about and walk as much as you are able. If the problem persists, a rubber tube may be put through your nose and into your stomach for 24 hours. The doctor may also order pain medication. If you have trouble urinating, you can be given a medication to stimulate natural voiding. If the problem continues, you may have a catheter inserted to empty the bladder. The ability to urinate spontaneously returns usually within a week's time.
- *Pain:* If you have pain, your doctor may prescribe a pain medication. Many times pains involved with abdominal surgery are gas pains.
- *Other:* Depending on the operation and your condition, the doctor may order antibiotic drugs, intravenous fluids and medications, blood transfusions, and enemas.

Are there any common problems I can expect from my operation?

There is a wide variation of side effects from operations, again depending upon the operation and your own condition. Many people never experience any serious problems. However, some of the symptoms are:

- *Nausea and vomiting* due to the anesthetic, drugs, or the operation. The doctor may not allow you to eat or drink for 24 hours or may pass a tube into your stomach.
- *Gas pains* sometimes follow stomach operations. They usually disappear in a few days. Sometimes for severe cases, a tube is inserted in the rectum or in the stomach. Usually by the third day, the bowel begins to function normally.
- *Soreness* in the wound area. Medication can be ordered.
- *Dizziness and weakness.* If they occur, they usually disappear within a week or two without treatment.
- *Headaches* may occur when spinal anesthesia is used. The doctor may order a special medication plus lots of fluids. The headaches may last a week or two.
- *Tiredness.* Many people complain that they have little energy and feel like sleeping. It is important for you to nap when you feel tired and to limit visitors if you do not feel up to seeing people.

How can I be sure I am getting the right medication in the hospital?

If your doctor orders medicines for you on a regular basis, learn to recognize the ones he has prescribed, and if an unfamiliar capsule or liquid is offered to you, ask about it.

What will the nurses be checking me for during the first few days after my operation?

They will be checking your general color and appearance and your blood pressure, pulse, temperature, and rate of breathing. They will observe if your reflexes are getting back to normal and if you are swallowing properly. They'll come in to give you your medication and other things you may need. They will make you move in your bed, sit up, dangle your legs over the side of the bed, or walk—depending upon what your doctor has ordered for you. They will be checking for proper elimination of both urine and stool. For the first few times after the operation, they will help you get out of bed.

Will I get any help for deep breathing?

That depends upon the operation and your physical condition. It is important that you begin deep breathing early after an operation to prevent pneumonia and other complications. If your breathing is shallow, the air sacs around the edges of your lungs don't fill out. You may be made to blow into a special machine to help with your deep breathing.

What if I have soreness around my incision?

There is some soreness generally around an incision, but if there is unusual soreness let your doctor or nurse know at once.

When will the dressings be changed?

The time for changing dressings varies widely depending upon the operation. Usually if the wound is clean without a drain it is left alone until the doctor takes out the stitches. Draining wounds or those which become infected might need to be changed every day. If it is the kind which would be painful, you may get a pain-relieving medication before the dressing is changed.

When will the stitches be taken out?

They are usually taken out from the sixth to the tenth day, depending on where the operation is. If it is in an area where there is tension on it or if it is not healing firmly, it will be left in for a longer time. Sometimes metal clips are used instead of sutures. These are usually taken out on the fourth to sixth day.

The nurse does not seem to want to answer my questions. What should I do?

It depends upon the kinds of questions you are asking. There are some questions which the nurse cannot answer. But you should realize that the nurse in the hospital (and in the doctor's and radiation therapist's offices) is one of your best sources of information. If she can't answer the questions herself, she might be able to get you the answers. It is helpful to write down your questions so that when you do see the doctor you can ask those that the nurse has not been able to answer for you.

What does surgery for cancer cost?

Surgery costs vary greatly from one area of the country to another, from one doctor to another, and from operation to operation. The one rule you should follow is to have a full and frank discussion of the costs of surgery before you go into the hospital. Extra charges may be made by the hospital for such items as x-rays, special drugs, medications and treatments, blood transfusions, anesthesia, the use of the operating room, the use of laboratory facilities, fees for consultations and/or second opinions while hospitalized, etc.

chapter 7

Radiation

Radiation therapy is the second most common treatment for cancer, following surgery. The National Cancer Institute estimates that more than half of all cancer patients receive radiation treatment sometime during the course of their illness.

Questions to Ask Your Doctor

- Exactly what type of radiation treatment will I be getting?
- Who will be responsible for my radiation treatment?
- Whom should I notify if I have questions about my radiation treatment?
- Can I continue to work during these treatments?
- Is there a more convenient place where my treatments can be given?
- How long will it take for each treatment? for the whole series?
- What side effects can I expect?
- What should I do if these side effects occur?
- What side effects should I report to the doctor?
- How much will it cost?
- How much of a risk is involved?
- What is the alternative?
- What if I don't have this treatment at all?

Radiation Terminology

Type	Definition	Use	Other Terms
External beam	Machine delivers x-rays or gamma rays to tumor on or in patient's body. Machine usually some distance from patient's body. Neutron beam is a new experimental type of external beam therapy.	Most frequently used kind of radiation	X-ray machine, linear accelerator, cobalt machine, superficial x-ray, orthovoltage machine, supervoltage equipment, megavoltage machine, cobalt 60 machine, betatrons, cobalt therapy
Internal radiation	Radioactive material such as radium placed directly into or on area to be treated. It is either sealed in a container and inserted into a body cavity or given orally or injected with a syringe.	Breast, vagina, bladder, mouth, tongue, prostate, thyroid	Radioactive cesium, radium needles, radium seeds, radioactive iodine, liquid radioactive gold, radioactive phosphorus, radium, cobalt 60, gold 198, phosphorus 32, iodine 131, iridium 192, interstitial implant, intracavitary implant, needle implant

Do I have a choice as to where I will have my radiation treatments?

Usually, the doctor will advise you where your radiation treatments will be given. It is a good idea for you to have a frank discussion with him about why he advises a specific radiotherapy department or a specific radiotherapist. You may want to explore whether it would be advantageous for you to use a large medical center versus a small hospital closer to home. You must weigh for yourself the advantages of convenience versus the technology and expertise a larger medical center usually has to offer. Radiology is a science which has made many advances both in technology and in application, and the radiologist will be playing an important part in your treatment.

Is radiation therapy used alone?

Yes, it can be used alone. However, many treatments for cancer today include more than one form of therapy, and radiation is often used in combination with surgery or chemotherapy.

Is radiation therapy called by any other names?

You will hear it referred to by many other terms, such as radiotherapy, radiology, x-ray therapy, x-ray treatment, irradiation, radiation treatment, and cobalt treatment.

Is there more than one type of radiation treatment?

Radiation treatment is usually divided into two basic kinds: external-beam radiation and internal radiation.

What is external-beam radiation?

When external-beam radiation is used, a machine delivers x-rays or gamma rays to a tumor on or in the patient's body. The machine is usually some distance from the patient.

What is internal radiation?

This is when the physician places some radioactive material such as radium directly into or on the area to be treated. Sometimes, this is called a radium implant. Usually the radioactive materials are put into small metal tubes or needles which are then placed surgically within or near the cancerous tissue. The tubes or needles are usually removed after the required radiation dose has been given. Sometimes internal radiation is used alone; other times it is used in addition to external-beam radiation.

What are the categories of radiation treatment?

Again, as in surgery, there are three general categories: primary or curative treatment, palliative treatment for control of symptoms (not expected to cure), and treatment used as an adjuvant to other therapies.

What is curative radiation?

Curative radiation is when radiation is being used as the primary treatment to cure the cancer. It is the treatment of choice, for example, for some stages of Hodgkin disease and cervical, skin, and head and neck cancers.

When does the doctor choose radiation as a curative treatment rather than surgery?

The doctor usually chooses curative radiation instead of surgery when:

- The tumor is the type that is especially susceptible to destruction by radiation.
- Radiation has as good a chance of success as surgery but will preserve function and appearance better than surgery will.
- The tumor is impossible to reach by surgery without destroying vital tissues, as in the case of some brain cancers.
- Radiation is clearly the treatment of choice in tumors of the lymph system such as in Hodgkin disease and in some lymphomas.

What is palliative radiation?

Palliative radiation is when the treatment is not used to cure the patient but to treat other symptoms, such as to relieve pain or to shrink tumors.

How is palliative radiation used to relieve pain?

Sometimes radiation is used to relieve pain caused by tumors pressing on vital organs. By shrinking metastatic tumors, for example, radiation can relieve the pressure placed upon nearby structures, especially nerves. Radiation can also relieve headaches resulting from a metastatic tumor in the brain. In addition, it may also relieve other symptoms due to brain metastases, such as nausea, vomiting, and double vision. For some persons with bone metastases, if the bone where the tumor is growing is a weight-bearing bone (such as leg bone), radiotherapy may be used to avoid a fracture caused because part of the bone has been weakened or destroyed by the tumor growth.

How is radiation used to relieve tumors blocking other bodily functions?

It may be necessary to shrink a tumor that is blocking a passageway in the body, such as a large blood vessel, the breathing tube, the swallowing tube, or the intestines. Some tumors ulcerate and bleed. Radiotherapy can sometimes shrink these tumors and occasionally stop the bleeding.

When is radiation used as an adjuvant treatment?

Radiation is used as an adjuvant treatment when chemotherapy or surgery is the treatment of choice and radiation is being used in addition, with the hope of curing the patient or giving the patient a long disease-free survival. Radiation is used as a preventive measure in those cancers where research has shown that although they cannot be seen on the microscope, cancer cells may have already spread to other parts of the body. Sometimes, radiation is used after surgery if the operation was unable to take out all of the tumor or if the doctor feels that the tumor has spread to other parts of the body. It is also sometimes used before surgery to reduce the size of the tumor so it will be easier to remove. Or it can be used to treat the lymph-node area to which a cancer drains when it is possible to operate on the tumor itself but not on the draining nodes.

How does radiation treatment actually affect the cells?

X-ray treatments actually injure the cancer cells so they can no longer continue to divide or multiply. With each radiation treatment, more and more of the cancer cells die. The tumor shrinks because the dead cells are broken down, carried away by the bloodstream, and excreted by the body.

Isn't radiation only for people who have advanced cancer?

No. That is not true. Of those cancers treatable by surgery, radiation was originally used after the operation to get rid of any cancer cells the surgeons had left behind. At that time, it was difficult to treat the cancer cells without also destroying a great number of normal cells. Thanks to new technology, the use of radiation treatment has changed dramatically. The new machines give off rays which are capable of penetrating deeply into the body tissue. They give high doses of radiation to the tumor area with less injury to the surrounding tissue. Radiation may be used for very early stages of cancer of the mouth or larynx, so that the voice box need not be removed. Radiation is also used for some cancers, such as lymphomas, which are not treatable by surgery.

What is a cancer which is radiosensitive?

A radiosensitive cancer is susceptible to destruction by radiation.

What is a cancer which is radioresistant?

This means that the cancer, because of the type of cells from which it originates, is not usually destroyed by radiation that is within a dose range safe to surrounding tissues. Since some cancers are known to be radioresistant, radiation treatment is not used for them.

What is a tumor which is not amenable to radiation therapy?

This means that the cancer, either because of its location, size, or previous treatment, would not best be treated by radiation. Conventional radiotherapy would harm overlying vital organs, or the tumor may not be radiosensitive. Thus some other kind of treatment would be used.

What is localized radiation?

Localized radiation is radiation that is being used to treat one specific site. Sometimes radiation is given to a number of different sites or areas. Sometimes whole-body radiation is used, indicating that the radiation is delivered to the entire body.

Why isn't radiation treatment used for every cancer patient?

Each kind of tissue, each kind of cancer, and each patient have a different sensitivity to the effects of radiation. Some kinds of radiation treatment work better for some cancers than others. Different cancers spread and grow in different ways. The general theory in using radiation is that the radiation dose must be large enough to destroy the cancer cells but not so great as to seriously damage surrounding normal tissues. Sometimes the dose required to kill the cancer would also do permanent damage to the surrounding normal tissue. This is the major limitation in the use of x-rays and radium in the treatment of cancer.

After an operation, when is radiation therapy started?

If indicated, radiation therapy can be started as early as two weeks after surgery, or when the wound has healed, usually by six weeks. Of course, this schedule varies depending upon the condition of the patient, the extent of the operation, the reason for the radiation treatments, and other factors.

Is radiation ever used both before and after an operation?

Sometimes in special cases, radiation is done both before and after the operation. This is called the "sandwich" technique.

Why does radiation work for some patients and not for others?

For many different reasons. Sometimes the tumor is too large for the radiation to have any real effect. Or it may be a tumor which for some reason is resisting the radiation. Or the cancer may have already spread too far for the radiation to be effective.

Is radiation therapy a new field?

Although radiation therapy is not a new field, research and improved technology especially in the past ten years has made it a major treatment area for cancer. It is an area which is rapidly growing and changing. Also, since information about other kinds of cancer treatment is also new and growing, new relationships are being found between the use of radiation treatment and the other treatments.

X-rays were discovered in 1895, and radium was discovered in 1898. Within a few years after that, scientists found that x-rays were capable of damaging body tissue. A little later researchers uncovered the curious fact that x-rays and radium did more damage to cancerous tissue than to normal, healthy tissue. The intricate details of the effects of these powerful radiations on living cells, especially cancer cells, are still being studied.

Is radiation more successful with some cancers than with others?

Yes, there are some cancers where radiation has been most successful. Hodgkin disease and some lymphomas respond well to radiation, especially when the disease is diagnosed and treated in the early stages. Certain cancers of the head and neck and cancer of the uterine cervix have had good cure records with radiation. Early cancers of the bladder, prostate, and skin and certain brain and eye tumors, and some bone tumors (particularly if surgery is not done) respond well to radiation. For some cancers, radiation is better than surgery because, besides having a high potential for cure, it causes little or no loss of function in the irradiated part. Psychologically it is better for some patients, since their appearance is not changed as it might be with surgery.

What if a person is getting radiation to one area of the body but the cancer continues to spread in other areas? Does that mean that radiation is useless?

Whether the radiation is useless depends upon three factors: the kind of cancer the person has, the exact area being treated, and whether the treatment is given to cure the disease or to relieve other symptoms. Some kinds of cancer continue to grow for a short time during radiation, but then they shrink or sometimes disappear altogether. Sometimes the cancer will continue to grow outside the area being treated (known as the field of treatment) even while it is shrinking inside the field of treatment. Sometimes the radiation makes the person feel better or experience less pain even if the cancer continues to grow elsewhere. There are cases where a particular tumor in a particular person proves not to respond to the radiation treatment. Of course, this cannot be predicted before the treatment starts. In these instances, other forms of cancer therapy, such as drug treatment, are often considered.

What kinds of machines are used for radiation treatment?

Several types of machines with different characteristics are used for giving radiation externally, but usually either an x-ray machine or a cobalt machine is used.

What is the difference between an x-ray machine and a cobalt machine?

Both the x-ray machine (such as a linear accelerator) and the cobalt machine use high-energy beams to destroy the tumor tissue. Both are usually referred to as x-ray machines. However, the beams are produced by different energy sources. The linear accelerator produces electromagnetic waves; the machine must be turned on for it to change the electricity into high-energy beams. The cobalt machine uses a metal (cobalt) which has been made radioactive. This is also called a radioactive isotope. The rays are beamed to the body from a source. The radioactive material is enclosed in a shielded unit and the beams are emitted through a shutter. In other words, the cobalt machine is "turned on" all the time. When the cobalt is moved into position in front of a window in the machine, the radioactive beam can be used. How far the beams penetrate in both instances depends on the speed at which the electrons hit the target; methods have been developed to accelerate the speeds by means of electromagnetic boosts.

How is the amount of energy of x-rays measured?

It is measured in electron volts (eV). The low energies are measured in thousands of electron volts, called kilovolts (KeV). The high energies are measured in millions of electron volts, called megavolts (MeV).

What is meant by superficial x-ray or orthovoltage equipment?

This equipment gives out low-energy rays; usually any machine with energy less than 1 megavolt (1 million electron volts) is called an orthovoltage machine. This machine gives radiation to the surface of the skin; the dose which can be delivered to a tumor which lies at any depth beneath the skin is limited by the tolerance of the skin to radiation. This type of equipment has limited use today; usually it is used only for skin cancer.

What is meant by supervoltage or megavoltage equipment?

This term is usually used to describe any machine with energy greater than 1 million electron volts or 1 megavolt. These machines give the maximum dose beneath the skin rather than on it. Therefore much higher doses of radiation can be given to deep-lying tumors. Some examples of supervoltage machines are linear accelerators, cobalt 60 machines, and betatrons. Megavoltage radiation can direct a more precise, intense beam to a tiny target area in the body with less scattering of radiation to surrounding normal tissue and less skin damage.

What do people mean when they say they are getting cobalt treatments or radium treatments?

Many terms such as these are used imprecisely by the public. Actually cobalt is a radioactive material that is usually used in supervoltage machines as a source of radiation. Often people say they are getting "cobalt therapy" when they are really getting external-beam treatment with a supervoltage machine. Radium is a radioactive material which is placed inside the patient and then taken out after a specific period of time. Many times, however, people say they are getting "radium treatment" when they really are getting x-ray or radiation treatments with an external beam.

What is neutron-beam radiotherapy?

This is a new, experimental kind of treatment. Sources of high-energy radiation in the form of subatomic neutron, proton, and pi meson particles have been developed and are being evaluated in studies supported by the National Cancer Institute. This therapy uses high-LET (linear energy transfer) particle radiation and requires a cyclotron, linear accelerator, or synchrotron to produce the particle beam and a beam application system to direct the radiation to the tumor. Experimental tests seem to show that it may be appropriate for cancers such as localized tumors of the head and neck.

Will my regular doctor be giving the radiation treatment?

No. This is a specialized field, requiring treatment from a doctor especially trained in therapeutic radiation. Your doctor will refer you to a specialist who can be called by several names: therapeutic radiologist, radiation therapist, radiotherapist, or radiation oncologist. We will be using the term "radiation oncologist" when we are referring to the physician who specializes in treating the cancer patient with radiotherapy.

What does a radiation oncologist do?

The radiation oncologist will thoroughly examine you and all the pertinent information about your case to decide whether or not radiation treatment would be of benefit to you. If you are to have radiation treatment, the radiation oncologist will decide what treatment should be used and supervise its administration. The radiation oncologist is well informed about the natural history of cancer and when radiation can be used in treatment. He carefully evaluates patients before treatment begins and at intervals during the course of the treatment to see whether the treatment is working. He knows how much radiation is enough to produce the best results while causing the least amount of damage to the normal organs near the tumor; he knows how much radiation is necessary for treating each kind of tumor as well as what radiation each normal organ can tolerate. He must be able to select the kind of radioactive energy best suited for the treatment of each case and to decide how to deliver it.

Is there a difference between a diagnostic radiologist and a radiation oncologist?

Yes. The diagnostic radiologist is a specialist in interpreting x-rays. The radiation oncologist is primarily a skilled clinical oncologist who is also an expert in the delivery of radiation therapy. The American Board of Radiology gives separate certification to these specialties.

Does the radiation oncologist have special training?

To be certified by the American Board of Radiology, the person must have graduated from an approved medical school, had four years of postgraduate training (three in pathology, nuclear radiology and therapeutic radiology), and have successfully completed the written and oral examinations given by the board. Thus this physician has had several years of additional specialized training in the treatment of human disease with radiation.

What other kinds of health professionals are on the radiation-therapy team?

It varies from place to place. But there are many other people whom the radiation oncologist depends on to help and support him in his work. The *radiation physicist* has had extensive training in planning treatments designed to deliver the desired doses of radiation; the *dosimetrist* is especially trained in calculating the doses to plan the treatment; the *radiation-therapy technologist* is trained in a certified school of radiation-therapy technology and has had additional hospital training and experience; the *radiation-therapy nurse* has specialized knowledge in the care of cancer patients receiving radiation.

What does the radiation oncologist need to know about me before treatment starts?

The radiation oncologist needs to have a complete understanding of you and your medical problem in order to determine whether radiation treatments should be used and to plan the best method of delivering those treatments. You will probably be referred to the radiation oncologist by your original doctor, who will have already discussed your particular problem with him. He will take a careful history, give you a physical examination, review all your previous records, such as x-ray films, pathology slides, and hospital records. You may also require additional special tests before your radiation treatment can be decided upon.

Will I have my first treatment at my first appointment with the radiation oncologist?

In many cases you will not. The doctor must first get all the information he needs about your case. Then the treatment plan must be set up. Remember that the treatment plan is different for each patient, so it may take several visits to the radiation oncologist before your treatment actually begins. Timing depends on the kind of cancer you have, the kind of treatments you have already had, the stage of your particular disease, your physical condition, and how complicated your treatment plan will be.

How is the dose of radiation decided on?

The dose varies with the size of the tumor, the extent of the tumor, the tumor type and grade, and its response to radiation therapy. Very complex calculations are needed to determine the dosage and timing of treatments. Sometimes a computer is used to help determine the best method of delivering the amount of radiation that is needed. Often a contour of the part of the body to be treated is made to help in planning. This can be done with a ribbon of plastic, lead wire, or some other device.

Why is the radiation therapy sometimes given from different angles?

One way of giving the maximum amount of radiation to the tumor and the minimum amount to normal tissue is by aiming radiation beams at the tumor from two or more positions. The patient or the machine is rotated; the patient and machine are placed so that the beams meet each other where the tumor is located. The tumor thus gets a high enough dose of radiation to be destroyed but normal tissues escape with minimum radiation effects since the beams take different pathways to reach the tumor.

How does the doctor decide exactly where to apply the radiation?

Since the area to be treated must be located with extreme precision, many different devices can be used to pinpoint the location. You may have to have a number of x-ray films of the area taken either with a special x-ray unit (called a simulator) or with the treatment machine itself. Sometimes radioactive isotopes, ultrasound equipment, and other specialized diagnostic apparatus may be used to locate the exact area. Since many tumors are located deep inside the body, when their exact location in relation to the outside surface of your body is found, it is marked.

Once the spot is found, how is it marked?

Generally, using your x-rays as a guide and with you lying or sitting on the treatment couch or chair, the radiation oncologist marks the exact area to be treated on your skin with indelible ink. Sometimes purple ink is used, sometimes blue or red. Some places use magic markers. Sometimes a few small black india ink dots are used to permanently indicate the treatment area. It is important that the spots remain so that the beam can be aimed at the same spot each time. Sometimes bands or casts of plaster of paris or plastic are used to secure you in a particular position so that treatments can be delivered precisely and consistently each time you come in.

Will my normal cells be affected by radiation?

All cells are affected by the radiation, whether they are normal or malignant. The normal tissues have a greater capacity to recover from the damage induced by the radiation than do the cancer cells. The radiation oncologist plans the treatment so that normal tissues are irradiated as little as possible. He also determines areas which are to be shielded and protected from the radiation, sometimes with the use of x-rays.

Can I wear my own clothes while I am having a radiation treatment?

It depends upon where on the body the treatment is being given. You will probably have to undress, so wear clothing that is easy to get on and off. You might even want to bring your own robe. Some patients wear old underthings because sometimes the colored ink used to mark the spot comes off.

What safety devices are used to protect me from unnecessary radiation?

There are many safeguards used to protect you from unnecessary radiation to the parts of your body which do not need treatment. All the machines are shielded so that the significant radiation is only applied to a specific area. The treatment field is usually lit with a light that will outline the surface through which the radiation will pass; a series of safeguards in the machine limits the radiation to this lighted area of your body. Shields, usually lead blocks, are placed on special trays suspended from the machine to shield small areas of your body not needing treatment.

What parts of the body are covered by the shields?

This depends upon where the radiation is being given. Lead casts and blocks or plastic molds are custom-made based on your own anatomy and are used to protect the vital organs and to maintain the proper treatment position throughout the treatment course. For example, in giving radiation to the ovary, lead blocks would be made to shield your kidneys. The shields are usually arranged on a wire-mesh or transparent plastic tray held securely above your body; they are placed in position just before your treatment starts.

How are the molds made?

You are put in the position you will assume during treatment. The area to be radiated is outlined by the radiation oncologist. The mold is made right on your body, using whatever material has been chosen. Small windows are cut into the mold to allow the beam to be directed to the precise area to be treated. The doctor can use the mold over and over again and will be sure that the beam is always directed to the correct area.

Do all patients need molds?

No, not all patients require molds.

How much do the molds cost?

The cost depends upon the material used and how complex it is. Costs can range from $20 to several hundred dollars. Each one is custom-made and is not transferable from one patient to another.

Where do I go for my radiation treatment?

You will usually go to the outpatient clinic of a hospital to get your external radiation treatment. Sometimes you will begin the treatment while you are in the hospital and then continue it as an outpatient. The actual treatment time is usually a few minutes, and you will normally spend about an hour in the therapeutic radiology department of the hospital. Many patients bring a book or some handwork to help them pass the time if they have to wait. You are normally able to walk or to drive to your appointment. Whether you can go alone or need someone to go with you will depend upon the treatment and the side effects you experience. It is always best to be accompanied by a relative or a friend for the first few treatments, until side effects, if any, are determined.

How many radiation treatments will I get?

The number of treatments depends upon the kind of tumor, the extent of the disease, the dose involved, and your physical condition. For some kinds of cancers a few treatments are needed over a few weeks; for other kinds the treatments may last for months. Sometimes the radiation is given over the period of several days; sometimes there will be a treatment followed by several days or weeks with no treatments.

Why is the radiation given over a period of time instead of all at one time?

This is because the radiation must be strong enough to kill the tumor and still allow the normal tissues to heal. The radiation oncologist determines the total radiation dose necessary and divides it into the number of single-treatment doses that will add up to the total dose by the time of the last treatment. In this way, although some of your normal cells will suffer radiation damage, they will recover between treatments. If the total dose were given all at once, many of the normal cells would be damaged beyond repair.

Why is it important to keep the appointments for radiation treatment?

Because the treatment plan is very precisely planned. Sometimes a lapse of time which is not part of the treatment plan means that the course of treatment must be started all over again.

Will I be able to drive myself to the treatment?

It depends upon how often you are having your treatments. Some patients have been able to drive themselves. Discuss this with the doctor before you start the treatments.

How often will I have my treatments?

It depends upon your particular illness and the treatment schedule your doctor decides on. Most often the schedule is for five treatments a week—Monday through Friday—with the weekends saved as a rest period so that normal tissues can recover from the exposure to radiation. Sometimes radiation is given twice a week or three times a week. Treatments vary in duration from as short a time as one day to five days to a number of weeks.

Will the treatment plan be changed during the course of treatment?

It could very well change. The plans for treatment depend on how you as an individual respond to the treatment as well as on other factors. Interruptions to allow for rest periods are common. The initial estimate of the time required to complete a series of treatments should not be taken as a rigid or fixed number of days.

Are any kinds of tests done when I go for my radiation treatments?

It depends upon your treatment plan. Usually tests such as blood counts are taken so that the doctor knows whether the radiation is doing damage to other structures. Sometimes x-rays and other tests are necessary to determine if the doctor should change the treatment plan.

What will actually happen to me when I have the radiation?

It depends upon what kind of radiation you are having and where on your body you are having the treatment. Usually you are put on a cot, which is wheeled under the machine's lighted cylinder. Technicians will measure and focus the machine and put in place any shielding devices necessary. When you have been properly positioned on the treatment couch, the x-ray equipment has been adjusted, and the controls have been set, the technicians will ask you to lie very still and will leave the treatment room.

How can the technicians tell what is happening in the treatment room if they are not in there?

The technicians are in the next room, monitoring you on closed-circuit TV. An intercom system lets you talk with them at any time and allows them to hear everything you say. The TV system lets them watch you during the whole time of your treatment.

Will I feel anything when I am receiving radiation?

Most people experience no sensation while the treatment is being given. Sometimes a patient says that a feeling of warmth or a mild tingling sensation is felt. However, you will feel no pain or discomfort and it will be unusual if you have any kind of sensation.

What should I do while the treatment is being given?

You should lie very still and try to relax. The treatment lasts only a few minutes.

How will I know when the treatment is finished?

Sometimes the machine will make clicking noises or a slight whirring sound when it is on. Each treatment lasts about one or two minutes.

Why can't the technicians stay in the same room with me while I am having my radiation treatment?

Because the machine, although pinpointing the beam at a specific part of the body, does scatter some of the radiation. Although the amount of radiation outside the beam is tiny during any single treatment session, over the months and years it could add up to a dangerous amount for the personnel. It is important for the personnel who are working with the radiation all day long not to be exposed to these scattered beams.

Does anyone monitor the amount of radiation hospital personnel are exposed to?

The Food and Drug Administration's Bureau of Radiological Health has the responsibility of monitoring radiation exposure. Maximum permissible doses have been set up for individuals who work with radiation. These are to protect anyone exposed to any radiation. Hospital personnel who work with patients who are getting radiation treatments must be carefully monitored with badges which measure the accumulated dose so that they will be able to tell when the maximum has been reached.

Is it safe for a pregnant woman to accompany me to my daily radiation treatments?

Basically, the levels in the radiation department should be acceptable for all people. However, some radiation oncologists feel that pregnant women should not take any chances, since even small amounts of radiation may affect the fetus.

Side Effects of Radiation Treatment

POSSIBLE SIDE EFFECTS	THINGS YOU SHOULD KNOW

All sites

Ink marks on skin where treatment is being given	Don't wash off the ink marks; they must stay on during the whole course of treatment, for they show the technicians where to aim.
	When taking a bath or shower, use lukewarm water only and pat skin dry. Do not wash treatment areas; let tepid water run over them. Gently sponge skin.
Dry or itchy skin; redness, tanning, sunburned look; skin may turn a shade darker than normal.	Ask nurse or technician to suggest lotion you can use.
	Don't wash area with soap or put on salves, deodorants, powders, perfumes, bandages, medications, cosmetics, suntan lotion, or other self-remedies during treatment or for three weeks after treatment unless specifically ordered by the doctor giving you radiation.
	Keep treated areas out of the sun. Be sure to prevent sunburn during treatment and after completion of treatment. You will always have to be careful about protecting the treated area from the sun. If treatment is to head and neck, wear wide-brimmed hat when outdoors.
	Do not apply hot or cold objects to the skin without doctor's permission. Do not use hot-water bottles, ice packs, hot-water compresses, electric heating pads, hot packs, or heating lights on treatment areas. Heat or cold may further shock your sensitive skin.
	Try not to rub, scrub, or scratch treatment area. Do not wear tight-fitting or irritating clothes over treated areas—no corsets, girdles, belts, or other articles of clothing that leave a mark on your skin. Do not shave the treatment area without asking the doctor or nurse. Use soft shirts and loose collars if radiation is in head or neck area.
	If skin blisters or cracks or becomes moist, be sure to tell the doctor. Remember these skin reactions are temporary and should disappear within a few weeks after treatment is stopped.
	In the future, after treatment is completed, the use of a sunscreen (such as Block Out) is recommended for the skin that has been irradiated to prevent further damage by the sun.

POSSIBLE SIDE EFFECTS	THINGS YOU SHOULD KNOW
Hair loss	Depends upon the site of radiation; sometimes occurs where hair is present within the area being treated. Areas affected are scalp, beard, eyebrows, armpits, and pubic and body hair. Hair usually grows back after three months; might be a little thinner.
Extreme fatigue; a weak or tired feeling	This is a natural reaction to radiation therapy and one of the most common complaints. Get more rest. Sleep when you feel like it. Don't try to force yourself to do things if you feel tired. Limit your visitors. Get extra sleep. Take a daily nap. Rest for an hour or so a day.
Loss of appetite	See eating hints in Chapter 22.
Sluggish bowels	See hints in Chapter 22.

Head; neck; upper chest; mouth; throat

Sore throat, red tongue, white spots in mouth, sore mouth, unable to wear dentures, lump-like feeling when swallowing, cough (rare)	Usually begins 2-3 weeks after treatment starts. Symptoms usually begin to decrease after fifth week of treatment and end 4-6 weeks after treatments stop. Make sure you report it to your doctor. See hints in Chapter 22.
Thick saliva	Usually occurs during third or fourth week of treatment. Rinse with club soda, which will refresh your mouth and can thin out the saliva. Check your local pharmacy for Xerolube (put two or three drops on your tongue and work it through your mouth). Use it as frequently as necessary.
Dry mouth	Usually occurs near end of treatment and lasts from several months to several years. See hints in Chapter 22.
Loss of taste or change in taste	Usually occurs during third or fourth week of treatment and returns to normal from three weeks to three months after treatment is completed; the x-rays may have destroyed some of the tiny taste buds on your tongue. Many patients prefer egg and dairy dishes instead of meat.

Side Effects of Radiation Treatment (continued)

POSSIBLE SIDE EFFECTS	THINGS YOU SHOULD KNOW
Problems with your teeth	If you have dentures, expect to remove them before each treatment. Have a complete dental examination before radiation therapy begins. Make sure your dentist talks with your doctor before removing any teeth.

Brush your teeth after every meal or snack with baking soda and a soft toothbrush. Don't use toothpaste.

Make sure there are no bits of food left between teeth. Gently use dental floss to clean between your teeth where food may be trapped. (Check with doctor first to be sure there is no chance of bleeding.)

Radiation treatments can increase your chances of getting cavities in your teeth. The dentist may order fluoride treatments. |
| Earaches | Ear and throat are closely related—sometimes ears can be affected by treatment. If your ears bother you, tell the doctor. Sometimes ear drops will be ordered. Sometimes radiation to brain results in hardening of ear wax, which can impair hearing. |
| Drooping or swelling skin under chin | Fatty tissue under the chin sometimes shrinks after treatment, leaving loose skin which droops or swells.

If you notice lumps or small knots on side of neck or in shoulder, tell the doctor. |
| Loss of hair | Whiskers, sideburns, and chest hair may disappear temporarily or permanently, depending on the dose and area treated. Do not use razor blades for shaving; you may shave with an electric shaver but not more than once a week. Radiation to brain area sometimes causes some hair loss. This is usually a temporary condition. Use a hairpiece or wig temporarily. See Chapter 8 for information on wigs. |

Breast

Dry, tender, moist, or itchy skin in armpit (axilla) or under breast	Can occur during third or fourth week of radiotherapy; if itchiness persists, ask the doctor for a spray to put on it.

POSSIBLE
SIDE EFFECTS   THINGS YOU SHOULD KNOW

Breast (continued)

If area is moist, be sure to talk with the doctor, who will give you a spray and have you expose it to the air several times a day.

Sometimes a yellowish discharge appears 2-3 weeks after the treatment is completed. Make sure you contact the doctor, who can give you medication for it.

Sometimes the side effects of radiation continue for 4-6 weeks, with skin reactions getting worse 2-3 weeks after radiation therapy. Do not be alarmed, but do discuss them with your doctor.

If you have had a breast removed, it is best not to wear an artificial breast (prosthesis) until a month or so after radiation treatment has ended.

Upper abdomen

Nausea, vomiting, feeling of fullness   See Chapter 22 for hints on eating.

Lower abdomen

Diarrhea

Feeling sick to stomach, cramps, rectal burning with bowel movement (rare), inflamed bladder (rare)

Usually occurs during third or fourth week of therapy. Varies from one to two soft stools a day to as many as ten watery stools a day. It is best to start diet with foods which are low in fiber early in treatment and not wait until you experience this side effect. See Chapter 22 for further information.

Does everyone have side effects from radiation?

The extent of the side effects in radiation, as in chemotherapy, varies. The health team involved with your treatment will discuss side effects with you and help you if you are having problems.

The side effects range from none to slight in some people to severe in a few instances, depending upon the intensity of the treatment, the location of the treatment, and the tolerance and condition of the patient. Some people go through their radiation treatments without suffering from side effects. Others do have serious problems with side effects. We have listed the side effects which have been experienced by people getting radiation treatment. It is important to remember that no one experiences all of them, that the doctors and nurses can help you minimize some of them, and that your own attitude plays a large role many times in determining how severe your side effects will be.

Are people usually very ill from radiation? Are they sick enough to stop the treatment?

Not usually. The common belief that people get very ill from the radiation is not true, although most patients complain about extreme fatigue. Very few people are unable to complete their entire treatments because of side effects. Sometimes the doctor will give you a rest from the treatments if a side effect is severe, or the doctor will decide to change the kind of treatment being given. It is very important that you tell the doctors, nurses, and technicians of the side effects you are experiencing.

Are there some general dos and don'ts for patients receiving radiation treatment?

Yes, there are some general guidelines. Later in this chapter there are comments on specific areas of radiation. But for any patient receiving radiation to any part of the body, here are some general recommendations.

- Do not remove the ink marks. They are very important to make sure you are getting the radiation in the same place each time. They must be kept on during the whole course of treatment.
- Do not wash or scrub the treatment areas; let tepid water (don't use hot water) run over the areas and pat dry. Do not rub them, or scrub them with a washcloth or a brush or scratch them.
- Do not apply any soaps, medications, powders, perfumes, cosmetics, suntan lotions, ointments, salves, bandages, tapes, or deodorants in treatment areas without checking with doctor or nurse. Stay away from talcum powder; it contains an abrasive. Adhesive tape should never be used because the skin is sensitive and may come off with the tape.
- Do not expose treatment areas to the sun during treatment or upon completion of treatment. You will always have to be careful about protecting the treated areas from the sun. After

treatment is completed, the use of a sunscreen (such as BlockOut) is recommended for the skin that has been irradiated.

- Do not wear tight or irritating clothing over the treated area (no corsets, girdles, belts, tight collars, or anything that leaves a mark on your skin). Use soft clothing. Make sure you keep the treatment area covered when you go outdoors. Don't wear nylon clothing over the treatment areas; it is not porous and tends to keep the skin wet, causing breakdown.
- Do not shave the treatment areas without asking the doctor, nurse, or technician.
- Do, if your skin becomes dry, ask the nurse or technician to suggest a lotion for you to use. Don't use any soaps, creams, lotions, or powders without asking the nurse or technician. They may interfere with your treatment or contain materials which would irritate the skin.
- Do expect your skin to turn a shade darker than its normal color; this is usually a temporary condition.
- Do not apply anything—cold or hot—to your skin without asking your doctor. Don't use hot-water bottles, ice packs, hot-water compresses, electric heating pads, hot packs, or heating lights on your treatment areas. Heat or cold may further irritate your already sensitive skin.
- Do expect there might be some hair loss, if hair is present within the area being treated. Areas that may be affected are the scalp, beard, eyebrows, armpits, and pubic and body hair. Usually hair grows back after three months but it might be thinner. If you are having radiation in the head and neck area, you might wish to buy a hairpiece before your treatment begins. See Chapter 8 for information.
- Do, if you are having problems with nausea and vomiting, ask your doctor about anti-vomiting medicine and about how often you should be taking it. Read the information in Chapter 22 about solving eating problems.
- Do, if your throat or mouth is sore, tell your doctor. He can prescribe a mouthwash medication which, when swallowed or gargled, can numb the mouth so that you can eat normally.

Will I feel tired from the radiation?

Probably, but it depends upon the person, the dose, and the area of radiation. Most people find they tire very easily. Some people complain of feeling tired a few hours after the treatment. Some who take daily treatments say they feel tired all of the time. If you feel tired, you should rest and take naps if you can. The feeling should start to wear off within a few weeks after the treatment ends. The following will help:

- Eat when you feel tired. Sometimes a small amount of food will give you the extra energy you need.
- Rest when you feel tired; some patients experience a tired feeling and need more rest during the course of treatments. Rest or sleep when you feel you need it. Don't feel that you must keep up your normal schedule of activities if you don't feel like it.
- Report any cough, sweating, fever, or pain to your radiation oncologist. Make sure you ask the radiation oncologist, technician, or nurse any questions you might have.

Will my skin get red or darker?

It depends upon the area of radiation and the condition and color of your skin. Usually about three weeks after your first treatment, you may find that your skin becomes red, or a shade darker than normal. You may get some irritation in the areas where you are being treated. Some people say their skin looks and feels sunburned. Be sure to tell the technician or doctor when you first note reddening of your skin.

What should I do if my skin gets irritated?

Some of this has already been covered in the list of dos and don'ts. However, the major points bear repeating. Try not to irritate the skin. Wear loose-fitting clothes. Gently sponge the skin while you are bathing or showering. Don't scrub your skin in the area of treatment with a washcloth or a brush. Because the skin in that area is more sensitive it needs more care in order to prevent irritation. Make sure you don't use soaps, creams, lotions, or powders on it without asking the nurse or technician. Don't apply anything hot or cold to it. Don't scratch or rub the skin in the radiation treatment area. Don't expose the area to the sun. If your skin looks like it is going to blister or crack be sure you report it to the doctor immediately.

Can I get a skin burn from the radiation?

Some patients are afraid of skin burns from radiation. In the past, with the old-style x-ray machines, this was a serious problem. But with today's radiation equipment, the painful skin burns sometimes associated with radiation almost never occur. Sometimes the skin in the area being treated turns a light pink after a few days. Sometimes it looks tan. Sometimes it turns a bit rough and might even peel slightly. You may find that your skin is not as flexible or as movable as before.

Does the skin redness always come in the area being treated?

Sometimes not. For example, some people who have treatments in the chest area find they have a sunburn effect on their backs. This is because the machine's beam focuses its energy on a specific area just underneath the skin's surface, but as it goes on through the body, the beam spreads and leaves the body through a larger area in the back. As it goes out, it leaves the skin a bit red or darker in color.

What happens if my skin gets a wet feeling?

This is something which should be reported immediately to your doctor. It sometimes happens as the radiation treatment continues. It is called "weeping" of the skin because the upper layers have shed. It is not a burn. Usually the doctor will stop the treatments for a while, or will prescribe an antibiotic lotion or cream for you to put on the skin. He will usually also tell you to expose the area to air. You will probably be taught how to wash the area twice a day, by just letting warm water run over it, patting it dry, and applying the cream or lotion.

Is there anything special I should do if I am getting radiation in the head and neck area?

Yes, there are several things you should know and some things you can do to minimize the changes in your system if you are getting radiation to the head and neck area (this includes radiation treatments in the area of the chest, mouth, throat, and head):

- Be sure you check with your dentist before you begin radiation treatments.
- You may be sore in the area of the mouth and throat. You

might notice your tongue is red or that there are white spots in your mouth. You might have a hard time swallowing, feel a lump in your throat, or feel your food sticking in your throat due to irritation of the tissues in your throat and swallowing tube. You might not be able to wear your dentures. All of these are temporary side effects which usually begin two to three weeks after treatment starts and usually begin to decrease after the fifth week of treatment. They usually end some four to six weeks after the treatments finish. Of course you should report any of these side effects to your doctor.

- Smoking and drinking make your mouth and throat sorer. Don't use tobacco, alcoholic beverages, or hot, spicy, rough, or coarse foods like pepper, chili powder, nutmeg, vinegar, etc.; they can irritate your mouth.

- If your mouth is irritated, frequent mouth care is needed, as often as every one to four hours depending on your need. Use a mouthwash made of 1 teaspoon of salt or 1 teaspoon of salt and 1 teaspoon of baking soda to 1 quart of warm water. A mixture of equal parts of glycerin and warm water is also effective. Do not use a commercial mouthwash without your doctor's permission. Do not use hot water; let it cool before using.

- Don't breathe in strong fumes such as paints and cleaning solutions.

- Brush your teeth with a soft toothbrush. Use dental floss to clean between the teeth.

- Don't shave with razor blades in the areas being treated. You may shave with an electric razor. You may find that whiskers, sideburns, eyebrows, head hair, hair under your armpits, or chest hair fall out temporarily, depending on the dose of radiation and the area being treated. Some men with much hair on their chests getting chest radiation will find that the hair in the treated area falls out within a few weeks; it may grow back after about three months, sometimes a little thinner.

- Make sure if you are having radiation in the head area that you wear a wide-brimmed hat or scarf when you are out in the sunshine. Don't use any sunburn product on your skin during the course of your treatments.

- Don't use starched collars if you have radiation in the head and neck area; wear soft shirts and loose collars to prevent irritation to the treated area.

- See Chapter 22 for hints about eating during this period.

Will anything happen to my teeth?

If your field of radiation extends up to your mouth area, you might develop dental problems. Your doctor may tell you to see your dentist because the loss of saliva may make you more prone to cavities and may contribute to periodontal disease. The dentist should not pull any teeth without checking with your radiation oncologist. Make sure you tell the dentist you are getting radiation treatment. Usually patients are told to rinse out their mouths five to ten times a day with a salt or peroxide solution. Since the effects of radiation on the teeth can occur one to three years after treatment, you need to be certain to continue to get good dental care.

Will my eyes be covered during treatment?

Again, it depends upon where the treatment is being given. The lens and the cornea of your eyes are sensitive to radiation. Therefore, the therapist will block these areas if at all possible, if the treated area is close to your eyes.

Can I get eye cataracts from radiation treatment?

This depends upon the location of the treatment and the dose being given. You should be aware that patients can develop eye cataracts from radiation treatment.

Are there any special side effects for persons getting radiation therapy in the breast area?

Usually, patients receiving radiation treatment in the breast area do not have any serious side effects or problems. Sometimes, if radiation is given to the lymph nodes along the breastbone, the esophagus (the tube which connects your mouth to your stomach) may be affected and you might have some difficulty swallowing. Follow the suggestions given for side effects of head and neck radiation.

Some persons develop either dry, itchy skin or moist skin in the armpit area (axilla), or under their breasts. If this happens, tell the radiation oncologist or nurse immediately so they can start treatment for it. In some cases, there may be a yellow discharge from the skin two or three weeks after the treatment has finished. If this occurs, call the radiation oncologist's office and discuss medication and treatment.

Many patients find it is better to wear a soft undershirt rather than a bra during the period when radiation therapy is being given to the breast area. It is important that nothing tight-fitting is worn to irritate the skin in the area of treatment.

Can I wear an artificial breast (prosthesis) during the time of my radiation treatment to the breast area?

If you have had a breast removed, it is best not to wear your prosthesis until a month or so after radiation treatment has ended.

Are there any special side effects I can expect if I am getting radiation therapy in the stomach area?

While some people do not experience any side effects at all, most experience some nausea, vomiting, and/or diarrhea during their course of treatment. Others experience one or two of these side effects but not all three. Side effects are related to the size of the field and the dose being given.

What can be done about the nausea and vomiting?

Nausea and/or vomiting usually come on shortly after the treatment and last a few hours. See Chapter 22 for information about eating during this period.

What can I do for diarrhea?

Many patients with treatments to the lower abdomen experience diarrhea, usually during the third or fourth week of treatment. It varies from one to two soft stools a day to as many as ten watery stools a day. Doctors feel it is best to start eating foods which are low in fiber early in the treatment and not to wait until you experience the diarrhea to begin your diet. There is further information on this subject in Chapter 22.

Can I become sterile from radiation treatment?

Whether or not you become sterile depends upon the location of the treatment and the dose of radiation being given. If your sex organs are in or very close to the field of radiation, the treatment can cause sterility in both men and women. If sterility is predicted, some males prefer to have their semen frozen and stored so that they can have children later on. You should discuss the question of sterility with your doctor before radiation treatment begins.

Should I tell the doctor if I have side effects from the radiation?

Absolutely. Your doctor will talk with you about possible side effects before you start the treatment. As soon as any side effects start, you should tell the doctor, the technician, or the nurse immediately so they can control the symptoms with medication if necessary. They may also wish to alter the treatment slightly. Some of the side effects might continue even after you stop the treatment. If any unusual symptoms or problems develop between your visits to the radiation oncologist, you should call the office to report them.

Can I take medicine for other illness while I am receiving radiation treatments?

You should make sure you tell your radiation oncologist what medicines you are taking, and if they are changed during your treatment period. If you are a diabetic and you eat less, your insulin dose may have to be changed.

Does my diet have to change when I am having radiation treatments?

No, your diet does not have to change. However, it is important for you to eat well to speed tissue repair. You should try to maintain your normal weight through a well-balanced, nutritious diet and sufficient rest. Your appetite may be affected, but it is important that you eat properly. Good nutrition is essential also for several months after treatment. You should be careful to have both good nutrition and plenty of rest to help your body repair and replace the normal cells. Try to keep emotional stress to a minimum. There is further information on diet in Chapter 22.

Can I continue my usual activity during treatment?

Continue normal activities as much as possible and do whatever you feel you can without strain. Many people find they can continue to work during the treatment period. Others find they can continue some activity but less than the normal amount. Your daily activity will be determined by how you as a person feel and how much you think you can do.

How long can the side effects of the radiation last?

After your radiation therapy is finished, the side effects of the radiation can continue for the next four to six weeks. Some of the side effects, especially skin reactions, may get worse after your treatment stops. Do not be alarmed. Follow the instructions given to you, or call the radiation oncologist's office if you need help during this period. (Since treatments are usually given in a hospital setting, nurses are available to answer your questions at any time.) You will usually be seen again by the radiation oncologist some four to six weeks after the completion of the treatment. At that time, he can usually tell the effectiveness of the radiation treatments.

Is there any special care I should take after my treatments are completed?

You should continue to bathe the skin in the treatment area in tepid water; wash gently, using a mild soap (talk to the nurse if you have questions about what kind to use). Do not rub or scrub. Ask the nurse or the technician to recommend a cream or ointment which you can use on the treated area after your therapy has been completed. Protect the treated area from the sun. Continue to wear soft clothing around the treated area. You can go back to other kinds of clothing after the skin has returned to its normal appearance. Gently wash off the marks. Do not scrub. The ink will wear off. Gradually return to your previous schedule of activity. If you notice any unusual sores in any of the treated areas, be sure to call the radiation oncologist's office and discuss them.

Is there usually followup done after I have finished my course of treatment?

After the treatment is finished, a complete report is sent to the physician who referred you. You will usually be asked to return for checkup visits with the radiation oncologist. It is important that you see both your primary doctor and the radiation oncologist at the intervals they suggest.

Is radiation expensive?

Yes. It is costly because of the equipment used in the treatment and the number of persons needed to give the treatment. Most major health-insurance policies cover the cost of radiation therapy, both the charge from the hospital or clinic and the professional charge by the radiation oncologist for the medical professional services. A course of radiation such as post-operative radiation for the breast or treatment for cervical cancer can range from about $1,200 to $1,500.

Is there any radioactivity left in me as a result of external radiation treatments?

No. There is no radioactivity left in you and you are not made radioactive by external radiation treatment. The radioactivity of external radiation is confined to the treatment beam itself. Neither the normal tissues nor the malignant tissues become radioactive. When the treatment is completed, no radioactivity remains in the body.

What are the different types of internal radiation?

There are two major kinds of internal radiation:
- Radioactive material which is sealed in a container and inserted into a body cavity at the site of the tumor. For example, a sealed tube containing radioactive cesium can be inserted into the vagina; radium needles are implanted in the tongue or breast; radium seeds can be used for prostate cancer.
- Radioactive material which is given orally or injected with a syringe; it mingles with body fluids and is transported to interior parts of the body. For example, radioactive iodine is swallowed and finds its way to the thyroid gland to attack a tumor there; liquid radioactive gold or phosphorus can be injected directly into the area of a tumor.

Why is internal radiation used?

The doctor is trying to put the radium or other radioactive material as close to the tumor as possible to control the growth. This also spares surrounding normal tissue. Because the radiation is concentrated in the tumor, it is possible to expose cancer cells to a higher dosage during a shorter period of time than would be possible with conventional radiation sources. For instance, it is known that radioactive iodine travels to the thyroid gland, and in some cases of thyroid cancer, the doctor can use it to destroy the gland and the cancer. Radioactive phosphorus is known to travel to the bone and is sometimes used to destroy metastases in the bone.

What kinds of radioactive materials are used as implants?

Some of the substances include radium, cesium, cobalt 60, gold 198, phosphorus 32, iodine 131, and iridium 192.

What kinds of devices are used in internal radiation?

Devices such as needles, plaques, seeds, wires, wax, molds, and capsules have been created to place the radiation source as close as possible to the cancer. For instance, "needles" made of such substances as radium or radioactive cobalt or gold may be inserted directly into the cancer. Sometimes, hollow, flexible plastic tubes are put into the tumor and filled with a radioactive solution. Other times, the radioactive materials may be applied against the tumor in some kind of applicator.

What is an interstitial implant?

An interstitial implant is a procedure in which tiny bits of radioactive isotopes are temporarily implanted in and around malignant tissue in a solid organ such as the breast. Interstitial-implant treatment is usually left in from three to five days. It is sometimes used in some cancers of the tongue, lip, breast, and prostate.

How is an interstitial implant done?

Technically, the doctor places several hollow steel needles into the tumor and the area surrounding it. Thin plastic tubes are then threaded through the needles and anchored into place. The radioactive substance, usually in the form of tiny seeds embedded in a thin, stiff nylon ribbon, is inserted into the tubes. The outer layer of the seed is a steel sheathing which blocks dangerous ionizing beta rays (electrons) but allows the escape of the high-energy gamma rays that destroy the tumor. Sometimes the patient receives external radiation as well as interstitial implant.

What is an intracavitary implant?

An intracavitary implant refers to the placing of radioactive material into a hollow space within the body. Intracavitary therapy is most commonly used in cancer of the uterus. Sometimes the radioactive elements, such as radium, cobalt, and iridium are used for removable implants; other times, radioactive elements such as radon, gold, and iridium are used for implants which are permanently left in the body. The removable implants are put into needles or plastic tubes which are fastened into the cancer.

What is a needle implant?

It is another term for an interstitial implant in a tumor using slender hollow needles in which a radioactive material is placed. Needle implants are used in the mouth and the tongue, for example.

How much radiation is given off by a needle implant?

This depends on the amount of radioactive material implanted and how long it is left in place, a decision made by the radiation oncologist who calculates this when planning the treatment.

Are needle implants in the mouth and tongue painful?

There may be some pain associated with needle implants in the mouth and tongue. Pain medication is prescribed if needed.

How will the doctor implant the radiation into me?

It depends upon where the implant will be. Usually you will be hospitalized and put under general anesthesia. If you were having a radium implant into your uterus, for example, the doctor would, in the operating room, insert a hollow applicator inside your vaginal canal and carefully pack it into position with medicated gauze. In some hospitals, the radioactive material is placed into the applicator in the operating room; in others the radioactive material is put into the applicator after you have returned to your own room.

How long is the implant left in the body?

This depends upon the site and on the treatment schedule. The implant is usually left in from one to six days. During this time you are kept in an isolated room and visitors are limited as to the number and times they may visit you. Sometimes the implants are used along with other kinds of therapy such as x-ray treatments; this would influence how long the implant is left in.

Will I be giving off radiation while the implant is in place?

It depends upon the implant. Usually, if you have radium or other radioactive materials introduced into the diseased tissues, the radiation will pass through your body into the surrounding area. However, if the implant is in a sealed source (needle or hollow applicator), neither you nor any of your body excretions such as blood, urine or stool become radioactive. Items you touch, such as bed linens, also do not become radioactive.

What happens once the implant is removed? Am I still giving off radiation?

No. Once the implant is removed there is no radiation to pass through your body, unless you have been administered a radioactive material by mouth or syringe. Then your body fluids do become radioactive, as do the bed linens.

Can the radioactive material which is put in the hollow applicator explode in my body?

No, you do not have to worry about that. The radioisotope is not explosive. The material will not explode.

Will I get regular hospital care when I have a radioactive implant?

Your hospital care will be a bit different than usual. The nurses and other hospital personnel are limited as to how long they can remain in your room and how close they can come to you and your bed. You might notice that they come into your room more often but for shorter periods of time. Your bed will probably be close to the window wall. The hospital personnel will probably not come close to the side of your bed, but will talk with you from the foot of the bed. They will probably be wearing film badges to measure the radiation. Naturally, the restrictions to the hospital personnel depend upon what part of your body the implant is in, the kind of radioactive materials used, and the dosage. Pregnant nurses will not be allowed to take care of you. Most times, you will be assigned to a single room. Although personal contact is limited because of the radiation implant, do not hesitate to call a nurse if you need her for any reason.

What about changing the bed and taking a bath?

Your sheets will probably not be changed routinely every day but only if they become dirty. The nurse will encourage you to take your own bed bath if you are well enough to do it yourself. If she must stay in your room for any length of time, she may use some kind of a lead shield for protection. If you have a vaginal applicator in place, the nurse will do as much as she can while standing at the head of the bed. When caring for a patient with seeds implanted in the head and neck area, the nurse will do as much of her work as possible while standing at the foot of the bed.

Will I be allowed to have visitors?

It depends. Usually visitors are restricted to persons over 18 years old, persons who are not pregnant, and persons who are not likely to become pregnant. Visitors are asked to keep a distance which allows for conversation but keeps them away from the bed. They will be allowed to stay only for a limited time to reduce their exposure to radiation.

How will the hospital personnel know I have a radioactive implant?

It depends upon what hospital you are in. A tag might be put on the front cover of your chart, at the foot of your bed, or on the door of your room—or in all three places. You will probably also be given a wristband which will say "radioactive precautions."

Will I be able to move around while the implant is inside me?

In most cases you must stay in bed while the applicator with the radioactive material is in place. (For breast interstitial implants, you will be allowed to be up and around in the room, but you will not be allowed to leave the room.) Depending upon the location of your tumor, part of your bed can be elevated. However, you must restrict your movements so that the radiation source will not become dislodged and harm sensitive organs. You will not normally be allowed to turn from side to side or turn over onto your stomach. The nurse can put pillows under some parts of your body, depending upon where the radiation source is located, so that you can be tilted or propped up. You will usually be given exercises to do with the parts of your body that you can move.

Can I eat while the radiation implant is in my body?

Yes, you will usually be given a special diet with lots of fluids. The nurses will place the food where you can manage it without having to move your body. If your implant is in the vaginal area, you will be given pills to discourage bowel movements while the applicator is in the body. Sometimes you will be given sleeping pills or other medication to relax you. It is important that you not touch the implant while it is in your body. Although the container is sealed, touching it could cause radiation damage to your skin.

Do I have to go back into the operating room to have the implant removed?

Usually not. The implant is usually removed right in the room. Normally you are given some pain medication about a half-hour before the doctor comes in to take out the applicator and the packing. You will then be allowed to get out of bed. Usually the nurse will help you move around until your strength comes back.

Will I have pain or feel sick while the implant is in?

Usually not. Some patients do experience a rise in temperature. Other patients complain of fleeting waves of burning sensations. If you feel hot or experience sweats, tell your doctor. Thyroid patients sometimes complain of a sore throat. Some patients are weak and tired from the anesthesia. Some patients find the applicator holding the implant to be slightly uncomfortable and lying flat for a period of time tiring. The doctor can order a sedative to relieve the discomfort. If you seem to have any side effects, be sure to tell the nurse.

Do I have to follow any special rules after my implant has been taken out and I go home?

You should avoid sunlight on the areas exposed to radiation. If you have dryness or itchiness, the doctor can give you a cream to relieve it. You should make sure you call the doctor if you have nausea, vomiting, diarrhea, frequent urination or bowel movements, a red vaginal bleeding or blood in the urine, a temperature above 100°, burning, or pain.

However, you should go back to your normal life. You can continue on your normal diet. You are no longer radioactive and are not a hazard to yourself or to anybody else. If you have had an implant in the gynecological area, you will be told not to take a tub bath, although shower baths or sponge baths can be taken. The doctor will also give you a list of other cautions; you may not douche, use tampons, or have intercourse for a time. You will be allowed to resume these activities gradually depending upon the condition of your vagina or cervix.

Will I feel tired?

Some people get tired easily and feel sleepy several times a day. If this happens, lie down and rest. It is better for you to do this than to get overtired. It is not unusual to take several naps the first few days.

Why is some radioactive material used in unsealed sources?

Some radioactive substances cannot penetrate casings, so they are used unsealed. The unsealed sources are usually liquids injected into the abdomen or the lung cavities. These liquids consist of particles that do not readily pass into blood and lymph; therefore they stay in one place. Another unsealed source is the iodine given by mouth to patients with thyroid cancer.

Are there any side effects from the liquids injected into the abdomen or the lung cavities?

Some patients may have nausea, vomiting, and diarrhea—similar side effects to those resulting from external radiation in the upper or lower abdomen. Also linens, dressings, and clothing can become contaminated if the unsealed source leaks. The patient's urine, feces, and vomit are not contaminated, since the liquids consist of particles that do not readily pass into blood and the lymph system.

Are there any special precautions if I am taking radioactive iodine therapy?

Yes. If you are taking iodine therapy, there may be a problem of contamination, since the body expels this substance through the kidneys, the salivary and sweat glands, and the stools. Therefore, the nurses will wear rubber gloves when handling bedclothes in case there is some urine on them; your bedpans will be thoroughly cleaned after each use and reserved for your use only; your urine will be stored in bottles placed in lead boxes. Even your tears and saliva will be radioactive.

How long will these special precautions have to be taken?

It depends upon the kind of radioactive material and the dose. The radioactivity of radioactive iodine decreases rapidly after a few days because of the decay in the activity of the substance and also because it is being excreted through the kidneys.

Will I be able to have visitors?

There will be restrictions as to how long and how close visitors can come, for anyone using unsealed-source radiation. Pregnant visitors will not be allowed to visit.

What is a permanent implant?

This means that the radioactive material is left in permanently. Often radioactive materials are permanently implanted in the tongue or the palate or floor of the mouth. Permanent implants are also done in the prostate. The radioactivity of the material diminishes each day so that after a few days there is very little radiation coming from the patient's body.

Do special precautions have to be taken around persons with permanent implants?

It depends upon where the implant is and the dosage of the radiation. In some cases, the patients are hospitalized for the days when they have the greatest amount of radioactivity. The materials selected for permanent implant do not usually entail hazards to family members or others once the patient is ready to be discharged. If there is a need for special precautions, both the patient and the family are given full instructions.

chapter 8

Chemotherapy

Questions To Ask About Chemotherapy

- Who will be giving me my chemotherapy treatments?
- What is the name of the drug/drugs I will be taking?
- What is the drug/drugs supposed to do?
- What are the possible undesirable side effects? What should I do if these side effects occur?
- Which side effects should I report to the doctor immediately?
- How will the drug be given to me? How often will the treatments be given?
- How long will each treatment take? How long will the whole series last?
- May I take other medication at the same time? May I drink alcohol?
- Is there any special nutritional advice I should follow?
- Are there any special precautions I should take while I am on chemotherapy?
- How much will it cost?
- How much of a risk is involved?
- What is the alternative? What if I don't have this treatment at all?

What is chemotherapy?

"Chemo" means "chemical" and "therapy" means "treatment";

thus chemotherapy is simply the treatment of cancer using chemicals (drugs).

What does chemotherapy do?

In simple terms, the chemicals destroy the cancer cells, either by interfering with their growth or by preventing them from reproducing. The various drugs work in different ways to interrupt the cell life cycle. Some affect the cell during one or more of its phases of growth and have no adverse effect on the cell during the other phases; others affect the cell throughout the whole cycle. The idea behind the use of chemotherapy is to lower the multiplying of cancer cells or to destroy the cancer cells themselves.

Has chemotherapy as a treatment been used for a long time?

Although the use of chemicals to fight disease has been known for a long time, chemotherapy has been used against cancer only in recent years. Until the 1940s, attempts to find drugs that would selectively destroy cancer cells were not successful. The observation at Yale University that the potent World War I gas nitrogen mustard produced selective damage to the lymphatic system and bone marrow led to interest in the use of chemotherapy for cancer. The first successful use of chemotherapy was at Yale in the mid-1940s. During the 1960s and 1970s the uses and successes of chemotherapy have expanded rapidly.

When is chemotherapy used?

Chemotherapy is used for many different reasons:
- It can cure some kinds of cancer.
- It can be used to achieve long-term remissions in some kinds of cancer.
- It can be used to reduce a large tumor, making it small enough to remove by surgery.
- It can be used after surgery to kill the cells which may have been left or are in another part of the body.
- It can be used to shrink tumors which cannot be operated on.
- It can be used to make radiation treatment more effective.
- It can prevent or relieve pain or control unpleasant symptoms.

Is chemotherapy usually used alone as a treatment?

Like other treatments for cancer, chemotherapy is sometimes used alone (for the leukemias and lymphomas, for instance). Most of the time chemotherapy is used in combination with another kind of treatment—radiation therapy or surgery.

What does chemotherapy do that is different from the other kinds of treatments?

The chemotherapeutic drugs enter the bloodstream either directly by intravenous injection or indirectly by absorption through the stomach tissues. Therefore, the drugs are transported wherever tumor cells may be growing. This is different from surgery and radiotherapy, which concentrate on a specific part or region of the body for treatment. Chemotherapy is used when there is the possibility that cancer cells may be deposited in a different place from the primary tumor or may be circulating throughout the body via the bloodstream.

Can chemotherapy ever cure cancer?

According to the National Cancer Institute, the drugs can produce cures in about 15 percent of clinical cancer. In many of the remaining cases, they often temporarily stop the growth, or relieve pain and allow the patient to live a longer, more comfortable life. In some cancers, in some patients, chemotherapy can cause the tumors to disappear. In other cases, chemotherapy makes the tumor shrink. When this doesn't happen, the drugs may at least stop the tumor from growing or make it grow more slowly. There are some cases, however, in which chemotherapy has no effect on the growth of the tumor.

Isn't chemotherapy used only as a last resort for advanced cancer cases?

During the early years, when chemotherapy was an investigative treatment, it was used primarily on patients after other treatments were no longer working. Today, many doctors are using chemotherapy to prevent the spread of cancer for persons with minimal disease. When the drug is used early, the main idea is to remove the micrometastases which are not yet seen under the microscope, but are believed to be present, especially in some stages of breast cancer.

What are the different types of chemotherapy?

Chemotherapy drugs are classified by their structure and function. They fall mainly into five classifications:

- *Alkylating agents* are known for their chemical action, which interferes with cell division. They are called non-cell-cycle-specific agents because they attack all cells in a tumor whether the cells are resting or dividing.
- *Antimetabolites* are drugs which interfere with the cells' ability to replicate. These drugs are designed to starve cancer cells by interfering with vital life processes. They fool the cell by introducing the wrong building elements or blocking synthesis of the right ones.
- *Natural products*, which include plant alkaloids and antibiotics. Plant alkaloids stop cell division at one of its phases. Antibiotics are made from molds like penicillin but are stronger and do not act in the same way as regular antibiotics. Rather, they interfere with cell division and damage more cancer cells than normal cells.
- *Hormones* are naturally occurring substances in the body that stimulate or turn off the growth or activity of specific cells or organs. In cancer treatment, the environment is changed either by adding or removing the hormones, thus antagonizing the growth-stimulating hormones that promote growth of cancer cells in certain tissues.
- *Miscellaneous agents* which don't fit into any of the other categories.

Who prescribes chemotherapy?

Chemotherapy should be prescribed by a doctor who has had special training in the use of drugs and drug combinations for the treatment of cancer. This may be a medical oncologist (chemotherapist) who is a specialist in internal medicine with special training in the overall care of the cancer patient or a hematologist who is a physician who specializes in blood diseases. Most chemotherapy drugs are too risky to be prescribed by general physicians without special training.

Do nurses play a role in actually administering the chemotherapeutic drugs?

Absolutely. There are specially trained chemotherapy nurses in many parts of the country, both in doctors' offices and in hospitals (outpatient clinics and inpatient facilities), who actually give the majority of chemotherapeutic drugs under the supervision of a physician. These nurses are well trained in the administration of the drugs, how to give them and what side effects to look for.

Why is it important to have specially trained personnel dealing with chemotherapeutic drugs?

Chemotherapy, and especially combination chemotherapy (in which more than one drug is used), may be a highly toxic form of cancer treatment. Patients who are not closely monitored could die from the side effects, because the drugs are very potent. In addition, it is a field of medicine that is very new and changing quickly. New forms of therapy may not always reach the doctors who are not specializing in this field. If you are living in a community that does not have a specialist to administer the drugs, you should make sure your doctor seeks a consultation with a cancer center, a medical school, or a large medical center for guidance from experts who know the latest drugs in use, the administration technique, how to adjust doses and what the side effects are on the normal cells.

Where are the drugs given?

Chemotherapy can be given either in a doctor's office or in a hospital—the latter either in an outpatient clinic or as a patient in the hospital. Most times oral drugs can be taken at home. Many times the first doses of the drugs are given in the hospital so that a trained health-care team can give them and closely monitor your reactions to them. This is usually only a one- or two-day stay with the remaining drugs given in the doctor's office or outpatient clinic. In other cases, the drugs are given in the doctor's office or outpatient clinic from the beginning. Occasionally, you may have to stay in the hospital overnight when drugs have to be given intravenously for a long period of time.

How does the doctor decide on what kind of drug to use?

The doctor must look at your general condition, the type of tumor you have, and the extent of its growth. He evaluates the responses of chemotherapy in similar patients and selects that kind of chemotherapy which is most likely to damage or kill the tumor. However, not enough is known yet about the effects of the anticancer drugs on various kinds of cancers and individual differences among patients to make this an exact science. Thus the medical oncologist cannot always specifically predict how the drug will affect the tumor of any given patient, although he can usually predict the amount of toxicity of the drug. It has been said that using chemotherapy is like trying to kill crabgrass without killing the whole lawn.

What is meant by combination chemotherapy?

That is when more than one drug is being used for treatment. Most often two to five drugs are used in combination. These combinations are often used in an attempt to kill cells in different phases of their reproductive cycle and to delay or prevent resistance of the tumor to the drugs from occurring.

Does each patient get the same dose of the drug?

No. The doses are based on many things, including body size. Some of the dosages are calculated in milligrams of drug per kilogram of body weight. Others are calculated in milligrams of drug per square meter of body surface area. More and more drugs are being based on surface area because the surface area changes less during the course of the treatment and thus allows a more constant amount of the drug to be given during therapy. When more than one drug is used in a combination treatment plan, the dose for each drug is usually lower than when it is used alone. What the doctor is trying to do for each person is to give him the "maximum tolerated dose"—that is, the amount of the drug which will give the greatest anticancer effect with the least amount of damage to normal cells.

Why is it that some of the drugs are given by intravenous injection while others are given in pill form?

It is because chemotherapy drugs differ in many ways, and this affects the form in which they are given. Some drugs are not absorbed when given by mouth and have to be given by injection.

How is chemotherapy given?

Chemotherapy can be given:
- *Orally,* by mouth as pills, capsules or liquid form (PO)

- *Intravenously,* either injected into a vein as a shot (IV push) or as a fluid drip (IV or IV drip)
- *Intramuscularly,* by injecting it into a muscle in the arm, buttocks, or thigh (IM)
- *Subcutaneously,* with an injection beneath the skin (SQ)
- *Intra-arterially,* by injecting it into an artery (IA)
- *Intrathecally,* by injecting it directly into the spinal fluid (IT)
- *Intracavitarily,* by injecting it into the pleural space (lung) or into abdomen (for fluid accumulation)

How is the method of administration decided?

Some drugs can be given only in one or two ways. Adriamycin, for example, can be given only intravenously or intra-arterially. If the drug can be given in different ways, the decision will hinge on the necessary dose, preferences of the doctor and the patient, what kind of cancer it is, and so on.

Does it hurt to get a chemotherapy drug?

It depends upon where and how it is being given. If you are taking it in pill, capsule, or liquid form or applying it as an ointment, it is no different from taking any other medicine in the same form. If you are getting a drug which is injected into the muscle, it is like getting a vaccination or penicillin shot. You usually feel a pinprick. If you are taking a drug which needs to be injected in the vein, the process takes longer than the muscle injection but does not usually involve pain. It is similar to having blood drawn for a blood test. A needle is put into the vein under the skin and the drug is pushed in or drips into the body from an intravenous setup. The time of the whole procedure varies from two minutes to one or two hours. Some people having certain drugs injected say they feel a temporary burning sensation in the area of injection. Others feel warmth throughout the body. Some patients say the needle insertion hurts. With a few drugs, extreme care must be taken when they are administered intravenously.

What determines how the chemotherapeutic drug will be given to me?

It depends upon the kind of drug being used, the kind of cancer you have, the extent of the disease, and the location of the cancer. For example, some drugs are given by IV (injection into the vein) because they reach the bloodstream better and thus reach the cancer cells better this way. IV is a way of making sure that the correct amounts of the drugs are carried to all parts of the body where the cancer may be growing. Some drugs are made only in a form which can be given in one manner.

Does one particular drug ever stop being effective in a particular patient?

Yes, sometimes the drugs lose their effect against the particular cancer. Scientists believe that in some cases the cancer cells are multiplying more quickly than the drug can kill them. Other times the doctors have to reduce the doses or stop giving the drugs entirely because they are producing side effects on the patients. Sometimes the cancer cells have undergone change and are now able to survive and even grow rapidly in the presence of the once-destructive drug. When this happens the cells are called "drug-resistant."

What is meant by regional perfusion?

That is when the drugs circulate in a closed circuit through the bloodstream of the cancer-affected region. A tourniquet prevents the drug from reaching and damaging sensitive organs beyond the cancerous area. The drug is injected through an artery to the cancerous area, is withdrawn from a vein by special tubes, and then recirculated through artery and vein by means of a pump oxygenator. Regional perfusion allows large doses of drugs to be directed to one spot in the body. It is especially suited to treating certain tumors in the arms and legs.

How long and how often will I be getting chemotherapy treatments?

The length of time and how often you will be having treatments depend upon the kind of cancer you have, the drugs being used, how long it takes your body to respond to the drugs, and how well you tolerate them. Treatment schedules vary widely. Chemotherapy may be given daily, weekly, or monthly. Some drugs are given every four to six weeks with other drugs given weekly in between. There are also drugs that may be given every day for a short time or drugs that may be taken orally once or twice a day over a long period of time. When used as a preventive measure (adjuvant therapy) chemotherapy may continue for one or two years depending on where the primary tumor is located. Some people have to stay on chemotherapy off and on for the rest of their lives.

How does the doctor measure whether or not the drug is working?

The nurse and doctor will use several methods for measuring the effectiveness of the drugs: physical examination, laboratory tests, scans, x-rays, blood counts, and blood chemistry tests. All patients on chemotherapy will have certain laboratory tests on a regular basis. Blood counts, for instance, will be used by the doctor to help adjust the doses of drugs. Other chemical tests will monitor your blood sugar and kidney and liver function. Scans and x-rays allow the health team to determine if the treatment is working. Team members will also be checking your weight, eating patterns, side effects, amount of pain you have, energy level, and how you are feeling in general.

Will I be able to continue working while I am having chemotherapy treatments?

Most people find that they are able to work and perform the physical activities to which they are accustomed, such as swimming, golf, tennis, etc. Often working people can be put on a program that doesn't interfere with work schedules, such as receiving the drugs just before the weekend or late in the day. Some patients, however, do feel tired when they are on drugs.

Does it make any difference what time of day the drugs are given?

It depends upon the drugs. Some drugs must be taken or given at a specific time in order to be sure that certain levels of the drugs are in your blood at all times. This is a subject that you need to discuss with the health team that is caring for you. It is important to follow your doctor's instructions very carefully.

I am taking my chemotherapy at home. What if I forget to take it?

You should set up a schedule so that you will not forget. Take the drugs at mealtime or at certain times during the day so it will be easier for you to remember. If you forget at any time, make sure you tell the doctor as soon as possible.

Will I be able to drink wine and cocktails while I am on chemotherapy?

Usually you can drink in moderation. That means not more than one or two cocktails daily or wine with your dinner. Double-check with your doctor first. In some circumstances it may be absolutely essential that you have no alcohol. If your platelet count falls, for example, or if you develop any bleeding, your doctor may advise you to stop drinking alcoholic beverages. Alcohol may interfere with your liver function and destroy vitamins when taken in large quantities. Chemotherapy may have to be stopped if this occurs.

Can I take other pills or drugs during treatment?

A few drugs may interfere with or in some way affect your chemotherapy, so to be safe you should tell your doctor the dose, frequency, and use of any medicine—pills or liquid, prescription, nonprescription, or over-the-counter—that you are taking. It would be most helpful if you bring your prescription medicines with you when you visit the doctor. If you begin taking new medicines while on chemotherapy, be sure to tell the doctor.

Some of the drugs which can interfere with your chemotherapy include antibiotics, anticoagulants, blood medicines, anticonvulsant (anti-seizure) pills, aspirin, barbiturates (such as Seconal and Nembutal), blood-pressure pills, cough medicines (including Robitussin), Darvon, diabetic pills, hormone pills (including birth-control pills), sleeping pills, tranquilizers (nerve pills), and water pills.

Will I be able to have dental work done while on treatment?

Generally you will. Again it depends upon your illness and the drugs you will be taking. Regular teeth cleaning and cavity repairs are not usually a problem. However, be sure to tell your dentist that you are on chemotherapy drugs. If the dentist is going to perform oral surgery, take out a tooth, or give you an injection, tell your doctor so that blood counts can be taken a few days before the dental work is going to be done. If the counts are normal, your dentist can do minor surgery as he would if you were not receiving the drugs.

A friend of mine on chemotherapy has to weigh herself every day. My doctor never told me to do this. Should I?

As has been noted earlier, there are many different kinds of drugs being used to treat many different kinds of cancers. People respond to the treatments in different ways. You cannot compare what is happening to you with what is happening to anyone else, even if that person seems to have the same kind of cancer you do at the same stage. For instance, some of the drugs destroy many cancer cells, which results in large amounts of body wastes. These wastes must be eliminated from the body by the kidneys. Your friend may be taking her weight daily to determine whether or not her kidneys are getting rid of this extra waste. For other drugs, your weight loss may not have anything at all to do with kidney function.

Do all chemotherapy drugs give some side effects?

The extent of the side effects (you will sometimes hear the word "toxicity" used when referring to side effects) varies greatly from patient to patient and from drug combination to drug combination. The side effects range from slight in some people to severe in a few instances. Some drugs have more noticeable side effects than others. Some people go through their entire chemotherapy treatment without suffering from side effects. Others do have serious problems. We have listed the side effects as known for each drug. It is important to remember that no one experiences all of them. Remember too that the doctors and nurses can help you minimize some of them. Your own attitude plays a large role many times in determining how severe your side effects will be. Many patients who have a relaxed attitude toward chemotherapy experience milder side effects.

Why does a patient get side effects from the chemotherapy?

The drugs that kill the cancer cells may also harm the normal cells, especially those cells that are growing fast or are not fully developed. The mouth, stomach, and intestines, the hair follicles (roots), and the bone marrow are areas of the body which normally have fast-growing cells and are thus affected by the chemotherapy. To allow the normal tissues to repair themselves, drugs are generally given in cycles to provide drug-free intervals. The drugs work against cancer over the long term because the normal cells repair themselves faster than the malignant ones.

Are the side effects of all the drugs the same?

No. Each drug has its own possible side effects. When drugs are combined, the side effects can change. You should talk with your doctor about what the side effects are for the kind of treatment you are getting.

What can be done to fight off the side effects?

It depends upon the drug, the dosage being given, the tumor being treated, the stage of the disease, and the severity of the side effect. Sometimes, as in the case of some cancer where there are several different kinds of drugs which can be used, as soon as a sign or a symptom is noticed, the drug is discontinued and another given in its place. In other cases, the dose may be decreased to just below the symptom level. Or the doctor may prescribe medicines to lessen the side effects if he feels it will not interfere with the chemotherapy drugs. There are several suggestions in this chapter (and in Chapter 22) of ways to deal with side effects.

How long do the side effects last?

Most of the problems last a few hours to a few days. For example, the nausea and vomiting will usually disappear in a few hours. At the other end of the scale of side effects is hair loss, which may not disappear until the chemotherapy treatments are finished.

Do the side effects mean that the drugs are working?

There does not seem to be any relationship between the side effects and what is happening to the tumor. Neither the appearance of side effects nor the absence of them seems to have any relation to the effectiveness of the drug. A patient may have no side effects and yet the drug may be making the tumor shrink greatly. Another patient's tumor may also be shrinking greatly but that patient can be experiencing considerable side effects. It depends upon the individual's tolerance to the drugs being given and the responsiveness of the cancer cells to them.

Are there any serious side effects for which I should call my doctor immediately?

You should promptly report the following to your doctor:

- Fever over 100°
- Any kind of bleeding or bruising
- Development of any rash or allergic reaction such as swelling of eyelids, hands, or feet
- Shaking chills
- Marked pain or soreness at the chemotherapy injection site
- Any pain of unusual intensity or distribution, including headaches
- Shortness of breath or inability to catch your breath
- Severe diarrhea
- Bloody urine

Any new, unexpected symptoms, especially severe ones, that arise during chemotherapy should be promptly reported to the doctor.

Major Chemotherapy Drugs: Their Uses and Most Common Side Effects

DRUG	KIND OF CANCER COMMONLY USED FOR	HOW GIVEN	COMMON SIDE EFFECTS	OCCASIONAL, DELAYED, OR RARE SIDE EFFECTS
Alkylating Agents°				
Busulfan (Myleran)	Chronic leukemia	Oral	Nausea and vomiting; diarrhea	Bone-marrow depression, chronic lung problems, skin darkening, hair loss, breast enlargement, impotence, sterility
Chlorambucil (Leukeran)	Chronic lymphocytic leukemia, lymphomas, breast, ovary	Oral	—	Bone-marrow depression
Cis-platinum (Cis-diamminedichloroplatinum, CDDP, platinol)	Testicular, ovarian, head and neck	Intravenous	Severe nausea and vomiting	Bone-marrow depression, kidney damage, hearing problems
Cyclophosphamide (Cytoxan, Endoxan)	Lymphomas, breast, ovary, myeloma, lung	Intravenous; oral	Nausea and vomiting	Bone-marrow depression, hair loss, bloody urine (can be prevented by drinking lots of fluid), sterility (may be temporary), chronic lung problems, skin darkening

°*Can cause gonadal dysfunction [sterility] and long-term use can lead to a slight increase in leukemia.*

Major Chemotherapy Drugs: Their Uses and Most Common Side Effects (continued)

DRUG	KIND OF CANCER COMMONLY USED FOR	HOW GIVEN	COMMON SIDE EFFECTS	OCCASIONAL, DELAYED, OR RARE SIDE EFFECTS
Mechlorethamine (HN2, Mustargen, nitrogen mustard)	Lymphomas, lung, mycosis fungoides	Intravenous (for mycosis fungoides, local instillation, and topical)	Severe nausea and vomiting, irritation of veins	Bone-marrow depression, hair loss
Melphalan (phenylalanine mustard, Alkeran, L-PAM)	Breast, ovary, myeloma	Oral	Mild nausea	Bone-marrow depression, especially platelets
Triethylenethiophosphoramide (Thio-TEPA)	Breast, ovary, bladder	Intravenous; intracavitary (to prevent fluid accumulation); local instillation for bladder	Nausea and vomiting, local pain	Bone-marrow depression, loss of appetite
Antimetabolites				
Cytarabine (ara-C, cytosine arabinoside, Cytosar-U)	Acute leukemia, lymphomas	Intravenous; intrathecal; subcutaneous	Nausea and vomiting, diarrhea	Bone-marrow depression, mouth sores, liver damage

Drug	Used For	Administration	Common Side Effects	Other Side Effects
5-Fluorouracil (5-FU, Adrucil, Fluorouracil)	Stomach, colon, pancreas, liver, ovary, breast, bladder, prostate (basal-cell skin cancer—used as a cream)	IV push; oral less dependable	Nausea and vomiting, diarrhea	Mouth sores, bone-marrow depression, skin darkening (sensitive to sun), hair loss, skin rash, poor muscle coordination, nail loss or brittle nails.
6-Mercaptopurine (Purinethol, 6-MP)	Acute leukemia	Oral	Occasional nausea and vomiting	Bone-marrow depression, liver damage, mouth sores, skin rash
Methotrexate (MTX, Amethopterin)	Choriocarcinoma, acute leukemia, lymphomas, sarcomas, head and neck, breast, colon, lung, testicular	Intravenous; oral; intramuscular; subcutaneous; intraarterial; intrathecal	Nausea, diarrhea	Mouth sores, GI problems, bone-marrow depression, liver damage, kidney problems, cough or fever, hair thinning
6-Thioguanine (thioguanine, Tabloid)	Acute leukemia	Oral	Occasional nausea and vomiting	Bone-marrow depression, possible liver damage

Natural Products (Plant Alkaloids and Antibiotics)

Drug	Used For	Administration	Common Side Effects	Other Side Effects
Bleomycin (Blenoxane)	Squamous cell cancer of head and neck, penis, vulva, cervix, skin, anus, lymphomas, soft tissue sarcomas, testicular	Intravenous; intramuscular; subcutaneous; regional arterial infusion	Nausea and vomiting, fever, chills	Skin rash, darkening, discoloration, peeling or tenderness, chronic lung problems, mouth sores, hair loss, headache, swelling and pain in joints, unusual taste sensation, loss of appetite

Major Chemotherapy Drugs: Their Uses and Most Common Side Effects (continued)

DRUG	KIND OF CANCER COMMONLY USED FOR	HOW GIVEN	COMMON SIDE EFFECTS	OCCASIONAL, DELAYED, OR RARE SIDE EFFECTS
Dactinomycin (actinomycin D, Cosmegen)	Testicular melanoma, choriocarcinoma, Wilms tumor, neuroblastoma, rhabdomyosarcoma, Ewing sarcoma	Intravenous	Nausea and vomiting, swelling of vein	Mouth sores, hair loss, bone-marrow depression, skin rash
Doxorubicin hydrochloride (Adriamycin)	Breast, bladder, thyroid, lung, ovary, acute leukemia, sarcomas, neuroblastoma, Hodgkin and non-Hodgkin lymphomas, Ewing sarcoma	Intravenous	Nausea and vomiting, red urine, burning pain where needle put in (if drug leaks out during IV), diarrhea	Bone-marrow depression, hair loss, mouth sores, liver damage, heart problems (dose related); skin darkening (nails, creases), can reactivate skin reactions from past radiation, kidney problems, fever, chills.
Mithramycin (Mithracin)	Testicular	Intravenous	Severe nausea and vomiting, diarrhea	Bleeding, bone-marrow depression, liver and/or kidney damage, mouth sores
Mitomycin (Mutamycin)	Gastric, pancreas, colon, breast, head and neck	Intravenous	Nausea and vomiting, burning pain where needle put in (if drug leaks out during IV), fever	Bone-marrow depression, mouth sores, kidney problems, hair loss

Vinblastine (Velban)	Hodgkin, lymphomas, leukemias, testicular	Intravenous	Nausea and vomiting, burning pain where needle put in (if drug leaks out during IV)	Bone-marrow depression, hair loss, mouth sores, loss of reflexes, severe constipation
Vincristine (Oncovin)	Lymphomas, breast, acute leukemias, Wilms tumor, brain, childhood tumors	Intravenous	Burning pain where needle put in (if drug leaks out during IV)	Pain in arms, legs, jaw, stomach, numbness or tingling in hands or feet, foot drop, hair loss, bone-marrow depression, severe constipation
Hormones				
Calusterone (Methosarb)	Breast	Oral	Nausea and vomiting	Fluid retention, masculinization, lowered blood calcium
Cortisone acetate	Lymphomas, leukemias, breast	Oral	Fluid retention, weight gain	High blood pressure, loss of potassium, increased risk of infection, diabetes
Dexamethasone (Decadron)	Lymphomas, leukemias, breast	Oral	Fluid retention, weight gain	High blood pressure, loss of potassium, increased risk of infection, diabetes
Diethylstilbestrol (DES)	Breast, prostate	Oral	Nausea and vomiting, cramps	Fluid retention, lowered blood calcium, feminization, bleeding (uterine)

Major Chemotherapy Drugs: Their Uses and Most Common Side Effects (continued)

DRUG	KIND OF CANCER COMMONLY USED FOR	HOW GIVEN	COMMON SIDE EFFECTS	OCCASIONAL, DELAYED, OR RARE SIDE EFFECTS
Dromostanolone propionate (Droblan)	Breast	Intramuscular	–	Fluid retention, masculinization, lowered blood calcium
Ethinylestradiol (Estinyl)	Breast, prostate	Oral	–	Fluid retention, lowered blood calcium, feminization, bleeding (uterine)
Fluoxymesterone (Halotestin, Ora-Testryl)	Breast	Oral	–	Fluid retention, masculinization, jaundice, lowered blood calcium
Hydroxyprogesterone caproate (Delalutin)	Endometrial, kidney, breast	Intramuscular	Local abscess, pain	Jaundice, lowered blood calcium
Medroxyprogesterone acetate (Provera, Depo-Provera)	Endometrial, kidney, breast	Oral; intramuscular	Local pain and abscess (when given intramuscularly)	Nausea (when taken orally), fluid retention, lowered blood calcium
Megestrol acetate (Megace)	Kidney, uterus	Oral	–	None reported

192

Drug	Uses	Route		
Prednisone (prednisolone, Meticortin)	Lymphomas, leukemias, breast	Oral	Fluid retention, weight gain	High blood pressure, loss of potassium, increased risk of infection, diabetes
Testolactone (Teslac)	Breast	Intramuscular	—	Lowered blood calcium
Testosterone propionate (Oreton, Neo-hombreol)	Breast	Intramuscular	—	Fluid retention, masculinization, lowered blood calcium
Tamoxifen (Nolvadex)	Breast	Oral	Nausea	—
Miscellaneous				
Carmustine (BCNU, bischlorethyl nitrosourea)	Brain tumors, lymphomas, multiple myelomas, lung	Intravenous	Nausea and vomiting, swelling of vein	Delayed blood-count depression
Dacarbazine (DTIC, Imidozole carboximide)	Hodgkin, melanoma, sarcomas	Intravenous	Severe nausea and vomiting	Bone-marrow depression, flu-like symptoms, hair loss, kidney problems, liver damage
Hydroxyurea (Hydrea)	Chronic myelogenous leukemia, acute leukemia, head and neck	Oral	Nausea and vomiting (mild)	Bone-marrow depression, skin darkening, skin rashes, mouth sores

Major Chemotherapy Drugs: Their Uses and Most Common Side Effects (continued)

DRUG	KIND OF CANCER COMMONLY USED FOR	HOW GIVEN	COMMON SIDE EFFECTS	OCCASIONAL, DELAYED, OR RARE SIDE EFFECTS
Lomustine (CCNU, cyclohexyl chloroethyl nitrosourea, CeeNU)	Brain tumors, lymphomas, renal, lung	Oral (3-4 hours after meals, preferably at bedtime)	Nausea and vomiting	Delayed blood-count depression, mouth sores, hair loss
Mitotane (o,p'-DDD Lysodren)	Adrenocortical carcinoma	Oral	Nausea and vomiting, diarrhea	Mental depression, tremors, visual disturbances, skin rash, lethargy, drowsiness
Procarbazine (Matulane)	Lymphomas, lung, brain	Oral	Nausea and vomiting, mental depression	Bone-marrow depression, mouth sores, skin rashes
Investigational°				
5-Azacytidine	Acute granulocytic leukemia	Intravenous	Nausea and vomiting, diarrhea, fever	Blood-count depression, liver damage
Daunomycin (daunorubicin, rubidomycin)	Acute leukemia	Intravenous	Nausea and vomiting, fever, red urine	Bone-marrow depression, heart problems, hair loss

°All side-effects information is preliminary; additional or more severe adverse effects may be reported.

Drug	Used for	Administration	Common side effects	Other side effects
Ftorafur	Breast, colon-rectal, lung	Intravenous	Nausea and vomiting, diarrhea	Mouth sores, GI problems, loss of muscle coordination, skin darkening
Hexamethylmelamine	Lung, ovary, breast, lymphoma	Oral	Nausea and vomiting	Bone-marrow depression, mental depression
ICRF-159 (Razoxane, razoxin)	Lymphomas, acute leukemias, lung, GI	Oral	Mild nausea	Bone-marrow depression, hair loss
L-asparaginase (Elspar)	Acute lymphoblastic leukemia, some lymphomas	Intravenous; intramuscular	Nausea, fever, allergic response, abdominal pain, diabetes	Liver damage, pancreatitis, mental depression, clotting problems
Semustine (methyl-CCNU)	Melanoma, gastrointestinal, lymphoma, brain tumor	Oral	Nausea and vomiting	Lowered blood count
Streptozotocin (Streptozocin)	Malignant insulinomas, carcinoid	Intravenous	Nausea and vomiting, local pain	Kidney damage
VP16-213 (epipodophyllotoxin)	Lymphomas, monocytic leukemia, lung cancer	Intravenous; oral	Nausea and vomiting	Bone-marrow depression, hair loss

*All side-effects information is preliminary; additional or more severe adverse effects may be reported.

Is there anything I can do to control nausea and vomiting?

First of all, you need to understand that nausea and vomiting will vary from person to person. It can also vary in severity and in timing depending on the drugs used and the dose of the drugs given. In addition, the effectiveness of the drugs given to counteract its effects can vary depending on the drug used. See Chapter 22 for information on what to do for nausea and vomiting.

Can I take drugs at different times of the day to help control nausea and vomiting?

It depends upon the drug. Some must be taken or given at specific times or else they will not be effective. However, most nausea and vomiting seem to occur two to four hours after the treatment and last less than 24 hours. For some drugs, and some people, getting the drug early in the morning (along with antinausea medicine), then taking the antinausea medicine again four hours later and eating a light meal, allows them to eat a large meal at dinnertime, free of symptoms. Others say taking their treatment late in the day along with antinausea medicine and a sleeping pill seems to work. These people say they can sleep through the night and feel only slightly nauseous in the morning. Talk with your doctor or nurse to see if there is any way to experiment with the times you take your antinausea medicine, depending upon the drugs you are being given.

Do nausea and vomiting usually occur at specific times?

Generally there seem to be three different kinds of nausea and vomiting experienced by cancer patients on chemotherapy:
- Nausea and vomiting which start a few hours after treatment and last a short time (this is the most common)
- Violent nausea and vomiting which is of 12 to 24 hours' duration
- A feeling of nausea which seems to be always with you (with this symptom you must force yourself to eat)

Is it true marijuana can reduce nausea and vomiting?

There are presently studies being conducted in some cancer centers around the country to test the effectiveness of marijuana—or more accurately the active chemical compound called THC (tetrahydrocannabinol)—to reduce pain and control nausea. The researchers feel that the drugs used in chemotherapy often cause the patient to feel nauseous by triggering a response in the brain rather than a response in the stomach. Marijuana, they theorize, acts on the brain to block or at least suppress the response. Some of the early studies seem to prove that this is true. THC is being given to the patients in the study in the form of pills—not as marijuana cigarettes.

Sometimes the nausea takes away my appetite. Other times, even when I am not nauseated, I don't feel like eating. Is there something I can do?

It is important for you to eat well—especially a diet high in protein—during your treatment period. Your appetite may be poor but you need to make sure you are eating a balanced high-protein diet in order to maintain your strength, to prevent body tissues from breaking down, and to rebuild the normal tissues that have been affected by the drugs. See Chapter 22 for additional information.

Will I lose my hair?

Many people find this the most upsetting side effect of chemotherapy. The rapidly growing cells that make up the hair roots (follicles) are sensitive to chemotherapeutic drugs. Not all drugs cause hair loss, however. There are several important things to remember. The hair loss is temporary. All body hair will return once the chemotherapy drug is stopped. Occasionally, the hair will begin to regrow while you are still being treated with the chemotherapy drug. Complete baldness occurs generally within two to three cycles of the drug. When your hair begins to regrow it will be thick and soft and sometimes even better than before.

If I am bald to begin with, will I grow hair when chemotherapy stops?

No. If you are already bald before starting your chemotherapy treatments, there will be no new hair growth.

Will I lose my hair in places other than on my head?

The hair follicles of the beard, eyebrows, mustache, eyelashes, armpits, legs, and pubic area are all rapidly growing cells and are sensitive to some of the drugs used in chemotherapy. Sometimes the loss is partial, but many times there is a complete loss of scalp and body hair.

What should I do to get ready for the hair loss?

You should buy a hairpiece, a wig, or a toupee before you start the treatment. Eyebrow pencil and false eyelashes may be needed. Some people find that horn-rimmed glasses or other glasses that are fitted with rims coming just in front of the eyebrows can conceal this hair loss. Turbans, hats, or scarves can be used instead of a wig but most patients feel more comfortable if they have made the effort to buy a wig before their hair starts to fall out. Wigs are tax-deductible medical expenses and may be covered by some medical insurance policies. Some hospitals and some American Cancer Society units have wig banks where you can get them free.

If you have long hair, cut it short before it begins to thin. If you buy a hairpiece, use it as the hair begins to thin out. Some black patients find they can delay hair loss by braiding their hair instead of vigorously combing it. Some doctors have found that some of the hair loss from vincristine can be prevented by using a scalp tourniquet during the administration of the drug when it is given by IV. The tourniquet, which is kept in place ten to fifteen minutes after the dose for maximum effect, is said to protect the hair follicles from high concentrations of the drug. Often the patient is responsible for having the tourniquet available and for putting it on. Some centers are experimenting with ice-packed caps during treatment to lessen hair loss.

When hair falls out from radiation or chemotherapy treatments, does it fall out gradually or all at once?

Though it differs from patient to patient, and from drug to drug, don't be surprised if your hair falls out in huge hunks, and your head becomes sensitive. Your scalp may also become flaky and irritated. A mild dandruff shampoo or some olive oil rubbed into the scalp may help.

Do you have any general hints about buying wigs and hairpieces?

Yes, we have a few hints.

- Buy the wig before you start losing your hair. This is very important. It is really best to go before you start having the chemotherapy treatments if at all possible.
- Buy the wig yourself; bring a friend with you if you like, but don't send someone else to do it for you. It is essential that the wig or hairpiece fits you well, looks nice on you, and pleases you.
- The less-expensive wigs tend to look synthetic. If this is the kind you are buying, dust it with a little baby powder to take away the shiny look.
- Get your first wig the same color as your hair. You can start wearing it while you lose your hair.
- Many people find it's useful to buy more than one wig. That helps you especially if you tend to perspire.
- Buy a good synthetic, rather than a real-hair wig, because it washes better, is less expensive to maintain, is cooler, and is cheaper than the real hair wigs.

Is there any kind of wig that is better if I am only going to have partial hair loss?

If your doctor expects you to have only partial hair loss, it is better to get a capless wig.

Will it be hard to hold the wig on my head if I have complete hair loss?

It may be. It is generally recommended that you use beautician's tape folded upon itself to hold the wig in place. Tape it to the crown and the temple areas of the wig. You should also have the wig styled to fit your face. Styling is usually included in the cost of the wig, but if it isn't, you can have it done at a beauty parlor. If you are expecting complete hair loss, make sure that the inside of the wig is smooth.

Can I wear a headband underneath my wig?

Yes, if you prefer. People who wear headbands under their wigs usually like cotton scarfs instead of silk or synthetic scarfs. Cotton is cooler and helps keep the wig from sliding.

How often should I wash a wig if I am wearing it every day?

People who wear wigs all the time usually wash them every week. Wigs tend to trap dust, and then they become hotter to wear. You should use shampoo to wash your wigs. Deodorant soaps will leave a coating on them.

How will my hair fall out?

It depends upon the drugs you are taking and the reaction your body has to them. In some cases, the hair falls out gradually. With some drugs, the hair falls out by the handful.

Are there specific hints for things I can do while losing my hair?

You can wear a soft fabric nightcap to catch the hair. If you use a nightcap, make sure it is a soft one, not a stiff netting type. Check the elastic on it so it will be comfortable for your head size.

What about when my hair starts growing in again?

As your hair starts growing in, shampoo it often. You might also want to go back to a hairpiece rather than wearing your full wig while your hair is growing back.

What can cause my urine to change color while I am on chemotherapy?

Some drugs can temporarily change the color of your urine. Some may turn it red, orange, or bright yellow. This is a temporary side effect and is not due to blood in your urine. The doctor can tell you if your drug can cause this side effect.

What can I do for bloody urine?

It depends upon what is causing it. If it is due to infection, the doctor will need to provide medication. However, if it is a side effect of your drug, you can do some things yourself to help. You can avoid it by drinking about 2 quarts of nonalcoholic beverages every day, if you are on a drug such as cyclophosphamide where this can be a problem. The bloody urine (or cystitis) caused by drugs is due to irritation of the lining of the bladder. This gives you discomfort or bleeding when urinating. Usually the doctor will tell you that if you are taking the particular drug at home daily, you should take it early in the morning. If you are taking it twice a day, take one in the morning and one in the early afternoon so that you will have plenty of time to drink a lot of fluids and flush your bladder well before bedtime. Otherwise the urine and drug will be sitting in your bladder for several hours. If you see blood in your urine or have a burning sensation and the urge to urinate often, increase your fluid intake and call your doctor's office.

What can I do about the sore spots inside my mouth?

Good mouth care such as brushing your teeth several times a day and frequent use of a mouthwash can help lessen the soreness. Even if you do not now have mouth sores, it is a good idea to take extra care of the mouth as a preventive measure when taking these drugs. Salt, glycerine, or peroxide mixed with water can be used several times a day as a rinse. Commercial mouthwash usually irritates the sores. A soft-bristle brush or swab can be used to clean your mouth if your regular toothbrush is too stiff. Topical anesthetics, such as those used for teething children, may be soothing. You might ask your doctor to prescribe a topical anesthetic to use before meals. If your mouth is sore, try to plan your menus around bland, nourishing foods that are heated only to a medium temperature. There are additional hints in Chapter 22.

Will I get tired?

It depends upon you—your physical condition and how your body reacts to the drugs. Some people do complain about being tired easily. Some people find they can continue their normal daily activities. Do whatever you feel like doing at your own pace. Understand that increased cellular activity is taking place as cancer cells are being destroyed. If you find you are getting tired, plan rest periods during the day. Don't get overtired. The fatigue will gradually decrease as your therapy progresses. Don't get discouraged or alarmed if you find that you are getting tired; it is a normal reaction and it does not mean that you are getting worse. Patients say they continue to have a fatigued feeling for a period of time even after the treatments have stopped. The feeling gradually goes away.

What is meant by temporary damage to the bone marrow?

Many types of chemotherapy, while stopping the growth of

tumor cells, also stop the growth of cells in the bone marrow. The bone marrow is where your body manufactures:

- *White blood cells* (leukocytes), which help fight fungal and bacterial infections. They capture, destroy, and remove germs from your body.
- *Red blood cells*, which help carry oxygen to the various parts of your body. They also bring back waste products such as carbon monoxide.
- *Platelets*, which help blood to clot where there is a cut. They act as a tiny plug that stops the flow of blood.

Why are these cells particularly sensitive to chemotherapy?

Since bone-marrow cells duplicate rapidly in order to maintain normal blood counts, these cells are particularly sensitive to chemotherapy. Bone marrow is responsible for producing most of the blood cells, and thus you may experience a drop in some of your blood counts while on chemotherapy.

What does the doctor mean when he says he is going to take a complete blood count?

When the doctor takes a complete blood count (CBC) he will test some or all of the following:

- *White blood count*, which gives the number of white blood cells per cubic millimeter
- *Differential count*, which refers to the distribution of the various types of white cells in the blood, usually expressed in a percentage
- *Platelet count*, which gives the number or quantity of platelets per cubic millimeter in the blood
- *Hemoglobin*, which gives the amount of oxygen-carrying protein present in a known volume of blood, expressed in grams per centigram
- *Hematocrit*, which is the percentage that red cells occupy of the whole blood volume
- *Retic or reticulocyte count*, which is the percentage of young (non-nucleated) red cells present in the blood

What is meant by the term "bone-marrow depression"?

It refers to the decreased ability or inability of the bone marrow to manufacture the platelets, red blood cells, and/or white blood cells normally produced there.

What is a drop in the blood count called?

It depends upon which cells it affects. A drop in the white blood cell count is called leukopenia. A drop in the red blood cell count is called anemia. A drop in the platelets is called thrombocytopenia. If all of them drop it is called pancytopenia.

When does the doctor check my blood count?

Your doctor generally will be checking your blood count before he gives you any chemotherapy. If your counts are slightly low, he may hold up giving you your next dose of chemotherapy or wait and check your counts in a few days. This is not a bad sign, it simply means the effects of the drugs are still in your system.

What if my blood count falls very low?

If your blood count falls very low, you will be carefully followed and in some cases you may be admitted to the hospital for observation and for transfusion of blood cells, either white blood cells, red blood cells, or platelets.

Is there anything special the doctor will tell me to do if my platelet count is low?

Too few platelets will affect the clotting of your blood. This means that your blood will clot more slowly than usual so that bleeding may be prolonged following a cut or injury. If you should cut yourself, apply pressure over the cut for at least five to ten minutes. If the cut is on an arm or leg, elevate it to slow the bleeding. It is best to avoid situations which might result in an injury—such as contact sports or heavy work. Be especially careful when using knives or razors. Avoid noseblowing or forceful sneezing. For shaving, an electric razor is safer than a straight razor.

A lack of platelets may also cause small red dots called petechiae on your skin. These spots are not harmful but you should tell your doctor about them. You may also notice that you bleed easily from your nose or gums. Applying pressure or using ice or cold water will usually stop bleeding. If it lasts more than 15 to 20 minutes, call your doctor.

You will be given injections only if absolutely necessary. Your chemotherapy drugs might be suspended until your bone marrow recovers. Your doctor will probably suggest that you avoid sun, alcohol, and aspirin and any other medication unless approved by him. If severe bleeding develops, platelet transfusion may be necessary.

How does a shortage of red blood cells affect me?

A lack of red blood cells makes it difficult for your body to get enough oxygen to do its work. This may cause you to have the symptoms of anemia: tiredness, dizziness, pale skin color, and a tendency to feel cold.

What should I do if I have symptoms of anemia?

Even though you may have some of the symptoms of anemia you can still be fairly active. You'll need to have a balance of rest and activity in your day. Don't get overly tired. Set aside rest periods during the day. Allow yourself seven to nine hours of sleep a night. If anemia gets too severe, your doctor may transfuse you with packed red blood cells to correct your condition and decrease your symptoms.

What kind of problems will I have if my white blood count is too low?

Low white blood count makes it difficult to fight infection. Even the common cold can be a problem.

If your white blood count is low you should take precautions such as:

- Try to stay away from crowds and people who have cold and flu; this is particularly important the first ten days after receiving your drugs, because your white blood count will automatically drop before it goes back up.
- Keep cuts and scratches clean with an antiseptic such as alcohol and keep the area clean with soap and water until the sore heals.
- Inspect your body for signs of infection in your nose, on your lips, in your eyes, or in the rectal area. If an infection should develop, tell the doctor about it right away.
- If you contract a cold or flu, ask your doctor for advice. Do not take any medicine that has not been prescribed by the doctor, including aspirin, cough medicine, vitamins, antibiotics, painkillers, or any other type of medicine.

When I have a low blood count, are there any special symptoms I should watch for?

You should be alert to the following symptoms and report them to your doctor at once:

- *Signs of infection:* fever, sore throat, cough, sputum (phlegm), cold symptoms, chills or sweating, burning on urination and/or increased frequency of urination and/or voiding small amounts, wounds that do not heal or that become red and swollen, boils and pimples that do not clear or vaginal discharge or itching
- *Signs of bleeding:* oozing gums, nosebleeds, bruising (especially without known injury), cloudy, pink or red urine, black or bloody stools, vaginal bleeding, long menstrual periods or too heavy or too frequent flow
- *Signs of anemia:* extreme weakness or fatigue

When I have a low white blood cell count are there any special symptoms I should look for?

You should be alert to the following symptoms and report them to your doctor's office at once:

- An area of redness, swelling, or increased warmth on a part of the body
- Increased bruising and bleeding from your mouth or rectum; blood in urine or sputum; black bowel movement
- Extreme weakness or fatigue; a rise in temperature, runny nose or cough; chills or diarrhea.

Are special isolation rooms used for patients with lowered blood count?

Special isolation rooms are in hospitals and are sometimes used for people who need to be protected from infection. Although still regarded as experimental, special germ-free rooms are used for patients while they receive massive doses of cancer drugs.

What is a laminar-air-flow unit?

This is an enclosure in which the patient is surrounded with a steady stream of sterile bacteria-free air, giving him sterile air to breathe and at the same time protecting him from contamination from the environment and from the attendants. All persons who enter wear a sterile gown, cap, mask, gloves, and shoe cover.

Sometimes patient isolation systems are called life islands with the hospital bed enclosed in a plastic canopy.

What is leukapheresis service?

This is another way of controlling infection in cancer patients. Patients who are treated intensively with drugs which produce a dangerously low white cell count can be given white cell transfusions. Doctors remove white blood cells from healthy donors for transfusions into patients who need them. In some study projects, the white cells are being given regularly to patients who have not yet developed an infection, as a preventive treatment.

What are some of the nerve and muscle effects one can get from chemotherapy?

They include numbness and tingling in the hands and feet. Some patients describe the feeling as similar to having one's hand "fall asleep." Some people experience a clumsiness in movement. Sometimes there are weakness and lethargy in moving the muscle. In rare cases, some people have problems with keeping their balance. They are temporary effects of the medicine on nerve cells.

What can I do about irregular menstrual cycles?

There is little you can do except to know that it is common for women who are still having menstrual periods to develop irregular menses, to stop flowing, or to have some menopausal symptoms such as hot flashes as a result of the drugs. However, conception may still be possible, and because of the unknown effects of many chemotherapeutic drugs on the unborn child, conception during chemotherapy is not advised. Once chemotherapy is stopped, conception and normal pregnancy may be possible. Menstrual periods may return after the drug is stopped.

If you are of childbearing age, it is wise to discuss family planning with your doctor before you start your chemotherapy treatments. He will be able to help you decide on birth-control methods while you are on chemotherapy and will discuss with you your future family planning.

Will males become completely sterile from chemotherapy?

Chemotherapy in men often results in reduced sperm count and reduced viability of the sperm, thus resulting in infertility. However, this will not interfere with erection or intercourse in any way. Because men on chemotherapy have fathered children and because of the possible effect of chemotherapy on the sperm, contraceptive measures are advised. Production of sperm may return to normal when chemotherapy is stopped. However, it is possible for the fertility of the male to be permanently curtailed by some treatment programs. If your treatment program has this potential, your doctor can discuss with you the possibility of freezing and storing your sperm for future artificial insemination.

Can I have sexual relations during my period of chemotherapy treatment?

Yes. Treatment usually does not interfere with your ability to continue normal sexual relations.

What will the doctor recommend if I am retaining fluids?

He will probably tell you to avoid salty foods and to cut down the amount of salt you are using in your foods.

Can I expect side effects from hormone therapy?

Men taking estrogens sometimes get enlarged breasts and/or decreased sexual desires. Women taking androgens may find that their voices deepen, hair growth increases, and sexual desire increases. Women who are menopausal may have bleeding. You should discuss any of these symptoms with your doctor or nurse. These changes usually disappear when you stop taking the drugs.

Are skin rashes common during chemotherapy?

This side effect is not seen very often. Sometimes a drug will cause a slight rash around the injection site. It usually disappears within 30 to 90 minutes. Localized or generalized rashes are usually red and sometimes very itchy.

I have dry skin. Is that a result of the chemotherapy?

Dry skin can be a side effect of chemotherapy. Sometimes the cells of the skin become sensitive to the drugs. You may notice changes in skin color. The change may be in one small area or may cover a large area of your body. Both color changes and dry skin are temporary effects. Your skin should return to normal once you are off the medication.

What kind of personality changes might a cancer patient on chemotherapy expect?

Again, this is not a very common side effect. It is difficult to differentiate personality changes due to disease from those due to drugs. However, sometimes the person will experience changes in emotions, such as depression, because of the drugs. There are many things in life which affect your moods, but it is important that you and your family recognize that some drugs may cause depression so that you will be prepared for unusual feelings and keep them in proper perspective.

What flu-like symptoms do some patients experience?

Some of the drugs may cause a flu-like reaction after they are given. Many people experience fever and chills, aching bones, and a general tired feeling. Like other side effects, these should be reported to your doctor.

Is the metallic taste in my mouth a common side effect?

No, but it can happen to people on some of the drugs. Patients often try washing out their mouths frequently to try to mask the taste. Some also suck on citrus fruits or hard candies as a remedy.

What can I do for heartburn or pain in the upper stomach?

This side effect can usually be relieved by taking a half-glass of milk or one or two tablespoons of an antacid preparation; if it is severe and unrelieved, contact your doctor's office.

Is it unusual for dark circles to form on my fingernails?

Some drugs cause darkening of the fingernails. This is a harmless side effect and will usually disappear when the drug is stopped.

Do veins ever get darker when a patient is on chemotherapy?

Sometimes the drugs will irritate the veins and some discoloration may develop along the pathway of the vein. Sometimes it looks as if someone has marked it with a dark-brown felt-tipped pen. The darker your skin, the darker the vein becomes. Exposure to the sun makes the vein even darker. Don't be alarmed—veins are not damaged and the coloring fades within a few weeks.

Do patients sometimes suffer from irritation where the drug is being injected?

This may happen. If it is a rash it normally disappears in 30 to 90 minutes. However, tissue burns from leakage of medications at the site of the injection should be reported to the person giving the drug immediately. He may prescribe cold compresses such as ice and pain medication to help alleviate discomfort.

Do any of the drugs cause a gain in weight?

Some of the drugs, such as prednisone or dexamethasone, do increase your appetite and cause weight gain in some patients. Sometimes your blood pressure also gets higher. If this happens the doctor will probably tell you to not add salt to your food and to avoid salty snacks such as pretzels.

Will I experience constipation if I am on chemotherapy?

It depends upon the drugs you are being treated with. Most of the pain medications are likely to make you constipated. For some drugs, such as vincristine, constipation can be an early symptom of a more serious problem. Try to prevent constipation before it occurs by drinking lots of water (at least eight glasses a day) and fruit juices. Eat raw fruits and vegetables if your diet allows. A glass of prune juice or a few tablespoons of bran in the morning may help you. Keep active with hobbies and light exercise such as walking. You can try a stool softener such as Metamucil or milk of magnesia, both of which you can buy at a drugstore without a prescription. If you do become constipated, discuss it with your nurse and doctor. They may tell you to take a regular laxative or prescribe something for you. It is important to discuss the side effects with the health team taking care of you so they will know if there is anything unusual happening. There are additional hints for dealing with this problem in Chapter 22.

Will I experience diarrhea?

The patients who get diarrhea are usually those taking antibiotics and antimetabolites. You should try a diet low in roughage, high in constipating food like cheese and boiled milk. Diarrhea can easily cause you to lose fluid and become dehydrated. It is important that you drink plenty of fluid every day. If you have tenderness in the anal area, use a substance such as a medical ointment. If it does not stop in one or two days or if you have more than two or three loose stools a day, be sure to talk with your doctor. You should not take any medicine for diarrhea without your doctor's permission. There are additional hints for dealing with this problem in Chapter 22.

What can I do about sensitivity to the sun?

You should be careful when going outside, even if you are walking outdoors. Wear a hat, and use sunblock lotion. Be careful when you are at the beach. Be sure to wear sunblock lotion that contains para-amino benzoic acid (PABA).

What is meant by the term "Leucovorin rescue"?

This is an experimental technique which is used to spare normal cells from the toxic side effects of high doses of methotrexate. Methotrexate has been used in low doses for many years to treat cancer. It is now being tested in high doses for the treatment of several diseases, including head and neck cancer, leukemia, and osteogenic sarcoma. Large amounts of methotrexate are given for a prescribed period of time, followed by the administration of another drug, citrovorum factor (Leucovorin) at a predetermined time. The Leucovorin rescues or protects the patient against the life-threatening effects of high doses of the methotrexate. Because this treatment differs markedly from the standard regimen, doctors who wish to use it must obtain an investigational new drug license from the Food and Drug Administration. The doctor must explain the technique to the patient and an informed-consent form must be signed by the patient before the treatment can be given.

Are cancer patients on chemotherapy at a higher risk for getting shingles?

Cancer patients, especially those with lymphomas, are more susceptible to shingles. Other patients receiving chemotherapy drugs which suppress the immune system are also at a higher risk.

Shingles (or herpes zoster) is a painful viral infection of certain sensory nerves that causes a skin rash along the course of the affected nerve.

Is there any drug which can be used in a cancer patient against shingles?

Recent research in at least one cancer center has shown that an antiviral drug, given intravenously, can be used effectively to speed the healing of shingles without toxic side effects. The drug, adenine arabinoside (ara-A), has increased the speed of healing of shingles in cancer patients included in the study.

Can I be vaccinated or take flu shots when I am on chemotherapy?

Vaccination can be dangerous for patients with lymphomas. It is important that you check with your doctor before taking any type of immunization shots.

What does the doctor mean when he says a breast or prostate cancer is "hormone-dependent"?

He means that the cancer is depending on the hormones in your system to make it grow. It is not clearly understood how this mechanism works. But it is known that about 40 percent of the breast cancers and over half the prostate cancers fall into the "hormone-dependent" category. In the case of hormone-dependent prostate cancers, sometimes the testicles are removed to take away the hormones which are supporting the growth and the female hormone estrogen is given to change the environment. In the case of breast cancer, particularly in younger women, the ovaries may be removed to change the environment. In three out of ten cases, the tumor will actually be reduced in size and occasionally will disappear. Tests (called estrogen receptor tests) have been devised to determine whether or not the tumor is hormone-dependent.

Why are female hormones used to treat prostate cancer and male hormones used to treat breast cancer?

Scientists are uncertain as to the exact mechanism by which hormones influence the growth of cells. Some cancers of the breast, prostate, and uterus occur in tissues which are influenced by hormones; sometimes they appear at a time of life when hormonal activity in the body has changed, such as after menopause. Cancer that starts in tissues such as the breast in women and the prostate gland in men depends for its growth on the presence of the hormones to which these tissues normally respond. Scientists feel that treatment with hormones may affect these cancers through changing the normal environment. Thus androgens (male hormones) are sometimes used to treat women with breast cancer. Older women who have passed menopause sometimes respond to treatment with doses of estrogens (female hormones). Female hormones help to suppress the growth of cancer of the prostate. Other hormones used are corticosteroids such as cortisone and prednisone for certain types of leukemia and lymphomas. Doctors also sometimes remove glands which secrete hormones (such as the ovaries or testicles) to help slow down malignant growth.

How many different kinds of chemotherapy drugs are there now in use?

Over 50 different chemotherapy drugs have been developed that are useful in the treatment of some kinds of cancer. Some of them are still in the experimental or investigational stages.

Who discovers these new drugs?

The National Cancer Institute sponsors an international cooperative chemotherapy program, involving many research laboratories of the federal government, the universities and medical schools, and the pharmaceutical industry. This program encourages scientists of all kinds to search for drugs to cure cancer. Chemotherapy is now the most heavily studied area in cancer treatment. Scientists are creating new chemical compounds, studying plant specimens, and extracting antibiotics from natural fermentation products and soil samples. At the same time, many of the world's top chemists are searching for ways to improve the activity of known drugs.

How many new materials are tested each year?

According to the National Cancer Institute, each year about 50,000 materials are tested including chemicals, antibiotics, natural products, and newly synthesized compounds related to known drugs. Of almost equal importance is the testing of new doses and schedules which alter the antitumor activities of some of the older drugs.

How are the new materials tested?

The first series of tests for new materials are performed on animals. They are tested against particular kinds of cancer in rats and mice that have been shown to predict antitumor activity in man. If the drug appears to work in the small rodents, it is then tested in larger animals such as monkeys and dogs to see what kind of side effects it produces and to make sure that the drug kills cancer cells without damaging normal tissues excessively. If the drug passes these tests, it is then put through a series of tests on human patients.

How are the drugs tested in patients?

After a new cancer drug comes out of the laboratory testing, there are several years of careful, step-by-step "clinical trials" before it can be approved for general use. Before a new drug may be used in clinical studies with cancer patients, the Food and Drug Administration (FDA) must license the compound as an Investigational New Drug. The National Cancer Institute coordinates these clinical trials, using investigators who participate on a voluntary, cooperative basis. These scientists determine the suitability of candidate drugs for evaluation in the treatment of one or more malignant diseases. Only one out of every 2,000 drugs originally tested is considered promising and safe enough to be studied in patients.

What are the phases of drug evaluation?

- *Preclinical:* This is the phase in which drugs are tested in rodents, and if they pass those tests are then tested in large animals.
- *Phase I:* This phase involves patients with advanced disease who have exhausted other forms of treatment. The first trials are usually begun at one-tenth the dose that produced side effects in the most sensitive animal species. The drug is usually used on patients with a wide range of cancers. During this phase the dose is gradually increased in subsequent patients until the dose that produces tolerable side effects is

reached. Effects on the tumor are also evaluated. The data collected in this part of the study indicate the side effects which can be expected in humans. The drug can be used only if the person gives informed consent and can stay nearby to be closely monitored during the first few treatments.

- *Phase II:* The anti-tumor activity of the drug is determined in several specific cancers during this phase. Tumor masses are measured and x-ray studies are done so that the effectiveness of the drug can be evaluated before the decision is made to continue the trials. Again, the tests are performed on patients having advanced disease who have no effective treatment available. During this phase, the types of tumors which respond to the drug and how often they respond are closely measured to determine the effects of various dosages and how frequently they must be given to produce good results.

- *Phase III:* If the drug is found to be effective in the Phase II trial, this phase establishes whether the drug is more useful and/or has fewer side effects than other drugs already being used. The drug is tested on patients on a large scale, comparing it with the best standard therapy (drugs currently being used) to determine which is better.

The doctors say they are going to use a "Phase II" experimental drug. Should the word "experimental" scare me?

The words "experimental" and "investigational" are used when the new anti-cancer drugs are in the research stages. They are understandably alarming words unless you understand the stringent guidelines which govern drug development. The experimental drugs are only available through persons working under the auspices of the National Cancer Institute, using U.S. Food and Drug Administration regulations governing the use of experimental drugs. If your physician is using a Phase II drug, it has already gone through several phases in the preclinical and Phase I evaluation.

How do I know whether or not my doctor is using an experimental or investigational drug?

You will know because you must sign a consent form. The person giving the investigational drug must clearly explain to the patient both the potential value and the possible risk. This procedure allows the patient to weigh the advantages against any additional problems it might create. A patient may receive an investigational drug only if he qualifies under very specific criteria. Before any of the investigational drugs are administered, the doctor must have a diagnosis (from a biopsy), x-rays to determine the extent of the disease, and studies to determine the patient's blood picture.

Who is allowed to give investigational drugs?

The federal regulations allow only qualified oncologists (cancer specialists) to prescribe investigational cancer drugs. This is to ensure that the patient will receive every possible benefit with a minimum of risk.

Does the doctor giving the investigational drug have to follow any rules and regulations?

Yes. All drug investigations have written guidelines, called protocols, which spell out the overall plan, the criteria for selecting patients, and requirements for monitoring patients, and they give general directions to the investigators. The three distinct phases of drug evaluation on patients are carefully controlled experiments which reveal dosages, side effects, and anti-tumor activity.

During a Phase III drug evaluation, does the doctor or the patient know which patients are getting the experimental drugs and which are getting the drugs already considered standard therapy?

It depends on several factors. The drug evaluation may be done in what is called a randomized trial. In some, neither the doctors nor the patients know whether the drug which is being given is the new experimental drug or the standard therapy. These are called "double-blind" studies. In others, the persons giving the drugs and sometimes the patients know whether they are getting the new drug or the standard therapy.

How am I, as a patient, protected in these investigation trials supported by the National Cancer Institute?

All patients participating in the National Cancer Institute-supported research programs are protected by Department of Health, Education and Welfare regulations (45 CRF, Part 46) pertaining to studies with human subjects. The institutions in which the research is carried out must have review committees of medical scientists who decide whether the importance of the knowledge to be gained outweighs the risks to the patients who participate. In addition, the patients must give their informed consent to participate. The major elements of informed consent as noted in the regulations include:

- A fair explanation of the procedures to be followed and their purposes, including identification of any procedures that are experimental
- A description of the discomforts and risks reasonably to be expected
- A description of the benefits reasonably to be expected
- A disclosure of any appropriate alternative procedures that might be advantageous for the patient
- An offer to answer any inquiries concerning the procedure
- A disclosure that the person is free to withdraw his consent and to discontinue participation in the project or activity at any time without prejudice to the subject

Do the hospitals using the investigational drugs have any say in what drugs are being used?

All investigational drugs used in accredited hospitals must be approved by a committee (usually called the human investigations committee or the human experimentation committee) which usually includes administrators, pharmacists, and physicians. They study all available information on a drug to decide whether or not it is appropriate for use with patients in their institution.

I hear the word "protocol"—what does that mean?

"Protocol" is the term used to describe your treatment program. It means a predetermined treatment plan for groups of patients with similar medical problems. It is usually used when referring to treatment with experimental drugs.

What does the term "randomization" mean?

Randomization is part of being on a clinical trial. Some protocols have several treatment groups or "arms." People are assigned to an arm on an unbiased basis—this is called randomization. This is the best way to remove bias on the part of the doctors and to clearly establish if one treatment is better than another. These studies are not done unless there is a question as to whether one treatment is better than another.

How expensive is chemotherapy?

The cost associated with chemotherapy varies depending upon the drugs being used, how often they are given, and even where they are being given. At the present time, Adriamycin is one of the most expensive drugs, running in the vicinity of $65 to $125 for the cost of the drug each time it is administered. To this must be added the cost of the visit to the doctor, the tests involved, and the charge to administer the drug.

Will my insurance cover chemotherapy?

It depends. Some major medical policies cover chemotherapy. In most places in the country, Blue Cross/Blue Shield only covers chemotherapy if it is given in a hospital or an outpatient clinic. It normally does not cover chemotherapeutic treatments in a doctor's office. Before you agree to the treatment, it is important that you discuss the costs with your doctor.

chapter 9

Immunotherapy

Questions to Ask About Immunotherapy

- What type of immunotherapy will I receive?
- How long will the treatments take?
- How long will the series last?
- Will I be likely to have side effects from the treatments?
- If the vaccine type, will I have scars from the vaccinations?
- Where will the scars be and how prominent are they?
- What are the risks involved?
- Is this an investigational treatment?

Is the National Cancer Institute supporting any research on immunotherapy?

There are several clinical cooperative groups studying new ways to treat cancer with immunotherapy. Studies include cancers of the breast, cancers of the gastrointestinal tract, leukemias, cancers of the lung, head, and neck, lymphomas, melanomas, and cancers of the ovary. If your doctor wishes more information, he should get in touch with Coordinator, International Registry of Tumor Immunotherapy, National Institutes of Health, Bethesda, Md. 20014.

What is immunology?

Immunology is the study of the body's defense system, which is called the immune system. The body uses this mechanism to protect itself against infection and disease.

How does the immune system work?

The immune system is a complex natural watchdog. If you get a cut, for instance, as bacteria invade the system and infection starts, the body is warned by its immune system. It mobilizes cells to survey the invading agents and then to form specific neutralizing proteins (called antibodies) as well as specific cells able to engulf, destroy, or neutralize. Another example of the work of the immune system is in diseases such as measles or smallpox. It has been known since early times that people who recovered from such diseases were nearly always safe (immune) from getting the disease if ever exposed a second time. This protective mechanism is the immune system.

How does the immune system recognize these foreign bodies?

White blood cells—some of which are lymphocytes—are constantly circulating through the blood and lymph system. These lymphocytes recognize cells that are different and foreign, such as bacteria and viruses. When the lymphocytes recognize the foreign cells, they multiply and attack and kill them. The lymphocytes essentially are a surveillance system—they watch over the body cells and try to get rid of those which do not belong in it.

Does the immune system recognize cancer cells?

One of the most important recent advances in this field is the demonstration that the lymphocytes recognize tumor cells in much the same way they recognize bacteria and viruses. It seems, however, that in some persons the immune system may not work perfectly and fails to recognize cancer cells or to respond appropriately to them, allowing them to grow. Some scientists feel that the changes in the surface of cancer cells are not as foreign to the body as viruses or bacteria, since cancer cells are closely related to normal body cells. Many scientists feel that cancer cells occur in our body more often than we realize, and that most of us repel these early cancers without ever being aware of it.

Why does the immune system let cancer cells grow?

Researchers have found that cancer cells often have a way of hiding from the immune system. They may add a biochemical disguise that prevents the system from knowing they are foreign bodies. Scientists also feel that by the time the body's defense has been mounted in some persons, there are already too many cancer cells formed. The body's immune system is capable of destroying only limited numbers of cancer cells. Doctors have found that cancer patients often have a deficient immunological response to agents (antigens) against which normal individuals generally show strong reactions. Although specific responses to cancer-cell-surface antigens have been harder to demonstrate, it is believed that they are also likely to be defective in the person with progressive cancer.

What is meant by "spontaneous tumor regression"?

When tumors in untreated patients get smaller for no apparent reason or disappear completely, it is called spontaneous tumor regression. In some rare cases when a tumor disappears spontaneously it may remain undetectable for long periods. It is more usual, however, for the tumor to shrink temporarily, for the patient to get better, and then for the tumor to grow back again. Scientists feel that it seems logical to assume that the immune system is responsible for these regressions. However, it is possible that the supply of nutrients to the tumor or other factors play a role in this phenomenon. The phenomenon of spontaneous tumor regression has stimulated much research into possible immunological mechanisms.

What is immunotherapy?

Immunotherapy is the management of cancer by making use of the body's own immune system. In immunotherapy the patient is given either a vaccine or a stimulating material which may boost the patient's ability to make antibodies or to send lymphocytes and other cells capable of killing the cancer cells. In other words, immunotherapy is an attempt to strengthen the immune system of the patient to fight off the disease. It is important to understand that as a treatment, immunotherapy is in an investigational stage and is being used only in major medical centers around the country.

Is immunotherapy ever used alone?

Sometimes. More often immunotherapy is used in conjunction with other treatments—surgery, radiation, and chemotherapy. After the surgeon or therapeutic radiologist has removed the bulk of the tumor, immunotherapy may be started, sometimes in addition to chemotherapy. Sometimes it is given alone, especially in those cancers that are particularly resistant to chemotherapy, such as melanoma. The aim is for the immune response to be boosted sufficiently to kill tumor cells wherever they may be in the body. There are times when more than one immunotherapy agent is used in this treatment.

Why is immunotherapy used in combination with other treatments?

The immune system works best when there are only a few cells that it is required to eliminate. When many millions of cells are present, it is more difficult for immunotherapy to achieve good results.

What are the different kinds of immunotherapy?

There are three general ways in which immunotherapy may be given:
- *Active immunotherapy* uses vaccines either prepared from the patient's own tumor or from other individuals' tumors to stimulate the immune system of the patient.
- *Adoptive immunotherapy* takes advantage of the immune response in one individual to improve the defenses in another. This usually refers to cells like lymphocytes or derivatives of reactive lymphocytes like information molecules (RNA) or transfer factors.
- *Passive immunotherapy* involves the transfer of serum antibody from one reactive individual to a patient who may lack this antibody.

What is specific immunotherapy?

Specific immunotherapy is a kind of active immunotherapy. The patient is immunized with a vaccine produced from his or her own tumor or from another patient's tumor cells of the same type as the treated patient's. Tumor cells may be used directly, or made unable to divide by heavy irradiation or treated with chemicals to increase their ability to produce an immune response. For instance, a tumor is taken from a patient. It is reduced to a suspension of single cells, which are given radiation in order to make them unable to divide anymore. These cells are reinjected into the same patient directly, or after incubation with enzymes or chemicals. Although the cancer cells are now harmless, they still may stimulate the immune mechanism to work more actively than it was working before.

What is nonspecific immunotherapy?

Nonspecific immunotherapy is used to stimulate the immune system in a general way. It uses agents which are strong stimulants of the immune system. The agents are injected under the skin, into the tumor itself, or, less frequently, intravenously. They are not related specifically to the tumor itself. Rather, the strong, generally heightened response may also include heightened reactivity against the tumor.

What is a cross-transplant or cross-transfusion immunotherapy?

This is a kind of adoptive immunotherapy which has been used on an investigational basis. It involves two patients with the same tumor type and the same blood type. Cancer cells are taken from patient A, made incapable of further growth, and implanted in patient B and vice versa. After a period of time required for immunization, blood is taken from both patients: red cells are given back to the donor and white cells (including the lymphocytes which attack and destroy cancer) are given to the other patient. This may immunize each patient to the other patient's tumor and allow for further adoptive or passive immunotherapy.

What is transfer factor?

Transfer factor attempts to transfer the immunity of one person to another. It is a kind of adoptive immunotherapy being tried on an investigational basis. Transfer factor is extracted from the white blood cells of one person (called the donor), when the donor's lymphocytes are shown to be reactive in tests against the patient's tumor. Blood is taken from the donor, and the white blood cells are collected, separated, and extracted. This extract is injected into the nonimmune patient. This chemical extract is called "transfer factor" since it appears to transfer specific immunity from one person to another. Transfer factor has been reported to have some success in treating infections, and preliminary studies have been carried out in some cancers. It is now under clinical trial, but until long-term controlled studies are conducted, both transfer-factor and cross-transplant immunotherapy will be used only on an investigational basis.

What are some of the agents used in nonspecific immunotherapy?

There are several different kinds of agents being tried. Some are living microorganisms. Others are vaccines of dead organisms. Still others are synthetic materials. You will hear names such as BCG, *C. parvum,* MER and lavamisole.

What is BCG?

BCG stands for Bacillus Calmette Guerin and was named after the two scientists responsible for discovering it. It is a material which consists of live mycobacteria, very much like the living germ which causes human tuberculosis. The agent is prepared so as to reduce its ability to cause an infection in man, while preserving its stimulation of immunity. It has been widely used to immunize children against tuberculosis in other countries.

How are the various kinds of immunotherapy given?

Most immunotherapy is given by some kind of injection. Some use a method similar to smallpox vaccination, where the substance is pressed onto the skin at the surface with a pointed disc of needles (tine) leaving a rectangular or round vaccination mark. Sometimes the agent is scratched onto the skin with a needle. Some injections are given intravenously into the tumor itself, while others are injected under the skin, similar to a skin test.

Is immunotherapy usually given alone?

Sometimes it is given alone. In some trials it is being given in combination with chemotherapy.

What is *C. parvum?*

C. parvum (Corynebacterium parvum) is a bacterium that stimulates immunity through the cells.

What is MER?

MER (methanol extract residue of BCG) is the chemical remaining after exhaustive removal of fats from BCG. It is like BCG but is a dead virus rather than a live one.

What is Lavamisole?

Lavamisole is a chemical compound which can be taken by mouth. In some preliminary studies it seems to delay recurrence of disease after treatment by surgery or x-ray of some kinds of cancer. Like the other agents, it is an investigational agent.

Are there any complications or side effects from immunotherapy?

It depends upon the agent and on the way it is given.

BCG usually leaves patients with a very tired feeling, sometimes fever, chills, influenza-like symptoms, swelling of the lymph nodes, and inflammation around the area where it is given. Patients who experience these side effects say they usually last from one to three days, with most disappearing in 24 hours.

MER has side effects similar to those of BCG. Sometimes patients experience a very mild fever and a tired feeling during the 24 hours following treatment. The major problem is with local inflammation around the site. If it is very intense or there is an unusual reaction, the patient should tell the nurse or doctor. Sensitivity in this area seems to increase with continued vaccination. Some patients also complain of pain around the injection site, especially in the evening.

C. parvum has side effects such as mild fever, chills, and a tired feeling when it is injected under the skin. Sometimes there is a mild reaction at the site where it is given. When *C. parvum* is given intravenously, there are often fever, chills, and shaking that last from several hours to 24 to 36 hours.

Lavamisole has very mild side effects that usually do not last very long. They may include nausea and vomiting, loss of appetite, and a tired feeling.

Major Immunotherapy Drugs—Their Uses and Most Common Side Effects

DRUG	HOW GIVEN	COMMON SIDE EFFECTS	OCCASIONAL AND RARE SIDE EFFECTS AND UNIQUE FEATURES
BCG (Bacillus Calmette Guerin)	Usually like vaccination (scarification)	General tired feeling lasting about 24 hours; inflammation around area where treatment is given	Fever and chills, draining of vaccination sites, swelling of regional lymph nodes
MER (methanol extract residue of BCG)	Injected under the skin in 3 to 5 areas	Local inflammation (usually looks like large blind pimple or boil), local pain, usually more acute in evening	Draining of sites, nausea, vomiting or abdominal cramps
C. parvum (Corynebacterium parvum)	Intravenous	Fever usually within the first two hours after injection; chills, moderate to severe; headaches, flu-like feeling	Nausea and vomiting, high blood pressure, disturbances of the central nervous system
	Injected under the skin	Local pain at injection site with tenderness and hardness; general tired feeling, fever	
Lavamisole	Oral	Very mild side effects including nausea and vomiting, loss of appetite, fatigue; usually do not last very long	

Should the sites where the agent is injected be covered up?

The site may first be covered with a dry bandage or protective cup but the patient is instructed to uncover the site whenever possible to promote healing. The site should be kept clean and dry at all times. If the site is draining, the doctor will prescribe some medication.

Can I use lotions or powders on my skin when I am being treated with immunotherapy?

You should discuss this with the nurse or doctor giving you the injections. Usually you can use normal skin lotions 24 hours after the treatment. Some people find that calamine lotion helps with itching. Others find that talcum powder is good. Body lotions that are fragrance-free usually offer some relief to most people. The health-care team usually requests that you do not use any steroid preparation on the areas since it may interfere with the immune response.

How long does immunotherapy treatment continue?

As with the other kinds of treatments, the length of time immunotherapy is given depends upon many factors. If it is being used in combination with chemotherapy, for example, it is usually given for the same length of time, usually between the courses of chemotherapy. If used alone, following surgery or radiation which has eliminated all signs of the tumor, it may be given for long periods.

Does the treatment leave scars?

Yes, it may leave marks similar to smallpox vaccinations if the agent being used is given as a vaccination. A variety of sites may be selected and used in rotation. There is eventual healing from the vaccinations, even if the treatment lasts for years. In most patients, near-complete disappearance of the vaccination sites can be expected, but scarring is sometimes found, as with smallpox inoculations. Immunotherapy teams have developed many special approaches to the cosmetic problems of immuno-therapy and will be very happy to discuss them.

Is it true that chemotherapy and radiation interfere with or damage the body's own immune system?

It is true that radiation and chemotherapy can suppress the immune system. It is also true that some cancer patients seem to start out with an immune system which is not fully normal. It is thought that gaps in the body's immune system may allow emergence of cancers and that, at some time in the future, we will find ways to strengthen the body's own defenses so that drugs and radiation will no longer be needed. At present, when treatment must be given for established cancers, it is felt that the least immunosuppression occurs with the off-again, on-again therapy now being used, permitting immune defenses to recover and thus protect the body's other functions.

What do the scientists think is the future of immunotherapy?

It is really too early to tell. Trials of immunotherapy in cancer patients are underway in many major medical centers, and most of these experiments are still in the preliminary stages. Vaccination against cancer—a possibility that springs to mind with the very mention of immunity—remains a real hope. But an enormous amount of basic research remains to be done before immunotherapy of this sort can be understood and used on any wide scale.

Is immunotherapy new?

Although the idea that the immune system might hold the secret to the cure of cancer dates back to the 1800s, its use as a treatment for the disease is still in its infancy. Immunotherapy is a relatively new and experimental form of treatment with varying results. All forms of immunotherapy are considered investigational at this time, and clinical trials to evaluate these treatment methods are currently underway at a number of medical centers around the country.

How do I go about getting immunotherapy treatment?

This is a question you will have to discuss with your doctor, since the use of immunotherapy depends upon what type of cancer you have, the extent of your disease, and where treatments are presently being given. Information about the types of immunotherapy being studied and the names and addresses of investigators studying them can be obtained from Coordinator, International Registry of Tumor Immunotherapy, National Institutes of Health, Bethesda, Md. 20014. Or you can call your nearest Cancer Information Service (see Chapter 23).

chapter 10

Experimental and Unproven Treatments

Questions You Should Ask Yourself Before Agreeing to Investigational or Experimental Treatment

- Do I know exactly what the experimental treatment involves?
- Have I signed a consent form?
- Has the doctor explained the procedures to be followed?
- Has the doctor explained the purpose of the procedures and told me exactly which procedures are experimental?
- What are the risks involved?
- Will the treatment make me sicker?
- What are the benefits of the new treatment?
- What are my alternatives?

Questions You Should Ask Yourself Before Using Unproven Treatments

- Why do I want to use this kind of treatment?
- What do I think the treatments will accomplish?
- Am I jeopardizing my chances by using this type of treatment?
- Have I discussed these treatments with my doctor?
- Will the doctor continue to care for me if he knows about my plans?
- Is there some way my doctor and I can come to a compromise?

- Can I continue my regular treatments and try the unproven treatments at the same time?
- Is there some kind of investigational or experimental treatment that would give the same or better results?
- Is there some approved, alternative treatment I could try instead of my regular treatments?
- What will the costs be?

What is the difference between investigational or experimental treatment and unproven methods?

Investigational or experimental treatments are done under specific standards set up by the scientific community. The treatments have some basis for being tested in man—that is, they work against some tumors in animals. The term "unproven method" is used to describe cancer treatment in which either the substance or the treatment method has not been shown *scientifically* to be effective against cancer.

What are some of the investigational or experimental drugs and cancer treatments?

Many of them have been mentioned in the various other chapters in this book. In the area of chemotherapy, for instance, methyl CCNU, 5-Azacytidine, daunomycin, VP-16, and ICRF-159 are all investigational drugs. The adjuvant chemotherapy treatment for breast cancer, lumpectomy (taking out of the tumor alone) followed by radiation and/or chemotherapy for breast cancer, and whole body irradiation for lymphoma are all considered experimental. Hyperthermia (heat treatment) and the entire field of immunotherapy are all classified as experimental or investigational. The use of neutrons (atomic particles) for treating cancer of the stomach and pancreas is an experimental treatment. These treatments are all being conducted with investigational trials, using standard scientific methods.

What are some of the most common unproven methods?

There are at least 50 different unproven treatments. The best-known is laetrile, which is used by an estimated 50,000 to 75,000 Americans. There are many others, including a large variety of food cures, serums, and herbs. The American Cancer Society has published a book entitled *Unproven Methods of Cancer Manage-*

ment which provides information on both the most prevalent and most promoted unproven treatments.

Are there some treatments which were once known as unproven methods which have become standard treatments?

There are some treatment methods—the use of heat (hyperthermia), for example—which on and off for hundreds of years have been thought to have some effect on cancer cells. However, scientific evidence was scanty and inconclusive. New methods of producing and directing heat, such as using spacesuit underwear, radio frequencies, microwaves, and ultrasound, have brought the subject back into the forefront. However, the role of hyperthermia in the treatment of cancer is not fully established. The tests are in very early experimental stages.

What are the standards under which investigations of experimental treatments are usually done?

The standards under which investigations of experimental treatments are performed are the same type of scientific standards which are required to judge any claim. They include the following:

- The drug or therapy used should be tried and analyzed on experimental animals. These experiments must be able to be repeated by other impartial investigating groups or researchers with the same results under the same circumstances.
- The results of the treatment given should be compared with the natural course of the disease and with the usual treatment to be sure the new treatment is better or equal but with fewer side effects.
- The effects of the treatment should be studied on a large number of people who have a biopsy of proven cancer so that the nature and consistency of the results can be recorded.
- Other previous treatments and/or other treatment methods being used at the same time should be noted and analyzed in determining the effectiveness of the treatment.
- There should be clinical evidence—including seeing and examining treated patients, reviewing microscopic slides of biopsy, x-rays, and other *objective* evidence—which is open

for complete examination. ("Objective" means free from or independent of personal feelings and opinions.)

How are these standards usually applied to an investigational or experimental treatment before it is put into widespread use?

Drugs used in clinical chemotherapy trials are a good example of the rigorous testing that is required. The drugs, created in the laboratory, are first tested on rats and mice. If a specific drug works on tumors of these small animals, it is then tested on larger animals such as monkeys and dogs to see what kind of side effects the drug produces and to make sure that the drug kills cancer cells without damaging normal tissues excessively. If the drug passes these tests (and only one out of 2,000 drugs tested do), the FDA approves it as an investigational drug and allows it to be put through a series of tests on humans.

How is human drug testing done?

Human testing is done in three phases. The first two involve people with advanced disease who have exhausted other forms of treatment. All patients must have had a biopsy to prove that they actually have cancer, with appropriate tests to determine the extent of it. The first phase (Phase I) tests the amount of the drug which the patient can tolerate and side effects are studied. The drugs are then tested for their anti-tumor activity, for the types of tumors which respond to the drug and how often the tumors respond. These are all closely measured to determine the effects of various doses and how often they must be given to produce good results (Phase II). The drugs are then tested on patients on a large scale to see whether or not the drug is more useful or has fewer side effects than other drugs or treatments already being used. This phase (Phase III) is designed to compare the new treatment with the standard treatment and the normal course of the disease to see which treatment is more effective. There is more information about clinical trials in Chapter 8.

Who regulates the use of new drugs or substances for treating cancer?

The Food and Drug Administration (FDA) is the agency which regulates the introduction and clinical testing of the new drugs.

The National Cancer Institute or drug companies may be involved in conducting the tests, but neither the American Cancer Society nor the National Cancer Institute is a regulatory agency. The regulations governing the introduction and clinical testing of new drugs have been established and are administered by the FDA. These regulations require that certain standards of safety and effectiveness be met and that a carefully planned clinical study be undertaken.

Aren't American scientific standards very strict? Is it easier to get drugs approved in Europe?

Yes, U.S. standards are very strict. It is easier to get new drugs approved in Europe. The original U.S. Food, Drug, and Cosmetic Act of 1938 was amended in 1962, after the problems of the drug thalidomide became evident. Thousands of pregnant women around the world who took the drug produced deformed babies. The amendment requires a demonstration of the effectiveness of the drug as well as of the safety of the drug before it can be licensed for use in the United States. This means that there is a lag between the drugs which are used in the United States and in many other countries of the world. The new drugs in the United States must go through animal tests before they can be used on humans, and it takes five to ten years to do all the necessary testing before new drugs are considered safe and effective for use in this country.

Are the scientific standards used for investigational or experimental drugs also used in testing unproven methods?

No. Usually those who use unproven methods lead patients and their families to believe that the method can produce a cure— without the scientific evidence to back it up. There are several shortcomings:

- Usually the amount of experimental evidence is very small.
- Sometimes the treatment has shown little or no effect on animals, but the persons giving the treatment feel that it will work on people.
- Often there is no biopsy evidence available, or if it is available, it is found that the whole tumor had been removed by surgery or destroyed by radiation or chemotherapy before the unproven method was started.

- It is almost always difficult, if not impossible, for other scientists or doctors to obtain the drug for analysis and trial. The treatment used is not made freely available to other scientists in the field for independent trial under controlled circumstances.
- There is usually little or no attempt to follow up the patient. Complete objective records are not usually kept and the results of treatment are not published in accredited scientific journals for other scientists to evaluate.
- The results are often based entirely on subjective evidence (influenced by one's personal interests and emotions) such as how the patient feels rather than on objective scientific tests (biopsies, x-rays, blood tests) to show whether or not the treatment is working.

Will I know if the doctor is using an investigational or experimental treatment?

You will know if the doctor is using an investigational or experimental treatment because treatment being done under controlled scientific circumstances must be explained to you and a consent form signed. The consent form describes the treatment and the side effects in detail. Only qualified cancer specialists can prescribe the investigational drugs. On the other hand, unproven methods may be used without a similar explanation and without the signing of a consent form.

How can a person tell an umproven method from an investigational or experimental investigational treatment?

The American Cancer Society offers the following information which you can use to help distinguish unproven methods from investigational or experimental ones:

- The people involved in treating patients with unproven methods tend to be isolated from established scientific facilities and associates. Their treatment approaches have never been shown to be effective to the satisfaction of knowledgeable experts in cancer therapy. Those using unproven methods tend to avoid and to be avoided by competent medical specialists. The experimental or investigational treatment, on the other hand, is based on well established, universally accepted principles of observation and experimentation.

- Current, reputable scientific journals are not used for reporting scientific information. Instead of publishing findings in reputable journals or presenting them at meetings of their medical peers, those using unproven methods may take the publicity route and report findings to laymen who are in no position to evaluate statements critically and scientifically.

- Claims of persecution by organized medicine and science are often made. Investigation usually shows that papers are not published because the reports do not offer scientifically objective evidence of effective results. There are more than 200 medical and scientific journals where new developments are regularly communicated and thousands of regularly scheduled meetings of doctors and scientists at which to present well-documented scientific evidence.

- Records of unproven treatments are often scanty, inadequate, or nonexistent. Often no biopsy has been done to confirm the cancer. As a result, many of the claimed cures may not have been cancers in the first place.

- Often proven treatment is used along with the unproven method and if the patient reacts favorably, it is credited to the unproven therapy.

- Many of the cures are claimed by doctors with unrecognized degrees such as N.D. (Doctor of Naturopathy), Ph.N. (Philosopher of Naturopathy), DA BB-A (Diplomate of American Board of Bio-Analysts), and Ms.D. (Doctor of Metaphysics).

Is the subject of unproven methods new?

No. Unproven remedies for the treatment of cancer are as old as the disease itself. In 1748, the House of Burgesses of the General Assembly of Virginia, of which George Washington was a member, passed a resolution appointing a committee to make a trial of Mary Johnson's "receipt of curing cancer," consisting of garden sorrel, celandine, persimmon bark, and spring water, and to report on its effect. In 1754, the committee, after hearing the testimony of many witnesses who had taken the remedy that they had been cured of cancer, put the report into the minutes of the House of Burgesses and voted Mrs. Johnson a reward of 100 pounds.

What is hyperthermia?

Hyperthermia is the use of heat to kill cancer cells. The treatment is highly experimental but considered to be worth further study. The degree and intensity of the heat must be closely controlled and accurately applied to the area. Both the effectiveness and the possible harmful side effects of heat treatment remain to be evaluated.

Why do the scientists think that hyperthermia may work?

The idea of using heat for the treatment of cancer has been around for a long time. Some say it goes back to 600 B.C. However, no one has yet produced consistent, good results in scientific studies under controlled conditions. The new studies, which are in very early experimental stages, are attempting to produce the needed scientific evidence for this treatment. Scientists note that heat seems to stimulate the immune system and enhance the anticancer activity of drugs. Recent evidence from studies of cancer cells in culture and of animals bearing various tumors indicate that hyperthermia has definite anti-cancer effects.

Is more than one kind of heat treatment being investigated?

Yes. There are basically two kinds of heat treatments under investigation: local and total-body. Local hyperthermia tries to raise the heat in a specific part of the body. Among methods being investigated for local hyperthermia are the use of radio-frequency waves (similar to those used in radio broadcasting), microwaves (similar to those used to relay TV signals), ultrasound (high-frequency sound waves), and perfusion (heating the blood going to one particular organ). Whole-body hyperthermia raises the heat of the entire body, usually using a suit similar to those worn by the astronauts. Also under investigation is the use of heat in combination with other treatments such as radiation, chemotherapy, and immunotherapy.

Where is hyperthermia being tested?

Hyperthermia is being tested in several medical centers in the country and at the National Cancer Institute. Most patients being treated are those for whom all other standard treatments have been tried. See Chapter 23 for a listing of some areas where this investigational work is being conducted.

What is interferon?

Interferon (also known as human leukocyte interferon) is a protein substance which is taken from whole body cells. It occurs naturally in the body and is produced by white blood cells and other types of cells that have been exposed to certain viruses. In test animals, the substance has shown some activity against tumors. The supply of human interferon is scarce, since only small amounts can be made from large numbers of human white blood cells or other human cells grown in cultures.

Is the National Cancer Institute or the American Cancer Society involved in human trials using interferon?

The National Cancer Institute has started limited investigations of interferon as a treatment in patients with non-Hodgkin lymphoma and advanced breast cancer. The American Cancer Society is giving major financial support to interferon trials (Phase II controlled clinical trials) on approximately 100 to 150 patients at several major institutions, including Columbia University College of Physicians and Surgeons (New York City), Johns Hopkins University (Maryland), M.D. Anderson Hospital and Tumor Institute (Texas), Memorial Sloan-Kettering Cancer Center (New York City), Mt. Sinai Hospital (New York City), Roswell Park Memorial Institute (New York), Stanford University Medical Center (California), University of California at Los Angeles Medical Center, University of Wisconsin Center for Health Sciences, and Yale University School of Medicine (Connecticut).

I have heard that Vitamin C is a good treatment for cancer. Are there any studies to back up the use of this vitamin?

Linus Pauling and others feel that Vitamin C enhances the natural resistance of patients to the disease and/or improves their well-being. Its relation to the treatment of cancer is presently unknown. The National Cancer Institute has funded a study which is being carried out at the Mayo Clinic in Rochester, Minn., to test Vitamin C. The study is to determine whether or not Vitamin C relieves symptoms and extends patients' lives. The patients who are included in the study have advanced cancer and can no longer benefit from standard therapy—surgery, radiation, and chemotherapy. They are being matched with a control group of similar patients who are taking a placebo (a pill made out of milk sugar). Neither the patients nor the doctors will know who is getting the Vitamin C and who is getting the placebo until the code is broken at the end of the study. All patients in the study are being asked about the relief of symptoms and their well-being. The length of survival is also being measured. The results of this study should be available in 1979. There are other studies going on to determine how Vitamin C might help in forming new white blood cells, which could contribute to improving the immune systems of cancer patients.

Is the drug thymidine being tested in humans?

Yes, it is. Trials are being conducted in two locations: the Stehlin Foundation for Cancer Research, 777 St. Joseph's Professional Building, Houston, Tex. 77002, and the National Cancer Institute facility at the Baltimore Cancer Research Program in Maryland. It is also being tested along with other drugs at the Sidney Farber Center in Boston and at the Memorial Sloan-Kettering Center in New York City.

Are there any other diet theories being tested by the National Cancer Institute?

In the NCI's newly established diet, nutrition, and cancer program, which is exploring the relationship of nutrition to cancer, the loss of appetite in cancer patients and ways to provide nourishment to them is being studied. This study, called Optimal Nutritional Support as an Adjunct to Cancer Therapy, is underway at 14 institutions in the United States. There are also studies of the way that normal cells and tumor cells compete for nutrients. The whole question of nutrition and cancer is being studied more closely than ever before.

Is mind control being used to treat cancer?

A great deal of experimentation and research is being done at present in this area, although there are few published valid studies which document the results of mind control in treating cancer. One of the leading experts in the field of psychosocial re-habilitation is Dr. Lawrence LeShan, an experimental psycho-logist who has written a book called *You Can Fight for Your Life* (New York: M. Evans, 1977). Another is *And a Time to Live:*

Toward Emotional Well-Being During the Crisis of Cancer, by Robert C. Cantor, M.D. (New York: Harper & Row, 1978). Some interesting experimental work is being done in the area of mind control under the direction of Dr. O. Carol Simonton and Mrs. Stephanie Simonton. Dr. Simonton is a radiation oncologist who applies the techniques of mind control in his practice. A tape recording explaining the Simonton method is available from the Cancer Counseling and Resource Center, 1413 Eighth Avenue, Fort Worth, Tex. 76104. Also available is a book by Dr. Simonton, *Getting Well Again: A Step-by-Step Self-Help Guide to Overcoming Cancer for Patients and Families* (New York: St. Martin's Press, 1978). A list of some of the rehabilitation research projects (which includes some psychosocial projects) funded by the National Cancer Institute is in Chapter 23.

Is biofeedback being used in treating cancer?

The nature of the measurable responses to biofeedback encourages further experimentation in the field of mind control. In biofeedback, people are taught how to control a body function such as heart rate, by being made aware of what their bodies are doing. The same principles are being experimented with to try to help control cancers.

What is laetrile?

Laetrile is a product made from apricot pits which contains a chemical called amygdalin. Amygdalin occurs in the seeds of many plants—it is abundant in the kernels of peaches, apricots, bitter almond, and apple seeds. A molecule of laetrile is made up of 2 parts sugar, 1 part benzaldehyde, and 1 part cyanide. Until the substance is dissolved in water and heated or placed in the presence of an enzyme called betaglucosidase (which is found in many parts of the body), the cyanide is locked into the formula.

How does laetrile work?

The explanation of the workings of the drug is based on a theory of the Scottish embryologist John Beard, whose work was published in the early 1900s. He felt that a malignant growth was a product of the fetal cells—cells which are released when the fertilized egg divides during pregnancy. These cells (known as trophoblasts) in the early months of development of the baby invade the uterine wall to form the placenta (the membrane which attaches the baby to the wall of the uterus). When the cells are no longer needed, an enzyme from the pancreas kills the trophoblasts. The people who support laetrile say that if the pancreas does not do this, the cells scatter throughout the body, lose their protective cover, and try to form a new fetus. This, according to the laetrile supporters, is the basis of cancer. And, they claim, laetrile can destroy the cells because it furnishes cyanide, which is the missing killer. The scientific community feels that this theory has no scientific evidence to support it.

Why do the supporters of laetrile feel it works?

They believe that cancerous tissues contain greater amounts of the enzyme betaglucosidase than do the healthy tissues and that the cancerous tissues release cyanide from amygdalin on a selective basis. Scientists say that there is no evidence to support this theory—that only traces of betaglucosidase are found in animal tissues and no more is found in cancerous tissues than in healthy tissues. Early research done at a major medical center shows that there is not enough of the betaglucosidase in the cancer cells to release the cyanide.

Are healthy tissues harmed by the cyanide?

Those who support laetrile say that the healthy tissues are protected from the action of the cyanide because they contain another enzyme (called rhodanase). They believe this enzyme protects the healthy tissues because it converts the cyanide to a harmless substance (called thiocyanate). The scientific community says there is no evidence that healthy tissues contain any more rhodanase than do cancerous tissues. They feel that cyanide, when released, affects normal cells as well as cancer cells—and that experiments with it show that cyanide action doesn't begin until there is a lethal dose.

Why must laetrile go through the FDA testing procedures?

The FDA defines any article "intended for use in the diagnosis, cure, mitigation, treatment or prevention of disease" as a drug. Therefore, if laetrile is to be used in the treatment of cancer, it must, under FDA regulations, undergo and abide by the regulatory rules. Under the FDA rules, a new drug must be approved by FDA on the basis of scientific evidence, including tests on animals, before its use can be justified for experimental tests on humans. A new drug can be distributed commercially only if it has been approved by the FDA as safe and effective after conclusive tests on both animals and humans.

Is laetrile a vitamin? I read somewhere that it is actually Vitamin B-17.

The supporters of laetrile began describing laetrile as a vitamin in the 1970s when it seemed that there would be difficulty in registering it as a drug. As a vitamin, rather than as a drug, laetrile would be exempt from the stringent drug laws enforced by the U.S. Food and Drug Administration. It was Ernst Krebs, Jr., who apparently created the designation. The McNaughton Foundation, which sponsors laetrile research around the world, uses the designation Vitamin B-17 exclusively to describe amygdalin. The National Nutrition Consortium (which includes the American Institute of Nutrition, the American Academy of Pediatricians, and the Nutrition Board of the National Academy of Sciences) does not consider laetrile a vitamin. It says there is no scientific evidence for the existence of a nutrient identified as B-17.

Why is laetrile not considered a vitamin?

To be a vitamin, a substance must have certain characteristics:
- It must be an externally supplied organic substance that is vital to the life of the organism, and required in small amounts for the organism's health and well-being. It must serve a unique bodily function. (There is no evidence that laetrile is an essential nutritional substance. Laboratory animals have been kept alive and healthy for generations without having any of it in their diets.)
- If it is withdrawn, its absence must cause certain clearly defined diseases to afflict the organism—the organism would become diseased and die. The diseases must arise only because of the absence of the vitamin and must be entirely cured by supplying the vitamin. (There does not seem to be any scientific evidence that any specific disease—including cancer—has been linked to the lack of laetrile in any animal, man included, and no scientific evidence exists that cancer is arrested by supplying it.)

What are the names of groups that are supporters of laetrile?

The largest group is the Committee for Freedom of Choice in Cancer Therapy, Inc. Other groups include the International Association of Cancer Victims and Friends, the Cancer Control Society, and the National Health Federation. It is being used as treatment through the clinic run by Dr. Ernesto Contreras in Tijuana, Mexico, and at the Silbersee Clinic in Hanover, Germany, operated by Dr. Hans Nieper.

I have heard that the John Birch Society is behind the laetrile movement. Is that true?

There is no evidence that the John Birch Society itself is behind laetrile. However, some members of the organizations involved in supporting laetrile are also members of the John Birch Society, especially persons in the Committee for Freedom of Choice in Cancer Therapy, Inc.

Is there any truth to the claim that the laetrile supporters continually change their story on the use of the drug?

The opponents of laetrile make this charge. They say that first the drug was hailed as a cure for cancer. Then after many years of not being able to convince the medical community, laetrile supporters labeled the drug a vitamin which could be used in curing cancer. Today, the literature of the laetrile supporters themselves says that laetrile is not being promoted as a cure for cancer—that at best it is a control for cancer and that now it is regarded as a "metabolic agent or vitamin used in nutritional therapy and prevention."

Is laetrile taken as a pill?

Sometimes laetrile is given in pill form. It is also given by injection—an amber-colored liquid.

I have read that laetrile or a substance like it was being used back in the times of the ancient Chinese. Is that true?

The use of natural substances, which include cyanide, has been traced back to ancient China. However, laetrile first came into the modern treatment of cancer during prohibition in the 1920s when Ernst Krebs, Sr., a doctor in California interested in research, was looking at the role of the aging process in changing the taste of whiskey. In the course of research, he found that the apricot extract seemed to have some antitumor activity in experimental mice, but that it also killed many of the mice. In the 1940s, his son, Ernst Krebs, Jr., a biochemist, worked to try to purify the apricot extract to a substance which would be harmless to humans. He patented it in 1949 as a substance for possible use in human therapy.

Who is opposed to laetrile?

Most medical doctors are opposed to the drug because they feel that it has not been proved scientifically to work. The major cancer and medical centers, the National Cancer Institute, the American Cancer Society, and the Food and Drug Administration are also opposed to laetrile for the same reason. These groups feel that there are many risks in using the drug—the greatest one being that if laetrile is taken instead of proven remedies, it can be potentially fatal. They cite case histories of patients who had cancer in a treatable stage, but abandoned conventional treatment for laetrile. By the time the patients realized that laetrile was not working, their chances for recovery were poor or lost. These groups feel that the use of laetrile as a treatment stands in violation of basic patient rights against being duped and offered a false sense of hope. Patients, they feel, have the right to responsible, honest medical care of high quality for as long as they live.

What have been the results of the tests by the National Cancer Institute?

NCI has tested laetrile extensively in animals in institutions in different parts of the country. All tests have used laetrile or amygdalin. (Amygdalin is the generic chemical name.)

- In 1957, tests were conducted against three kinds of tumors. Laetrile was given to mice that had had tumors transplanted onto them (a common way of testing for anticancer activity). These test results showed that the chemical did not stop the tumor growth significantly, nor did it increase the life of the mice significantly.
- In 1960, a second experiment was run against three kinds of tumors. Laetrile was again given to mice with tumors transplanted onto them. Again, no antitumor activity was found.

- In 1969, a third laetrile test was run against leukemia in mice. This time laetrile was tested alone and also along with the enzyme betaglucosidase, which helps break laetrile down in the body. This test showed that the substance was ineffective both alone and in combination with the enzyme. When the drugs and the enzyme were given together the side effects increased.
- In 1973, amygdalin was tested alone and in combination with betaglucosidase against four kinds of tumors in rodents. It was found not effective, both alone and in combination with the enzyme.
- In 1975, a fifth experiment was conducted in mice against three mouse tumors. The amygdalin was tested alone or in combination with the enzyme. No anti-tumor activity was found.
- A sixth experiment was done in mice with breast cancer and colon cancer. Some of the mice were treated with amygdalin alone, some with the enzyme alone, and some with the combination. The scientists reported they found no difference in the growth of the tumors in the mice that did and did not receive laetrile.
- In addition, 11 series of animal experiments (23 experiments in all) were conducted to test whether amygdalin could kill spontaneous breast cancer or leukemia in mice. There is a discrepancy in the results of these tests. The scientists feel the discrepancies occurred because the experiments were evaluated by different methods. The tests which were favorable to laetrile had been evaluated by the observers' eyesight (size of tumor) rather than by objective tests. The tests which came out as unfavorable to laetrile were judged by more sensitive and objective tests called bioassays. Moreover, the findings from the favorable tests could not be reproduced a second time by other scientists. Scientists feel that if a substance actively works against cancer, it will do so consistently, no matter who is conducting the tests.

The supporters of laetrile dispute the results of the tests and have come up with their own evidence. However, no unbiased researcher has been able to duplicate the results of tests done by the laetrile supporters.

How did the National Cancer Institute conduct tests on patients using laetrile?

Several things have happened in the past two years:

- The National Cancer Institute launched a nationwide search for cancer patients who had benefited from using laetrile and whose case records could be used to document anticancer activity. Letters were sent to 835,000 doctors and 70,000 other health professionals, groups supporting the use of laetrile were contacted and the effort was publicized nationally. It was hoped that 200–300 cases would be found.

- As a result, some 90 patients signed consent forms to let NCI collect information from their medical records; 67 patients' records had enough information to allow their cases to be reviewed.

- A panel of 12 oncologists were asked to evaluate the results. The summaries of the 68 laetrile cases were mixed with 68 similarly prepared summaries of cases treated by conventional chemotherapy and 24 cases with no treatment. To prevent any bias, the oncologists were not told the actual treatment given.

- The panel found that 6 of the laetrile cases had some response: 2 showed complete disappearance of all evidence of cancer and 4 showed shrinkage of measurable tumor by 50 percent or more. In addition, 3 other patients were judged to show a longer survival than would normally be expected for their form of cancer (these cases were not considered evaluable because laetrile was used when no definite sign of disease was present).

- The National Cancer Institute noted that these results normally would *not* be sufficient to justify clinical trial of this drug over other drugs available for testing. However, because of widespread public use and interest in laetrile, NCI decided to pursue clinical studies, to be carried out in some of the major institutions in the country.

I hear that laetrile makes cancer patients have less pain and feel better. Is that true?

Those who support laetrile report that some patients say they have less pain. They say that a majority of the laetrile-treated patients report positive responses, ranging from an increase in feeling well to increases in appetite, and weight gain. Scientific studies show that 30 to 40 percent of cancer patients get pain relief when they take a placebo (a pill made out of milk sugar or pressed bread) which they are told is a painkiller. Studies show that even the color of a pill can change its effectiveness.

If I want to take laetrile, shouldn't that choice be mine to make?

That is the main question which is being asked these days, since the laetrile issue seems to be no longer fought on medical grounds. The questions now center around the issue of freedom of choice. But many scientists feel that letting down the bars for laetrile will also allow use of other remedies which have not been proved effective. They fear that drugs will be manufactured and distributed accompanied by all kinds of claims of benefits without having laboratory evidence that they really work, and that we will be returning to the days of the medicine men who could sell you anything and tell you it cured your ailment without having to give scientific evidence for its effectiveness.

But if I really want to do it, why can't I make that decision?

The choice or decision is always yours. But you should understand that the scientific community does not feel that this treatment is effective. If no proven treatment is available for your type and stage of cancer, other experimental treatments with more promise are available at the major cancer centers.

Is laetrile safe?

The supporters say that laetrile is not toxic and that it is safe unless it is taken in large doses. Most doctors usually agree that small amounts are not significantly detrimental. However, there is no body of scientific evidence to prove whether or not laetrile is safe. No one really knows what is being given—the FDA has strict guidelines for drugs so that each batch must be tested for purity and chemical compounds, but since laetrile is not licensed under the FDA, one cannot be sure what the drug actually contains. Laetrile does contain cyanide, and all agree that there is potential danger if large doses are given. Some patients have suffered serious drug reactions to laetrile, and poisoning has been described as a consequence of taking laetrile compounds by mouth. There have been known cases of children dying from swallowing doses of laetrile.

Is laetrile ever used in combination with other cancer treatments?

Sometimes patients use laetrile in combination with conventional treatments—surgery, chemotherapy, and radiation. In the clinic in Mexico, laetrile is sometimes combined with chemotherapeutic agents.

How expensive is laetrile?

The cost varies greatly depending upon where it is purchased. For example, it has been estimated that the cost of a month's treatment in a Mexican clinic can run from $1,500 to $2,500. A half-ounce of the liquid (used for injection) when smuggled into the United States has run up to $50 (it is about $9 when purchased in Tijuana).

Where in the United States is it legal to buy laetrile?

As of January 1979, 17 states have legalized laetrile: Alaska, Arizona, Delaware, Florida, Illinois, Indiana, Kansas, Louisiana, Maryland, Nevada, New Hampshire, New Jersey, Ohio, Oklahoma, Oregon, Texas, and Washington. Six states have rejected it, and it is pending in several states at this writing.

Does this mean that I can actually buy laetrile legally in these states?

The legalization of laetrile in these states means that the states are free to license drugs that are manufactured and used within their boundaries despite federal disapproval. In most of these states, however, it is not legal to manufacture the drug.

I understand that there is no scientific evidence supporting laetrile, but my mother's doctor has told her there is no hope left, that she is going to die, and I want to try laetrile. I live in a state where it is not legal. Is there any way I can get it?

In 1977, a judge in Oklahoma issued an order that said the Food and Drug Administration and the U.S. Customs Service could not stop the importation of laetrile and the transportation of it across state lines for any cancer patient who is terminally ill. Your doctor (M.D.) must submit an affidavit saying that the patient is terminally ill. He must specify the amount of laetrile the patient may import. The affidavit must be notarized.

Isn't it true that laetrile is being used in other countries and that there is scientific evidence that it is working?

Laetrile is being used in some other countries, but there is no evidence that it is working. It is difficult to find accurate statistics, but according to information that the American Cancer Society received from the U.S. Department of State, laetrile is unknown in 14 countries, is either prohibited or not approved in 10 countries, is neither registered nor available on the market in 38 countries, and its use is permitted in 2 countries. In those countries where it is being used, the control of drugs is much looser than in the United States.

Is it legal to use laetrile in Mexico?

In October 1976, the Mexican Department of Health banned laetrile in an action which could close down the manufacture of the substance by two laboratories. In banning the drug, the Mexican government stated that "no positive results were obtained in clinical research carried out at the Mexican Center General Hospital." One firm which appealed the ruling has lost. The other firm's appeal was still pending at this writing.

Where can I get information about laetrile and other unproven methods, so I can make up my own mind?

Information is available from a number of sources. The Committee for Freedom of Choice in Cancer Therapy, Inc. is the most active group. The address is 146 Main Street, Suite 408, Los Altos, Calif. 94022. The Cancer Control Society, 2043 N. Berendo St., Los Angeles, Calif. 90027, a nonprofit educational, charitable, and scientific society, publishes *Cancer Control Journal* and sends out a packet for a nominal fee. The National Health Federation, 212 West Foothill Boulevard, Monrovia, Calif. 91016, which describes itself as a noncommercial health consumer group, includes information on laetrile in its publications. There are numerous books that have been published, such as *Freedom From Cancer, the Story of Laetrile*, by Michael L. Culbert; *Laetrile: Nutritional Control for Cancer*, by Glen D.

Kittler; and *Cancer: How and Why It May Be Wiped Out,* by J. Gordon Roberts.

Have you heard about the use of cultured milk as a cancer cure?

A Florida milk producer, J. Gordon Roberts, claims that the use of *Lactobacillus* bacteria is useful in preventing cancer—but his theories have never been scientifically proved. Roberts' book is available through Roberts Cancer Research Publications Inc., P.O. Box 1662, Clearwater, Fla. 33517.

Don't some foods help to cure cancer? I have heard that asparagus is useful in cancer cures.

Many foods have been proclaimed as cancer cures, asparagus among them. Also in this category are nasturtium petals, mushrooms, violet leaves, red clover, cactus teas, and grapes. There is no scientific evidence that any of them have curative properties. However, the role that diet plays in causing, preventing, or curing cancer is a complex one that is just beginning to be studied. There is some tentative evidence to suggest that diets rich or deficient in certain factors may be implicated in certain types of cancer—for instance, it seems that women who have diets rich in fats are at a higher risk of developing breast cancer. In addition, certain chemical additives now pose a cancer-causing risk. The National Cancer Institute has established a diet, nutrition, and cancer program to study the role of diet and nutrition in the cause of cancer and in the treatment and rehabilitation of the cancer patients. At this time, however, there is no scientific evidence that any one food or any fad diet can retard the spread of cancer or serve as an effective treatment for cancer. Diets deficient in certain amino acids or vitamins seem to have anti-tumor effects and are being tested in men.

What are Hoxsey herbs?

A treatment called Hoxsey Herbs, the Hoxsey Method, or Hoxsey Chemotherapy was dispensed at two facilities known as the Hoxsey Cancer Clinic. One was in Portage, Pa., and one in Dallas, Texas, which later became the Taylor Clinic. The clinic in Portage was closed in 1958 by court action. In 1960 the Taylor

Clinic in Dallas was prohibited by court injunction from selling or dispensing Hoxsey medications. In the trial leading to the closing of the Hoxsey Cancer Clinic in Pennsylvania, the government presented scientific evidence that Mr. Hoxsey's claimed "cures" fell into three categories: patients who had never had cancer, patients who had been cured of cancer before they went to the clinic, and patients who had cancer and still had it or who had died while under the treatment. The FDA investigated the Hoxsey Method and found it of no benefit to cancer patients.

Who is Dr. Lawrence Burton and isn't he curing cancer in his clinic in the Bahamas?

Dr. Burton is associated with the Immunology Research Foundation, a private organization in the state of New York. He is a zoologist who says he has developed a treatment that is effective against cancer. Other problems such as skin diseases, circulatory ailments and rejuvenation of elderly people are also treated at the clinic he has established in Freeport, Grand Bahama. In newspaper interviews, Dr. Burton has described great success in treating patients with a serum created from a combination of agents of human blood. However, he has never formally reported his research results in the professional literature. The treatment materials have not been licensed for sale by the Food and Drug Administration and scientific evidence to confirm the anti-cancer properties of his products are lacking. Because Dr. Burton's research data have not been published, there has been no basis for evaluating or retesting his claims.

chapter 11

Breast Cancer

Women Most Likely to Get Breast Cancer

At highest risk:
- Women whose mother or sister or both have breast cancer
- Women who have already had cancer in one breast

At increased risk:
- Women who have continual breast problems such as lumps, discharge, or cystic breasts
- Women with a history of previous benign tumors
- Women aged 40 or over
- Women who have had two or fewer pregnancies; risk decreases as number of children increase
- Women who have not had any children
- Women who had first child after age of 30
- Women who began menstruating at 11 or younger
- Women who have experienced late menopause
- Women who are obese

Symptoms of Breast Cancer

- Hard lump in breast—may be fixed or movable
- Lump under arm
- Dimple in skin of breast
- Thickening or reddening of skin of breast

Symptoms of Breast Cancer (continued)
- Discharge from nipple
- Ulceration of nipple
- Inverted nipple, if nipple previously was erect
- Change in size of breast—swelling or shrinking
- Sore on breast or nipple that doesn't heal
- Persistent breast pain or sense of discomfort

To Find Breast Lumps As Early As Possible

PROCEDURE	EXPLANATION
Check breasts each month.	If you do this each month, seven days after the end of your period, you'll recognize a change as soon as it occurs. About 90 percent of breast lumps are found by the woman herself; about 80 percent of them are benign.
Make certain gynecologist, internist, or family physician checks breasts at least once a year.	This double-checks your examination and gives you the opportunity to make certain you are examining yourself properly. If you have cystic breasts, the physician check should be more frequent.
Look for changes in appearance of breast and call doctor immediately if any of these are present:	Cause for concern is any change from what is normal for you—and you are the one who can detect the changes fastest.
Any change in size or shape of the breast.	You are asked to do this by watching your breasts in a mirror as you raise your arms to determine if any area reacts differently from the comparable area in the opposite breast. This is usually found to be the result of fibrocystic changes—but it can signal the presence of cancer, and only the doctor can determine this.
Unusual pain or an area of unusual tenderness should be reported to the doctor if it persists after your menstrual period.	Pain is not usually one of the signs of breast cancer, but it is a common sign of a developing cyst and should be checked by the doctor even if there is no evidence of a lump.

PROCEDURE	EXPLANATION
Dimpling, puckering, or retraction of nipple or flaking of nipple skin should be called to the doctor's attention.	This may indicate the development of a cancer of the ducts beneath the nipple or of the nipple itself.
Nipple discharge is another cancer sign that should be immediately reported to the doctor.	Any noticeable nipple discharge should be checked. Any bloody discharge must be checked immediately because it indicates that there is some trouble in the nipple duct.
Have a screening mammography or xerography done if you are over 50 or if you fall into a high-risk group.	This will give the doctor something to check back on at a later date to determine if there has been a change, or to discover cancer at a very early stage.

If You Find You Have a Lump in Your Breast

STEP	EXPLANATION
Call the doctor for an appointment today.	This gives you the chance to tell the nurse that you have found a lump and that you want an immediate appointment. Delaying can prove to be a fatal decision.
Remind yourself that 8 out of 10 times the lump will turn out *not* to be cancer.	Don't naively assume, however, that since you feel well and the lump hasn't changed, you can afford to wait to see the doctor.
If the doctor suggests he will watch the lumps over a few months' time, discuss having a mammogram or a biopsy. Also think about asking for a second opinion.	Many physicians feel that having a baseline mammogram is important at this time because it gives him something to compare with at a later date. Also, it jolts the doctor into action, rather than passively deciding to wait and see.

Questions to Ask Your Doctor If You Have a Lump in Your Breast

- What does the lump feel like? What do you think it is?
- Should I have a mammogram? What does the mammogram show?
- What kind of biopsy do you do? Can it be done on an outpatient basis? Why not?

If he recommends a mammogram:

- Do you know how many rads I will be exposed to with the techniques being used by the radiologist you are sending me to?

Questions You Must Ask Yourself

- How important are my breasts to me?
- Am I willing to have a limited operation and later have a second operation if it is found that the cancer has spread? Can I live with that fear?
- Do I want to have breast reconstruction? (If you do, it is best if the doctor knows before he operates.)

Steps To Take If Doctor Suggests Biopsy

STEP	EXPLANATION
Arrange to have someone—husband, mother, sister, friend—come with you into the doctor's office.	Having a trusted person with you helps in getting answers to the questions you want to ask. It also helps to write down the questions before you go and the answers while you are there.
Ask the doctor if he believes in the two-step procedure—doing the biopsy separate from the operation.	This gives you several options which you will not have if the doctor proceeds with the biopsy and is given the okay to continue with removing the breast if he feels this is necessary.
Explain that you want the pathologist to have the full three or four days needed for a detailed study of the tumor and its spread.	Time is essential to the pathologist in determining the nature of the tumor.
Ask if you will be premedicated and semi-awake during biopsy and if it can be done on an outpatient basis.	This eliminates the hazard of going under anesthesia twice and leaves several options open to you.
Explain that you want to get a second opinion.	A second opinion at this point will help to establish a fuller view of what is involved and help you determine how you want to proceed.

Steps To Take If Doctor Suggests Biopsy *(continued)*

STEP	EXPLANATION
Make sure you have a mammogram before you have a biopsy.	After the biopsy, scar tissue will form inside the breast where the tissue was removed. A mammogram should be made before the biopsy so that any future changes can be compared with the original.
Make sure you have confidence in the doctor who will be doing your surgery. Find out how many breast operations he has done in the past month.	You are best off with a surgeon who specializes in breast disease—preferably a surgical oncologist. At least you should get a second opinion from such a doctor.

Steps To Take If The Biopsy Shows Malignancy

STEP	EXPLANATION
Ask the doctor his opinion about using radiation instead of removing the breast if the malignant lump is small and has not spread to other organs.	Many cases have been treated in this manner with success. This is very controversial with physicians but it should definitely be an option for discussion.
Ask the doctor what kind of operation he will be doing—a simple, modified radical, or radical mastectomy.	New evidence is showing that there is very little difference in survival statistics between women who had the most radical surgery (removal of breast and underlying and adjacent tissues, including pectoral muscles) and the modified radical (which does not remove the muscles of chest and fatty tissue under the arm). It is very important to discuss the operation with your doctor before surgery.
Ask the doctor about having an estrogen receptor test on the tissue.	If you have breast cancer that has spread, this test can help determine future treatment and should be done before chemotherapy starts.
Ask the doctor about breast reconstruction.	Though most surgeons find that reconstruction cannot be done at the same time as initial surgery, it is wise to let the surgeon know if you are interested in reconstruction before he operates so that the original surgery is planned with the future reconstruction in mind. Talk to him about seeing a plastic surgeon before the operation.

Tests For Breast Cancer

TEST	EXPLANATION
Physical exam	Includes clinical history, physical, routine blood, urine, and heart exams; close examination of breasts.
Mammography	Gives the doctor visualization of breast, showing natural contrast provided by fat content of breast. Sometimes possible to differentiate benign tumor from malignant. Allows doctor to see if additional tumors are present. Ultrasound mammograms being tested but have not yet been proved to be successful.
Thermography	Not as accurate in detecting preclinical cancers as mammogram, but is preferred by some doctors because it does not employ radiation. Graphic stress telethermometry, type of thermogram using heat patterns to detect lesions and distinguish benign from malignant, is now being tested. Early results very promising. Presently being tested at Memorial Sloane-Kettering Cancer Center.
Needle aspiration	Insertion of fine needle into lump to draw out fluid or tissue juice.
Surgical biopsy	Removal of sample (whole lump if small) of suspicious breast tissue to be examined for cancer cells. Minor surgical procedure, but only positive way of identifying malignant tumor. Can be done on an outpatient basis.

If Biopsy Shows Lump to Be Cancerous

Scans, bone and liver	Painless, routine outpatient diagnostic procedures similar to x-rays. Used to determine whether cancer has spread to bones and liver. Also known as metastatic workup.
Gallium scan	Sometimes used to determine if cancer has spread to more than one area of body. Capable of showing rapidly dividing cells.
Ultrasound scan	Sometimes used.
X-rays	May sometimes be part of workup.
CT scan	May sometimes be used.

Questions to Ask Your Doctor Before Agreeing to a Breast Operation

- How big is the lump?
- Where is it?
- What specific kind of breast cancer do I have?
- Do we have the opinion of more than one pathologist on that?
- Have you talked directly with the pathologist about my report? What did he say?
- Can you feel any lymph nodes?
- How fast does this type of breast cancer grow?
- Is there any evidence of metastases?
- What kind of operation do you plan to do?
- How often do you perform mastectomies?
- Have you ever performed a lumpectomy?
- Have you ever performed a simple or partial mastectomy rather than a radical mastectomy?
- Are there any alternative kinds of treatment for my case?
- Will you explain what the scar will look like?
- Will you do the operation with the thought that I am interested in having breast reconstruction?

What kind of doctor should I see if I have symptoms of breast cancer?

If you have a lump or other symptom of breast cancer, you should first see the doctor who normally takes care of you—your internist, family practitioner, gynecologist, or general practitioner. He will order whatever tests are necessary to determine whether or not your symptom is actually cancer. The doctors who specialize in treating breast cancer are usually surgical oncologists. Reconstructive breast surgery is the specialty of plastic and reconstructive surgeons. Since several options exist for treatment, make sure you get second opinions and read this chapter so that you can decide what options you wish to follow.

Is the National Cancer Institute supporting any studies on breast cancer?

Yes, the National Cancer Institute's clinical cooperative groups are presently supporting many studies on breast cancer, mostly

studying chemotherapy drugs but also comparing radical mastectomies with simple mastectomies and studying the use of
radiation for early breast cancer, hormonal treatments, and
immunotherapy. (See Chapter 23.)

What is the function of the breast?

The breast is a very complicated organ. It has tens of thousands
of tiny cells able to secrete milk on order, preparing itself
throughout pregnancy to supply the infant's nutrition, receding
when no longer necessary, prepared to start all over again when
called upon by another pregnancy. Each month, during
menstruation, changes occur in the breasts. The growth, matura-
tion, and function of the breast are the result of a sequential
stimulation by several separate hormones—secreted from the
ovary, anterior pituitary gland, adrenal cortex, and thyroid.

How are most breast cancers found?

Most breast cancers—over 90 percent—are found by the women
themselves, either during monthly self-examinations or by
accident when showering or looking in the mirror.

Are most breast lumps cancerous?

No, they are not. With all the information on breast cancer that
has been written in the past few years, it is important for you to
know that chances that a lump in your breast is *not* cancer are
really excellent. In fact, eight out of ten lumps are found to be
benign. However, it is important for you to know that lumps
found in post-menopausal women are more apt to be cancerous
than those found in women who are still menstruating. Ninety-
three percent of women never develop cancer of the breast.
Those are really very good odds. Further, the cure rate is 85
percent if the cancer is detected early.

Do men ever have breast cancer?

Yes. However, less than 1 percent of all breast cancers occur in
males. When they do occur it is usually at middle age or older. A

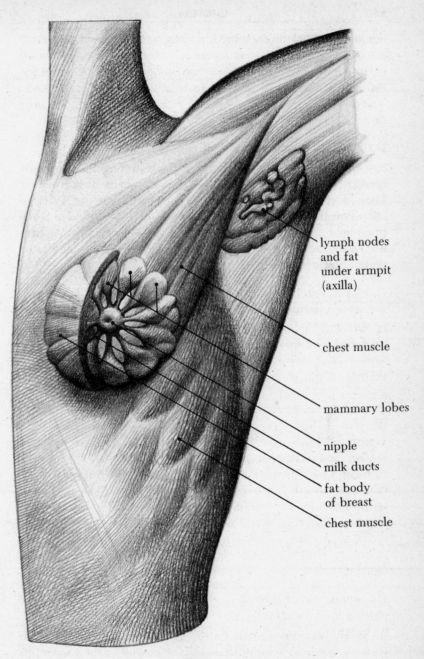

lymph nodes
and fat
under armpit
(axilla)

chest muscle

mammary lobes

nipple

milk ducts

fat body
of breast

chest muscle

Breast

modified radical mastectomy is usually recommended. Often the breast cancer in males is found in older men who are being treated for cancer of the prostate. Some doctors believe that the estrogen treatment often used in treating prostatic cancer may lead to the development of breast cancer. In some cases, the male breast cancer has metastasized from the prostatic cancer.

Is fibrocystic disease a form of cancer?

No. What is called fibrocystic disease (also referred to as lumpy breasts, cystic disease, or chronic cystic mastitis) is not cancer. Many doctors believe that it is not really a disease but a natural condition that is found in the breasts of many women at some times in their lives. Fibrocystic disease tends to involve both breasts, is seen chiefly in women 35 to 50 years of age, and often diminishes after menopause.

Can doctors tell the difference between these cystic lumps and cancerous lumps?

It depends upon many factors. Cysts are usually movable, spherical in shape, and relatively soft, unlike many malignant tumors. They are caused by a buildup of fibrous tissues which is related to the changes that normally take place in the breast during each menstrual cycle. These changes may be exaggerated if the menstrual cycle becomes irregular, particularly if there is a long time between periods. The lumpiness may disappear slowly after menopause. Fibrocystic lumps seem to appear and disappear with the menstrual cycle, while most cancerous lumps are stable. Many women have breasts with cysts of many sizes, giving the breast a "cobblestone" feel. Women with cystic disease should be examined frequently, and doctors often recommend that cysts that do not change in size be biopsied and/or surgically removed. If the cyst disappears after aspiration with a syringe and needle, this is a good sign it is benign.

Do women who have lumpy breasts have a higher risk of getting breast cancer?

A slightly higher risk exists for this group of women over women who do not have lumpy breasts. That is why women with this condition are urged to see their doctors more often—every three to six months—and be watched closely by a doctor who understands cystic breasts and can detect changes in the breast.

Do women with inverted nipples have a greater chance of having breast cancer?

No, not if this is your normal condition. Inverted nipples are subject to infection if not kept clean and dry, but there does not seem to be a relationship between inverted nipples and breast cancer. However, if your nipple is normally erect and retracts—or if you see dimpling or puckering in your breast—you should see the doctor so he can check this symptom.

Is discharge from the nipples of the breast a cause for alarm?

It is wise to call any discharge from the nipples to the attention of your doctor. If the discharge is bloody or has a green or brown color, this probably means that a small quantity of blood or other substance is being discharged and is reason for the doctor to look at it to determine the cause. Some young women may have a slight clear or yellowish nipple discharge at the time of menstruation; this is not unusual and should not cause alarm but should be mentioned to the doctor. Most discharges occur prior to menopause when other changes are taking place in the body and should be seen by the doctor to determine if there is a problem.

Why does the doctor try to see if the tumor will "move"?

Most cancerous tumors tend to invade breast tissue and cause the breast to form scar tissue in and around the cancer. This causes the lump to become "fixed." Benign tumors such as fluid cysts or solid fibrous growths tend to be more movable because they neither invade the surrounding breast tissue nor cause the breast to deposit scar tissue around them. However, in some cases, movable tumors have been found to be cancerous, and this is the reason why a surgical biopsy is necessary to determine the nature of most lumps.

Can blows or injuries to the breasts cause breast cancer?

No. But such injuries often draw attention to a lump in the breast even though the lump is not a result of the injury.

Do birth-control pills increase a woman's chances of developing breast cancer?

There is still no established link between the use of birth-control pills and breast cancer, although many studies are currently underway in this area. The pill has been widely used for about 10 years and it usually takes 15 to 20 years for most cancers to develop. However, it has been proved that both the administration of estrogen and the withdrawal of this hormone affect the rate of growth of breast cancers. Women who have had breast cancer or come from families with a high degree of breast cancer should be warned against the use of birth-control pills.

Is there any connection between breast feeding and breast cancer?

For many years, it was thought that nursing helped to immunize women against breast cancer. Later studies seemed to indicate that women who nursed were more prone to cancer. Today, the question remains debatable among doctors. It is a fact that although breast feeding has declined dramatically in the last 60 years, the incidence of breast cancer has increased. But whether or not this has any bearing when all other facts are taken into consideration is mere conjecture.

I try to examine my breasts but I'm not really sure what I'm looking for. What do I need to know?

The first thing you should know is that it is important to do the breast exam not just to look for problems but mainly to get to know your own breast tissue so that you will recognize a change when you feel it. The exam should be done once a month. If you are menstruating, probably the best time to do it is within the week following your period or on the last day of your period if that's easier to remember. If you are no longer menstruating or have had a hysterectomy, you need to pick a day of the month that you will always use. Some women pick their birthdate. Some feel that the first day, the last day, or the 15th day of the month is the easiest to remember.

When you have an appointment with your doctor, you should ask him to teach you breast self-examination after he has examined your breasts. Then you will know what your breast feels like when it is normal and he can answer any questions you have about what you are feeling. You can also get an illustrated pamphlet on breast self-examination by calling the American Cancer Society office near you or the cancer information service.

Just how should I examine my breasts?

Your breast self-examination should be done in three steps. First, look in the mirror with your arms down at your side. Make sure you have a good light that is not casting any shadows and a big enough mirror. Look at the shape of your nipples, and notice the contour of your breasts. The nipples are usually more or less equal and pointing outward. The contour of both breasts is

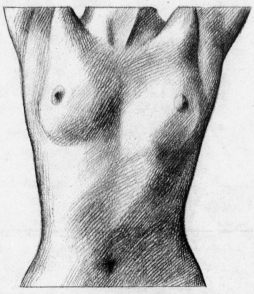

arms over head

Breast self-examination

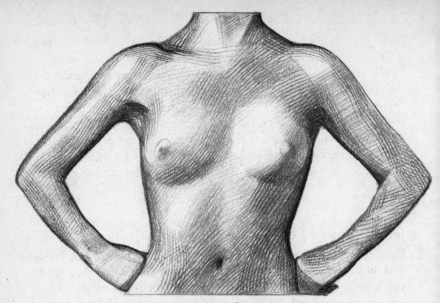

arms on hips

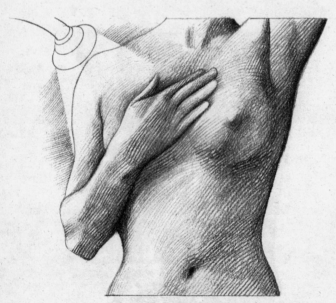

while body is wet

Breast self-examination

usually sloping downward. Although the shape and size of each breast may be different, the contour is usually the same. Now look at the same features with your arms over your head. Then rest the palms of your hands on your hips and press down firmly to flex your chest muscles. In all these views you are looking for any changes—a swelling, any dimpling of skin, nipples which have retracted, a change in contour. If you regularly inspect what is normal, you will have confidence in your examination and your ability to see something not normal.

What is the second step?

The second step is to examine yourself when you are wet—either during a shower or a bath, with soap on your breast. Some of the lumps most difficult to find can be picked up most easily in a soapy breast. Your hands will easily glide over your wet, soapy skin. With your fingers flat, move gently over every part of each breast. Use your right hand to examine the left breast and your left hand for your right breast. You are looking for any lump, hard knot, or thickening.

What is the third step of the breast self-examination?

Next you lie down. To examine your right breast, put a pillow or folded towel under your right shoulder. Place your right arm behind your head. This will distribute the breast tissue more evenly on your chest. With your left hand, fingers flat, press gently in small circular motions around an imaginary clock face. Begin at the outermost top of your breast (imagine that is 12 o'clock on the clock), then move around the breast (to 1 o'clock, 2 o'clock, etc., until you get back to 12). At the lower curve of your breast, you will feel a ridge of firm tissue. That is normal. Then move in an inch, toward the nipple, and keep circling to examine every part of your breast, including the nipple. This will require you to make at least three more circles. Now slowly repeat the same process on your left breast with a pillow under your left shoulder and your left hand behind your head. During this process you are again looking for lumps, hard knots, or thickening. Finally, squeeze the nipple of each breast gently

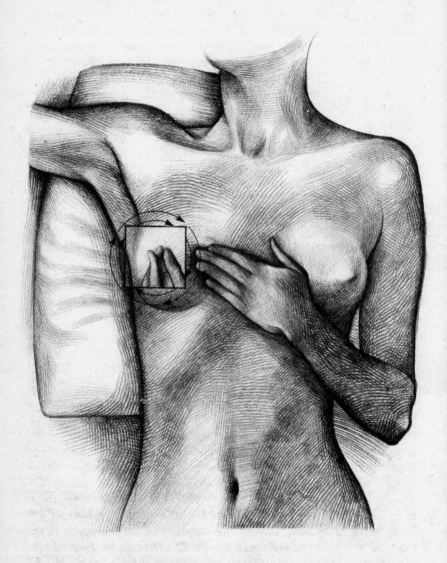

Breast self-examination (lying down)

between your thumb and your index finger. You are making sure there is no discharge. If there is any discharge, clear or bloody, you should immediately report it to your doctor.

My friend found a lump in her breast several weeks ago and won't go to the doctor. What can I tell her to make her go?

There are several things you can try.

- First of all, tell her that about 80 percent of the lumps which are found prove to be noncancerous. Her chances are eight out of ten that it it will prove to be nothing. For her own peace of mind, she should have a doctor evaluate the lump.
- Second, if the lump does prove to be cancerous, her chances of the cancer being arrested are much higher if it is found at an early stage than if she lets it continue to grow.
- Suggest that you or a family member make the appointment for her. It is sometimes hard for people to take the first step, to pick up the phone and call the doctor, to admit that something might be wrong.
- Offer to accompany her to the doctor's office or talk to a family member about going with her. If she is frightened, it could be very helpful for her to have someone go along with her to share the experience.

What happens after either the doctor or I find a breast lump?

There are numerous ways your case can proceed. This is an important decision point. You must prepare yourself to make a decision about how you want to proceed if, after the examination, the doctor suggests there is a possibility that the lump may be cancer. You need to decide, for example, whether you wish to have a second opinion on the kind of treatment you will have.

Is a second opinion important in breast cancer?

In our view, a second opinion is always important. It is essential in treating breast cancer simply because there are many options and differences of opinion in this area. A second opinion is important to help you think through your choices.

What will the doctor do if he has any doubts about my lump?

If the doctor has any doubts, he will suggest further studies. These may include a mammogram, a thermogram, aspiration of the lump with a needle and syringe to see if it is a cyst, or an excisional biopsy. These tests are used to make sure that the lump is *not* cancerous or to determine treatment if it should be cancerous. *Remind yourself again* that eight times out of ten it usually turns out that the lump is *not* malignant.

I am still confused. Tell me again what the steps are that would lead up to the operation for breast cancer.

Let us take it from the time when you find a lump or something unusual about your breast and go to the doctor. He will probably proceed as follows:

- He will look at what you have found and examine both breasts for lumpy areas.
- If he has any doubts, he may advise further studies, such as thermography, mammography, aspiration of the lump with needle and syringe to see if it is a cyst, a needle biopsy, or an excisional biopsy (taking out the whole lump for examination).
- If the biopsy shows that the lump is cancerous, the doctor will order a bone scan, x-ray of the chest, blood studies, and other tests to determine whether or not the cancer has already spread to distant parts of the body such as the bone, lungs, and liver.

What is a mammogram?

A mammogram is a soft-tissue x-ray of the breast. It shows breast masses and helps to identify those which may be malignant. Mammograms can show tiny concentrations of calcification or perhaps other abnormalities that may indicate a tumor in the breast. Tumors can often be observed by this x-ray technique before they can be discovered by physical examination.

Can a mammogram tell whether or not cancer is present?

Mammograms are diagnostic tools. They may indicate to a trained doctor whether cancer is present or not. They are used by surgeons to locate the site of the tumor and to check if there are additional tumors in the breast. However, they should never be used alone. They should be used in addition to a careful breast examination by a doctor who regularly treats breast cancer. In order to make a definitive diagnosis of breast cancer, a biopsy must be done of those suspicious areas seen on the mammogram.

What is a Xeroradiograph?

A Xeroradiograph is a mammogram which basically uses the Xerox techniques. It processes the x-ray image on Xerox paper. A selenium-coated metal surface is substituted for x-ray film, and after being exposed to x-rays, it is dusted with calcium carbonate powder. This produces an etching-like image. Many radiologists prefer this kind of mammogram because they feel it helps them see tiny irregularities more distinctly, shows more details, and is easier to interpret. The Xeroradiograph is blue and white. The mammogram is black and white. Sometimes this test is called Xeromammography.

Who performs mammography?

Radiological technologists who are specially trained in mammography normally conduct the tests and process the mammograms. The mammograms are then given to a radiologist, who studies them, interprets them, and reports the findings to your own physician. It is very important that you go to a qualified radiologist who reads many mammograms, for as with other diagnostic tools, the results are only as good as the skill of the person who conducts and interprets the tests.

What is contrast mammography?

This is an experimental form of cancer detection in which a water-based dye is introduced into the breast before the mammogram is taken so that the doctor can better study the pattern of the breast ducts.

Can mistakes be made in reading a mammograph?

Like any diagnostic tool, errors can be made in mammography or Xeroradiography. For instance, the position of the breast on the plate can distort results. The doctor reading the mammogram can make a mistake. This is why both the technicians involved in taking the films and the radiologist who reads them must be extremely qualified. Interpreting the films requires skilled and trained persons.

Why is it a good idea to have a mammogram before having the breast lump removed?

A mammogram of the breast before surgery can serve several purposes:

- It can be used as a record for the doctor to use in future comparison.
- It can tell if there are additional lumps in the areas of the breast which cannot be felt.
- It can sometimes help, used in conjunction with other findings, to determine if the lump is benign or cancerous.
- It will guide the surgeon during the operation.

What does the doctor look for in the mammogram to help him determine if the lump might be cancerous?

The doctor knows that benign tumors tend to show sharp edges in x-rays and are frequently surrounded by a halo of fat and seem to be homogeneous in density. Malignant tumors usually look as though they have tentaclelike tissue reaching into the surrounding areas. Fine, sandlike calcium deposits can be seen and the skin in the area is often distorted. Even with his expert eyes, however, the doctor needs other guidelines besides the x-ray to help him make a positive diagnosis.

What dose of radiation does a woman get when she has a mammogram done?

The dose of radiation for mammograms should be less than 1 rad per breast picture on a well-calibrated machine. You should ask when your physician makes the appointment for your mammogram or you should call the radiologist yourself before you have the examination. If the dose is more than 1 rad per exposure, try to find another facility with lower-dose equipment. Tests are now being conducted in several places around the country on techniques and equipment which are decreasing this exposure dose.

What does the mammogram tell the doctor that he can't get in some other way?

If the doctor finds a suspicious lump, the mammogram may give the doctor some indication as to whether or not the lump is cancerous. He will also see whether or not there are other lumps which might be cancerous in the breast and which cannot be felt by manual examination. This information is important to the doctor if he is to perform an operation on the breast. If the woman has large breasts or fibrocystic disease, mammography is especially useful.

There have been controversies about mammograms. Are they dangerous?

As noted earlier, mammograms use relatively low levels of radiation to create an image of the breast on film or paper. The controversy has not been over the use of the mammogram as a tool for diagnosing breast cancer in women who have symptoms. Rather it has been with the use of mammograms as a screening tool for women who have no symptoms.

Can the doctor tell definitely from a mammogram whether or not cancer is present?

A negative mammogram *does not* guarantee there is no cancer in the breast. A mammogram can identify certain lumps as benign. However, the mammogram is only one phase in the total picture. In most cases, surgical biopsy is necessary to finally determine whether or not a suspicious lump is cancer.

I have heard so much controversy over mammography that I don't know whether or not to have one.

The controversy on the question of mammography has been over the use of it for *routine* screening, to detect breast cancer. The concern over mammography grew from the risks involved in radiation. When it was first introduced, some of the techniques exposed women to 10 rads of radiation or more per exposure. (A rad is a unit of radiation that measures the amount of energy absorbed from radiation at a given point.) If mammography was given regularly as a routine exam over a 10- or 20-year period, there was fear that this exposure could be hazardous. However, newer techniques have been developed which have lowered the doses in some cases to a third of a rad or less for each exposure.

Because of the controversy, the National Cancer Institute has issued guidelines on the use of mammography to detect breast cancer. According to these guidelines, you should have mammography if:

- You have a lump or other symptom suggestive of breast cancer.
- You are over the age of 50. For women in this age group, mammography has proved its value as a screening device for breast cancer.
- You are between the ages of 40 and 49 and have a prior history of breast cancer yourself or if your mother or sisters had breast cancer.
- You are between the ages of 35 and 39 and have a personal history of breast cancer.

Does that mean that if I have a lump in my breast and my doctor tells me to get a mammogram that it is OK?

Yes, definitely. There is no question about the use of mammography in making a diagnosis when symptoms are present. In this instance, the true risk would be in not having the mammogram done.

What are the benefits of a mammogram?

According to the National Cancer Institute, at the ACS/NCI screening centers, mammography has helped detect 45 percent of breast cancers that were missed by the doctor when he examined the breast manually. For earlier cancers, called minimal tumors, which cannot be felt and are only detectable through mammography, cure rates of up to 95 percent are being reported.

I am still worried about getting too much radiation. What should I ask before I get a mammogram?

When making your appointment for mammography, be sure to ask what kind of techniques are being used and specifically how many rads you will be exposed to. A breast examination should require no more than 1 rad per film when proper equipment and techniques are used.

What preparations are necessary before having my mammography?

There are no special diets or other procedures. However, on the day of the examination you may be asked not to use any deodorant, perfume, powders, ointment, or preparations of any sort in the underarm area or on your breasts, since these can obscure the results of the Xeroradiographic mammograms. Also, it is more convenient to wear a skirt or slacks with a blouse or sweater, since it is necessary to undress to the waist for the examination.

What happens when I go for the mammography examination?

You will be asked to remove all clothing above the waist. Then you will sit, stand, or lie in various positions to obtain the best pictures of your breasts. Both breasts will usually be x-rayed, since it is important to compare images of each breast. The technologist sometimes uses a cone-shaped device, a sponge, large balloon, or a similar object to help position your breast for a better picture. The entire procedure usually takes about a half-hour. After the radiologist studies the results, he reports his findings to the physician.

How accurate is a mammogram or Xerogram?

It is accurate, but not as accurate as a biopsy—nothing is. The test is also not as reliable in young women because the density of the tissue makes it more difficult to forecast a malignancy accurately. The test is also not as accurate on women with very small or very large breasts. However, it can be an important part of the whole picture as far as a diagnosis of breast cancer is concerned. Radiologists feel that it has about an 85 percent accuracy rate. Furthermore, it should be in your records for future reference if you have any history of lumps.

What is ultra-sound mammography?

This technique, which is in the early stages of development, uses sound waves for the mammogram. It is considered at present an experimental diagnostic tool.

How much will a mammogram cost?

A mammogram usually costs between $70 and $125. It may or may not be covered by your medical insurance, depending upon your policy.

Is thermography used in diagnosing breast cancer?

Sometimes. Thermography uses infrared light to visualize the temperature pattern of tissues. The surface of the body has variations of temperature which can be recorded photographically using film sensitive to infrared light. Malignant tumors tend to produce more heat than normal tissues and thus show up darker on photographs.

Is thermography a proven diagnostic method?

At the present time, the reliability of thermography has not been proven. Other diseases besides cancer and other factors—such as infection—can cause increased temperature and heat patterns. Thus a positive thermogram is not enough proof, at this time, to make a positive diagnosis of cancer. Moreover, there is a significant number of false negatives with thermography—this means that the thermogram misses a number of cases of cancer. The results continue to provide an incorrect indication more than 60 percent of the time. Thermography should never be used alone as a diagnostic tool.

Is a thermogram a substitute for a mammogram?

Not at this time. Doctors feel that it is not as definite a diagnostic tool, although some studies have shown that thermography is capable of detecting some cases of breast cancer earlier than mammography. Its main advantage is that it does not expose the patient to radiation. However, since the reliability of thermography has not yet been proved, it is usually used in connection with other diagnostic methods.

Is anyone doing studies using thermography?

There are several places in the country where new techniques are being tested with this diagnostic tool. Memorial Sloan-Kettering Cancer Center in New York City is testing a new technique called GST (graphic stress telethermometry). Roswell Park Memorial Institute in Rochester, N.Y., has developed a new synthetic material which is easier to use in performing the thermogram. Researchers at the Massachusetts Institute of Technology are testing the use of microwave radio signals from within the body to measure temperature differences.

What is the breast screening test called GST?

"GST" stands for "graphic stress telethermometry." It involves studying the heat patterns of the breast tissue. The technique, which is experimental, is being tested at Memorial Sloan-Kettering Cancer Center in New York City. The test can detect both benign and cancerous breast lesions and can tell them apart. It does not impart any radiation and if it proves effective during the testing period it may be an ideal method for mass screening of women who do not have any symptoms of breast cancer.

How does GST work?

GST measures the difference between breast-tissue temperature and forehead temperature. The temperature of the breast is taken by passing a miniaturized infrared heat detector over nine sections of each breast. Areas that show a higher temperature than the forehead are considered suspicious. To determine whether these areas are benign or malignant, the patient's hands are immersed in cold water for 15 seconds. This causes the body temperature to fall, and the temperature-taking is repeated. If the lesions are benign, they will also cool off, but malignant tissue remains at a constant, higher temperature. The temperature differences are in tenths of a degree.

What is transillumination?

Transillumination is used by some doctors to further their knowledge of the nature of a lump. With the help of a powerful light beam, they interpret the contours of the lump. It is used mainly in addition to other clinical devices available to give the doctor further insight into the kind of lump being examined and can help distinguish a cyst from a solid tumor. Quite simply, in a darkened room, the doctor beams a powerful light through the breast area being examined. Though it cannot accurately distinguish a cancerous from a noncancerous lump, it can be another tool, when used with others, to help the doctor make his diagnosis.

What is a needle aspiration?

Sometimes, when the character of the lump and the mammogram suggest that the lump is a cyst, the doctor will take out the fluid with a needle and syringe (aspirate). The fluid which is taken out is examined by the pathologist for possible cancer cells.

What is a needle biopsy?

If the lump is solid—that is, if it does not have any fluid in it—the doctor may do a wide-bore needle biopsy. This needle is larger than the one used for taking out the fluid. It has a sharp cutting point which cuts a piece of the lump as it passes through the tumor. This test needs to be read by a specialized pathologist and thus is not often used.

What is a surgical or excisional biopsy?

Usually that means taking out the whole lump for examination. This will leave you with a scar, but it can be done in a way that disturbs the shape of your breast as little as possible. There is a fuller explanation of biopsies in Chapter 4.

Will I have to go to the hospital for the breast biopsy?

Breast biopsies can be done either on an outpatient basis or in the hospital. If performed on an inpatient basis, they can be done either as a separate operation or as part of a mastectomy. If the biopsy is done as a separate operation, it is known as a two-step procedure.

What kind of doctor will perform the biopsy?

Physicians who specialize in treating breast cancer are usually called surgical oncologists. Talk to your family doctor about whom he would recommend.

What is meant by a two-step procedure?

A two-step procedure means that the biopsy will be done separately, usually as an outpatient in the hospital or even in a doctor's office. A few days later, if the biopsy proves that the lump is cancerous, the mastectomy operation will be performed.

What is the alternative to a two-step procedure?

The alternative to the two-step procedure is to have both the biopsy and the mastectomy operation done at the same time. You go to the operating room and are put under general anesthesia as if the mastectomy were definitely going to be performed. The surgeon takes a biopsy and immediately sends it to the pathologist, who will determine whether or not it is cancerous from a test called a frozen section. If the biopsy shows that the lump is cancerous, the mastectomy will be performed immediately. Under this one-step procedure, a woman who signs the permission slip for surgery does not know whether she will wake up with or without her breast.

What are some good reasons for insisting I want a two-step procedure?

There are several.

- First of all, eight out of ten women will prove to have benign lumps. If you have a one-step procedure you will have been subjected needlessly to the danger of general anesthetic.
- Second, the one-step procedure uses a frozen-section biopsy, which does not tell the doctor as much as the regular biopsy and is not as accurate.
- Third, unless all the tests (such as bone and liver scans) are done before the biopsy, the doctor has no way of knowing how widespread the disease is. Doing this whole range of tests on every woman who needs a biopsy is unnecessary, since 80 percent of the women biopsied will be found not to have cancer.

Why should the bone and liver scans be done before operating?

These tests will help to tell the doctor the extent of the disease. Most doctors feel that doing a mastectomy on a woman who already has disease which has spread beyond her breast is performing needless surgery. Some statistics show that the removal of the breast and all the lymph nodes in these cases does not affect the cure rate. A woman who has positive bone and liver scans cannot be cured by surgery. Therefore, some doctors feel she need not be subjected to the trauma of a mastectomy when this may not provide a positive cure for her disease. The two-step method of determining the nature of a breast tumor seems like the only sensible approach. However, there is still much controversy over this subject.

What is the difference between a frozen section and a regular biopsy?

The main difference is in how much the pathologist can tell about the nature and the type of cancer. A full discussion of the two kinds of biopsies is in Chapter 4.

What if the doctor insists on a one-step procedure and I want a two-step procedure?

Our advice would be unequivocal: find another doctor, fast.

Do most doctors recommend a two-step procedure—that is, a time lapse between the biopsy and the removal of the breast?

Unfortunately, many doctors today subscribe to the belief that if a lump is found to be cancerous, the operation for removal of the breast should be done immediately. The attitude is changing, but many doctors are still recommending the one-step procedure.

Won't all this time delay mean that the cancer has more chance to spread?

No. There is no medical reason for doing the biopsy and the mastectomy in the same procedure. An interval of two days to a week between the two procedures is not a problem. Many medical professionals now agree that this time delay is perfectly acceptable and in most cases is a wise way to proceed. The advantages of getting all of the necessary information about the extent of the cancer far outweigh the advantages of performing a quick, disfiguring operation. It is surely worth the time lag to find a surgeon who will agree to the two-step procedure.

I feel I need some time to think, but everybody keeps pushing me to have the biopsy and the operation done right away. What should I do?

It is important to have the time to think and to look at the alternatives. You may want to talk it over with your husband and children, your sisters, your mother, or your friends. You may want to get a second opinion. It is all right to take a few extra days to make the right decision. It is better to take the time to study than to make a hasty choice. On the other hand, some people want to have it done and over with. If you are that kind of person, go ahead as long as you feel comfortable with your choice.

If I knew I could have a breast reconstruction, maybe the decision wouldn't be so hard to make. Is this something I can decide at this time?

Yes. This is something you should discuss with your doctor. You should ask your surgeon for a consultation with a plastic surgeon before the mastectomy if possible, even though the full extent of the reconstruction can't be determined until after the incision has healed. In some cases, the plastic surgeon can be in the operating room at the time of the mastectomy. Some women feel that the prospect of reconstruction makes a great deal of difference in their attitude toward the mastectomy. There is additional information on breast reconstruction at the end of this chapter.

What is meant by lymph-node involvement?

The doctors check to see whether or not the cancer which started in the breast has spread to the lymph nodes under the arm. This can be done during the biopsy stage. Treatment for breast cancer which has spread to the lymph nodes is different than localized breast cancer which has not yet begun to spread.

Can the doctor check whether there is any involvement with the lymph nodes if the biopsy is done as part of a two-step procedure?

Yes, he can.

What happens when a biopsy is done on an outpatient basis?

The patient is prepared for surgery and premedicated with a relaxant with an injection of morphine and scopolamine. A dose of Xylocaine or other local anesthetic is injected into the skin, the incision is made, and the lump is removed. There should be no pain. The sutures are carefully made, a pressure bandage is used to cover the incision, and the patient is taken back to her room and allowed to relax until the medication has worn off. Usually the operation is performed in the morning and the patient is ready to leave the hospital in the afternoon. The stitches are usually removed within three or four days, at which time the doctor will give the patient the result of the pathological report.

What if when I ask for a separate procedure for the biopsy, the doctor says that I will be doubling my risk of undergoing general anesthesia twice?

Your doctor, if he uses this argument, has overlooked the fact that a general anesthetic is not needed for a biopsy. In most cases, a biopsy can be performed under local anesthesia, with the patient fully conscious, or if she prefers, semiconscious. This entails only a one-day stay in the hospital. Some biopsies are now performed in an outpatient clinic (not even entailing a hospital stay) or even in the doctor's office.

What happens next if the pathological report shows that the tumor is cancerous?

Eight out of ten times, the lump will prove to be benign, but if the report shows the tumor to be cancerous, the next step will be for you to have a metastatic examination or workup. The workup will involve bone and liver scans to see if the cancer has spread. In addition, a chest x-ray, blood studies, and mammogram or thermogram—all of which have probably already been done— will be part of the decision-making process before the treatment is decided upon.

I am about to go into the hospital for a biopsy for a lump in my breast. I am very depressed. Is it normal for me to feel this way?

It is not unusual for women who are about to have a breast biopsy, and possibly face having their breast removed, to be very distressed. Studies show that women, particularly those who have had a friend or relative with cancer and are now facing that possibility themselves, tend to be depressed. On the other hand, there are some women who are optimistic in this situation, either feeling that the lump will be benign or that their doctor will be able to take care of it. It is important, if you can, to discuss how you feel with someone. Some people find it easy to talk with their husbands or their mothers, sisters, or close friends. Others feel more at ease talking with someone who is not close to them—such as one of the members of the hospital team. If you are in the hospital and feel you need this kind of discussion, ask for a cancer nurse, a doctor, the social-service worker, or the chaplain. There are also toll-free cancer information services around the country where trained volunteers can help answer your questions and discuss alternative kinds of treatment with you. (See Chapter 23.)

Understanding The Doctor's Terms

TERMINOLOGY	WHAT IT MEANS	REMARKS
Excisional biopsy	Removal of tumor only	Usually this operation can be performed under local anesthesia. If the lump proves to be benign—as in 8 out of 10 cases—no further steps are necessary. If the diagnosis is cancer, after the biopsy specimen is carefully studied, the type of treatment will depend on decisions you and your doctors must make.
Incisional biopsy	Removal of part of tumor	
Lumpectomy, limited mastectomy, tylectomy	Removal of tumor plus a wedge of surrounding breast	This is usually followed by radiation therapy in hopes of killing any other tiny cancers that might have been present in other parts of the breast. You should know that, according to some doctors, in terms of five-year survival rates, there is little difference between results of this sort of operation and results of radical mastectomies. Considered very experimental by most doctors.
Quadrant mastectomy	Removal of one quadrant of breast	Any of these terms may be used to describe operations in which the whole breast is not removed. These operations are all larger procedures than the lumpectomy. Many doctors still consider these experimental and not effecient operations for cancer, since the entire area is not explored. However, other doctors feel that this operation, followed by radiation therapy, is as effective as the more radical operation.
Partial mastectomy	Removal of part of breast	
Wedge resection	Removal of segment of breast	
Segmental resection	Removal of segment of breast	
Hemimastectomy	Removal of one half of breast	

Terminology	What It Means	Remarks
Simple mastectomy, total mastectomy, complete mastectomy	Removal of the breast. Lymph nodes and chest muscles left intact.	Not a simple operation at all. It means that the entire breast is amputated. Favored by doctors who believe more radical procedures slow down healing of the wound. Lymph nodes are left to help body fight off cancer cells that remain after operation. Usually followed by radiation therapy. If you are interested in breast reconstruction after surgery, be sure to explain this to the doctor so that it can be taken into consideration when he operates.
Modified radical mastectomy	Amputation of breast and lymph nodes in armpit. Chest muscles sometimes left intact. Variations: partial removal of lymph nodes in the armpit, partial removal of muscles of chest, complete removal of chest muscles, or a combination of these.	This operation is less disfiguring than a radical mastectomy but more disfiguring than the simple mastectomy. Range of arm motion after operation is greater than after a radical mastectomy, and though there is scarring of the chest and underarm there are no hollows in the chest.
Radical mastectomy (sometimes called the Halsted mastectomy)	Amputation of the breast, the fat under the skin surrounding the breast, the muscles on front of chest that support the breasts, and all the fat and lymph nodes that are contained in the armpit.	This operation, or the modified radical mastectomy described above, is the operation that most women in the U.S. with breast cancer routinely receive. Some doctors and patients are now questioning whether this extensive operation is really necessary, since statistics are beginning to show that there is little difference in five-year survival rates; women may not need to be subjected to the disfiguring operation.

TERMINOLOGY	WHAT IT MEANS	REMARKS
Extended radical mastectomy	Radical plus removal of internal mammary nodes and possibly thoracic nerve.	Insist on complete discussion of operation, disfigurement, and alternative treatments.
Supraradical mastectomy	Radical neck dissection or at least removal of supraclavicular areas in continuity with breast and armpit lymph nodes.	Same as above.
Radium implant	Radioactive material inserted into tumor area to kill cancer cells.	Used with small tumors; sometimes followed by external radiation treatment; breast is left intact; considered experimental.
Mammoplasty, subcutaneous mastectomy	Nipple and skin left intact; contents of breast removed; replaced with silicone pad insert.	Complicated operation usually done in two stages; considered experimental.

Actually, what are the various choices for treatment of breast cancer?

The treatment depends upon the extent of your disease. The basic kinds of treatment include:

- *Lumpectomy plus radiation and/or chemotherapy:* This means the doctor will take out the tumor itself and will use radiation therapy and/or chemotherapy to kill any other tiny cancer cells that might have been present in the breast. This experimental operation is usually performed when the breast cancer is small and there is no evidence of spread to any other part of the body. The procedure has also been done on women whose cancer has spread beyond the original site; in this instance radiation and chemotherapy are used after the lumpectomy to kill the cancer cells. Even with small tumors there is controversy among physicians as to the use of this treatment. It has been used for over ten years now, but on a relatively small number of patients, so it is still considered in the experimental category.

- *Surgery:* The surgical procedure for removing the breast is called a mastectomy. As you can see by the chart there are many different kinds of mastectomies. Many times radiation and/or chemotherapy are used in addition to surgery.
- *Radium implants:* Some doctors are using radium implants for both small tumors and large tumors which have spread. External radiation and/or chemotherapeutic drugs are often used in combination with this treatment. Again, this is considered experimental and there is disagreement among the doctors as to the use of this treatment.
- *Radiation:* External radiation is usually used in connection with other forms of treatment for breast cancer. In some rare instances external radiation is used alone, usually when surgery cannot be performed for some reason.
- *Chemotherapy:* Drugs are most often used to treat breast cancer after surgery and/or radiation treatment. They are usually used to kill the cancer cells which have spread to other parts of the body. Sometimes, if surgery is not possible, chemotherapy will be used as the primary treatment. Chemotherapy is used many times in breast cancer as a preventive treatment for patients who, even though the spread of the disease cannot be confirmed by tests, are at a high risk to develop metastases in other parts of the body. In this regard, the status of the lymph glands in the armpit is very important. The greater the number of lymph glands involved with tumor, the greater the chance of involvement. Sometimes immunotherapy is combined with chemotherapy.

Isn't it true that the more the surgeon removes of the breast and tissue, the more likely he is to get all of the cancer cells?

Research has *not* proved this to be true. Different treatment methods, involving comparisons of results over the years, seem to indicate that the results remain essentially unchanged.

What is the difference between a radical mastectomy and modified radical mastectomy?

In the radical mastectomy (also known as the Halsted mastectomy) the doctor removes the breast tissue, the lymph nodes under the armpit, and the muscle under the breast.

The modified radical, which many surgeons are now using, removes the breast tissue and the lymph nodes, but the muscle is left intact. The advantage of the modified radical is that it is cosmetically more attractive and does not handicap the motion of the arm. Studies done to date indicate that the survival rate for the two operations is the same.

Is the choice of what surgical procedure I will have up to me or to the doctor?

Of course your doctor is responsible for the surgery. But he cannot perform any operation unless you sign to have it done. You should have your doctor give you his complete explanation of what he recommends as his best judgment and ask him all the questions that concern you about the operation. Do not sign anything until you are certain you understand what you are signing. It is your right to refuse to sign the hospital form that gives blanket permission for a radical mastectomy. It is your right to refuse to sign the form that allows the hospital to do the biopsy and the mastectomy as a one-stage procedure. It is your right to modify the form in your own handwriting to indicate you are giving permission only for a biopsy.

What will happen to a cancerous breast lump if it is not removed?

That, in our opinion, is not a feasible alternative. Since cases differ, results differ. But the cancer will, in almost every case, continue to grow and spread, either in the breast area or to other parts of the body. Uncontrolled cancer of the breast is not a pretty or painless choice. In general, the life expectancy of women with untreated breast cancer is about two and a half years.

How does the doctor classify the stages of breast cancer when it is found?

Staging will usually include three sets of letters and numbers. The first two in the classification column grade the tumor size, the second two indicate the nodal involvement, and the third pair relate to whether or not the tumor has metastasized. The general categories of staging and more information on how it is done and what it means can be found in Chapter 3.

The General Stages of Breast Cancer

STAGE	OTHER CLASSIFICATIONS	EXPLANATION
Stage I:	T1a, N0, or N1a T1b, N0, or N1a, M0	Cancer located in breast only
Stage II:	T0 N1b T2a, N0 or N1a or N1b T2b, N0 or N1a or N1b, M0	Breast tumor and/or suspicion of node involvement, no spread suspected
Stage III:	Any T3, N1 or N2, M0	More extensive breast involvement but no known spread to other parts of the body
Stage IV:	T4, any N, any M Any T, N3, any M Any T, any N, M1	Cancer believed to have spread to other parts of the body

What size tumors are indicated by the "T" classifications?

T0 means there is no evidence of primary tumor. T1 refers to a tumor that is 2 centimeters or less in its greatest dimension. T2 refers to a tumor which is more than 2 centimeters but not more than 5 centimeters. T3 means that the tumor is more than 5 centimeters. A T4 designation indicates a tumor of any size with direct extension to the chest wall or skin.

Histologic Types of Breast Cancers

TYPE	PROGNOSIS	TREATMENT
Ackerman Type I: nonmetastasizing, noninvasive, intraductal carcinoma, papillary carcinoma, lobular alveolar carcinoma	Good prognosis. Multiplies slowly. Seems to be restrained by an anatomic barrier such as the outer membrane of a milk duct and does not tend to be spread to other parts of the body.	Usually only local tumor need be removed. Not necessary to remove breast.
Ackerman Type II: rarely metastasizes, invasive, colloid carcinoma, medullary carcinomas, lymphocytic infiltration, well-differentiated adenocarcinomas	Rarely spreads to other parts of the body, though they invade cells of breast area; have the power to penetrate the duct or alveolar membranes and continue growing outside the original area. Make up about 10 percent of breast cancers.	Requires more aggressive treatment. If spread over larger area, addition of radiation treatment or removal of entire breast recommended.
Ackerman Type III: moderately metastasizing, invasive, infiltrating ductal carcinoma, adenocarcinoma	This category constitutes about 65 percent of all breast cancers. May spread to liver, lungs, and bones.	Invades more rapidly than Types I or II. Usually cannot be eradicated by local treatment of breast and lymph nodes. Usually has spread to bloodstream. Immediate and prolonged chemotherapy beneficial.
Ackerman Type IV: highly metastasizing, invasive	Accounts for about 15 percent of breast cancers. Though breast tumor may be small, cells invade small veins within primary tumor, passing directly into bloodstream before tumor is found.	Immediate and prolonged administration of chemotherapy helps slow spread of cancer.
Inflammatory cancer	Rare. Affects less than 5 percent of cases. Spreads rapidly. Careful diagnosis essential.	Mastectomy *not* indicated. Attempts to remove cause further spread. Radiation plus chemotherapy is treatment of choice.

Is there more than one kind of breast cancer?

Cancer of the breast is not a single disease. There are at least 15 distinct varieties. The doctor and the patient need to know which variety they are dealing with before making the decision as to how to proceed. The varieties vary from slow-growing to highly invasive. One of the most controversial types, which occurs in perhaps as many as 30 percent of women at the age of 50, is referred to as "multicentric foci." Some surgeons feel that breasts containing these cell clusters (which grow in little islands whose cells are larger than normal cells and look like cancer cells but fail to develop into spreading tumors) should be removed for fear that they may later start growing and develop into true cancers. Many other physicians disagree with this approach. This same type of growth is often seen in the thyroid and prostate where it is not considered by physicians to be harmful or to indicate that surgery is required.

What does the doctor mean when he says he is going to do a simple mastectomy?

Watch these terms. Refer back to the chart showing the various surgical procedures. The terms involved with mastectomy operations are extremely confusing—and a simple mastectomy isn't simple at all. That means you will be losing a breast. It is not as extensive an operation as a radical mastectomy, but it is major surgery.

I am determined not to have a mastectomy, even if I find out my lump is cancerous. What steps should I take?

To make sure you will have that choice, it is most important to find a physician who will discuss the alternative methods of treatment with you and will give you the pros and cons for the various treatments in your case. There are times when mastectomies are the best treatment. If you do not know a surgeon who sees radiation treatment as an alternative, you can call the radiation therapy department at your nearest large medical center and ask for a radiation oncologist or a therapeutic radiologist—a specialist in using radiation as a treatment. Request a recommendation for a surgeon or physician who will consider this kind of treatment. In many cases, the radiologist will make an appointment to see you and after examination will recommend a surgeon to do the biopsy. Remember, however, that most doctors still consider anything other than a mastectomy an experimental treatment for breast cancer.

What about the use of radium implants instead of a mastectomy? When is that method used?

Though mastectomies have been favored by physicians as the surest route to survival in cases of breast cancer for several decades, other methods, such as radium implants, are being used by doctors at some of the larger medical centers in the U.S. and in Europe. Sometimes, if the breast tumor is still small—no more than 4 centimeters (1½ inches) in diameter—this method may be used. However, it is still considered an experimental method and most doctors will try to dissuade you from having it done. You must see a radiologist after your biopsy—but before your surgery—if you are to have this method of treatment.

How is the treatment done?

The first step depends upon where the treatment is being given and your own physical condition and type and size of tumor. Sometimes the whole tumor is removed. Sometimes radiation treatments are given. Usually larger tumors are left in place because their removal would destroy the shape of the breast.

For the second step, you are put under general anesthesia. Steel needles are drawn through the breast to make way for the insertion of plastic tubes, which are anchored in place by small plastic buttons at each end. These crisscross the cancer site. Radioactive material—usually the short-lived, man-made isotope iridium 192—embedded in a thin, stiff nylon ribbon is inserted into the tubes. The treatment lasts from three to five days. Then the buttons are clipped off, the ribbons are slipped out and the tubes removed. You may feel a little discomfort during the treatment, but there is little pain or scarring. Depending on the type of cancer and the spread of disease, there may be additional radiation or chemotherapy treatment. It is important to remember that this treatment is still experimental.

Exactly what will happen if I decide to have a lumpectomy?

If you have a lumpectomy, you will probably have the following steps:

- The surgeon will remove the entire tumor plus some tissue immediately surrounding it. He will probably also remove some of the lower lymph nodes under your arm to determine whether or not the cancer has spread through that route. Although you will have some scars, the shape of your breast will be changed as little as possible.
- After the operation, your breast will have a lot of gauze dressing on it and be bound in an elastic adhesive brassiere.
- The pathologist will examine the breast tissue and lymph nodes to determine the character of the cells and how they have spread.
- Radiation may be given to the breast.
- If the lymph nodes show involvement, chemotherapy may be used.
- If the cancer has spread to other parts of the body, chemotherapy and/or radiation therapy most likely will be recommended.

Why are so many doctors against lumpectomies? Why do they want to perform the mastectomy operation?

It takes a long time for the scientific community to accumulate the statistical proof that one method is better than another. Although lumpectomies have been performed for about ten years in the United States, there is not a large enough body of scientific evidence to convince most physicians that the lumpectomy plus radiation and/or chemotherapy is a better treatment than a mastectomy. Traditional treatments are relied upon by most doctors. In addition, many of the physicians are concerned about the long-range effects of the radiation treatment. Also, in some parts of the country there are no radiologists who are specially trained in this kind of therapy.

If you are interested in reading further about this form of treatment for breast cancer, get the book *The Breast: Its Problems—Benign and Malignant—and How To Deal with Them,* by Oliver Cope, M.D. (Boston: Houghton Mifflin, 1977.)

What can I expect to happen immediately before mastectomy surgery?

As for most surgical procedures, the area will be shaved and your breast washed with germ-killing soap. The nurse will administer a sedative that should relax you completely and put you into a drowsy, semiconscious state. An IV (intravenous) needle will be placed in a vein in your forearm or hand on the side opposite the side to be operated on, and the needle will be taped to your skin. The IV will be used for intravenous feedings, to administer anesthesia, and to administer blood if needed. There is more general information about what to expect when you have an operation in Chapter 6.

Why is a tight binding dressing used following mastectomy?

A mastectomy incision is usually large, and a tight dressing is used to help prevent fluid from collecting and to serve as a binding to reduce the pain when you turn or cough. A large collection of fluid at the site of the incision delays healing. That is why, in most mastectomies, the surgeon inserts a portable suctioning apparatus or other drainage tubes to help drain fluid away from the wound during surgery. This helps prevent swelling and pain after the operation. There may be a burning sensation where the vacuum tubes are attached. These will probably be removed after the third or fourth day.

Is it unusual for my chest and arm to feel numb after a mastectomy?

No, it is not unusual. This is a normal reaction. The entire operated side will feel this way for quite some time after the operation, sometimes for months, although the time varies from person to person. In a few persons, some numbness may be permanent. The numbness is the result of nerves injured or cut during surgery.

What does a mastectomy scar look like?

The appearance depends upon the extent of the operation and the doctor's personal method. Some doctors use a vertical cut, others a horizontal one. If you have a preference, you should discuss this with your doctor before the operation so your wishes can be considered and discussed.

How many days can I expect to be in the hospital for a mastectomy?

Usually from eight to ten days.

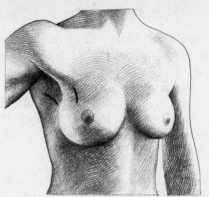

lumpectomy with axillary node dissection

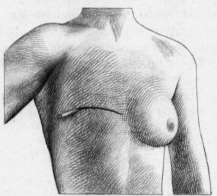

simple mastectomy

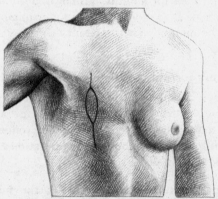

radical mastectomy with skin graft

Examples of breast operation scars

How long will the operation take?

It depends upon the operation. Simple lumpectomies require about 15 to 30 minutes, and many patients are sent home the same day. Radical mastectomies can take anywhere from two to four hours and the patient is encouraged to get out of bed the day following the operation.

How dangerous is a mastectomy?

Not dangerous at all as far as the surgery involved is concerned. Mortality rates referring to the mastectomy operation itself put it in the almost-no-risk category. It is a very safe operation.

How long will it be before the incision heals?

The incision for a lumpectomy will usually heal within a week or ten days. Wounds of more radical operations are usually healed within a month to six weeks after the operation.

Since both my mother and aunt died of breast cancer before they were forty, and since my breasts are lumpy and the doctor has done several biopsies with a diagnosis of precancerous condition, would I be wise to have both breasts removed?

This is a question which only the individual can answer. Much of the decision must be based on how worried you are about getting cancer, how important your breasts are to you, and whether you have gotten a second opinion on the biopsy findings. Today, the decision to have a double mastectomy is a much easier one to make, since reconstruction of the breasts is possible.

Questions You Will Want to Ask Your Doctor Following a Mastectomy

- What arm exercises can I do?
- When can I start to shower again?
- What restrictions do you put on my affected arm?
- When will I be able to drive?
- Will you arrange for a Reach to Recovery volunteer to see me?
- When will the stitches be removed?
- Are there any restrictions on sexual activity?
- What kind of therapy is prescribed?
- Why is it being prescribed?

- What will it do?
- Can I lift things?
- When can I start doing my household chores?
- When can I start active sports again?
- When can I get a permanent prosthesis?
- When can I have reconstructive surgery?
- Will I have to have any additional treatment such as radiation or chemotherapy?
- Why? Does that mean that the cancer has spread?
- How long will I have to have those treatments?

How shall I care for my incision?

Wash with soap and water. You may take a shower within two to three days after the stitches are removed. If the stitches are not removed before you go home, they will probably be covered with a gauze pad to protect them from irritation. Your doctor will tell you when they are ready to be removed. Do not use any medications—salves, creams or lotions—on your incision unless told to do so by your doctor. Watch for any signs of infection— redness, swelling, pus discharge, tenderness, or fever—and report them to your doctor as soon as possible.

One last word. Before you are discharged from the hospital, please force yourself to look at your incision carefully (even if you may not want to). This will help you to be alert to any changes that may occur. Ask the nurse for assistance and for guidance in evaluating it. It will appear swollen and red. This is normal. The swelling will go away, the color will return to normal, and the stitches will heal. But for your own sake, please don't avoid looking at the incision.

What is the role of Reach to Recovery?

This is a volunteer program sponsored by the American Cancer Society. It is based on the idea that women who have been through breast surgery and have experienced the pain, anxiety, and convalescence are able to help others through the initial period following the mastectomy. The program is set up so that only the surgeon or doctor, with the patient's permission, can arrange to have the volunteer visit the patient in the hospital.

Some doctors still do not know about Reach to Recovery or misunderstand its goals and methods, feeling that somehow it will interfere with the doctor-patient relationship. So, if you are interested, be sure to ask your doctor specifically if he will arrange for a Reach to Recovery volunteer to see you. Her visit offers help during the emotional, tense period of postoperative adjustment and allows you to talk frankly and honestly about a mutual problem. In addition to lending an understanding ear, the Reach to Recovery volunteer brings an invaluable kit with a realistically written manual of information and exercise materials as well as a temporary breast form and bra. She will demonstrate some of the basic exercises needed to facilitate recovery, and since she is a mastectomy patient herself, she is available to answer questions and give moral support.

Why is everyone so anxious to make me move my arm?

There are good reasons for this. First of all, it will help prevent swelling of the arm and help the drainage of the wound. Changing the position of the arm will limit shoulder pain and help you gradually build your affected arm back up to its fullest capacity as quickly as possible. Moving your arm is very important because it helps prevent the forming of adhesions which will later limit how much you can move it. Frequent exercising is necessary to relieve stiffness and a heavy feeling. Your doctor will tell you when you can safely begin to exercise. The amount and the extent of surgery will determine the problems you will have with your arm.

What kind of arm exercises should I do?

Your doctor will tell you when you can begin exercising and will probably give you his own list of exercises. A nurse or physical therapist will be happy to review them with you. You may feel some pulling and discomfort when you first do the exercises but gradually you will be able to have a full range of motion. Start exercising gradually and work up to doing each exercise three to five times a day. Here are some of the suggested exercises.

- Squeeze a ball, a rolled-up bandage, or a crumpled sheet of paper. You can start this one right away and do it as often as you wish. This helps strengthen the muscles in your hand and forearm.

- Brush your hair with your affected arm, gradually working your way around your entire head.
- Elevate your involved arm as much and as often as you can to prevent swelling. When you lie down, put pillows under your arm. When you sit on a couch, stretch your arm over the back of the couch.
- Keeping your elbow straight, palm down, lift your arm out in front of you and swing it to the side, then relax. Lift your arms high over your head with arms held as close to your ears as possible.
- Stand with your face to the wall, your feet apart with toes touching the bottom of the wall, your forehead resting against the wall. Place the palms on wall at shoulder level, elbows down. Slowly "walk" your fingers straight up the wall, then slide your palms back to shoulder level. Mark the spot on the wall and each day try to "walk" a little higher. The ultimate goal of this exercise is to be able to walk your arms so you can straighten them over your head, elbows straight.
- Use household chores as exercises to help restore the arm and shoulder movement: sweeping, vacuuming, pulling out and pushing in drawers, mopping the floor, washing and raising windows, hanging clothes, and buttoning clothing which is open in the back.

The booklet given to you by the Reach to Recovery volunteer also includes exercises for you to do.

Some people have swollen arms after a mastectomy. What causes that?

The lymphatic system which normally drains fluid from your arm is disrupted with mastectomy surgery. Your arm may be more likely to swell or to become red, warm, or unusually hard if you develop an infection. Therefore, it is important for you to take special care to avoid injury, infection, and swelling of the arm. You must always be careful what you do with the arm on the side where the mastectomy is performed, since the swelling can occur even several years after the operation.

When can I start using deodorant again?

It depends upon where the incision is made. You should wait until all the stitches are removed and the incision heals before using a deodorant.

What kinds of things should I watch for in order to protect the arm on the side where my mastectomy was performed?

- Do not allow blood samples to be drawn or blood pressure to be taken on the affected arm.
- Avoid injections and vaccinations on the affected arm.
- Do not wear tight jewelry or elasticized or tight sleeves on that side.
- Keep that side covered when you are out in the sun. Avoid insect bites by using protective insect repellent.
- Treat burns, cuts, and scratches immediately.
- Pamper your arm by carrying your purse or packages on the other side.
- Wear a thimble when sewing to avoid pinpricks.
- Wear gloves or mitts when gardening and working with sharp objects or hot objects. Use a mitt when taking hot dishes out of the oven. Use rubber gloves when washing with harsh detergents.
- Use an electric razor to avoid cutting this area. Underarm shaving may be a problem for a while because of the lack of mobility or numbness, so take great care.
- Never pick or cut cuticles or hangnails. Apply lanolin hand cream to hand and arm several times a day.
- If you do notice pain, swelling, or redness on your scar or arm, with or without fever being present, call your doctor.

What can I do if I have a swollen arm?

The swollen arm (edema) is due to the disruption of the lymph channels. It is very important that you do the exercises described (or similar ones which your nurse, physical therapist, or doctor has ordered) and follow the suggestions for arm care so that the swelling is prevented. If swelling does occur, elevating the arm on a pillow will help to reduce it. You may have to elevate your arm over your head while you sleep. If you continue to have swelling, an elastic sleeve can sometimes help (you can buy the elastic sleeves in a medical drugstore or the store where you get your prosthesis). The sleeve applies pressure, which helps, in some cases, to reduce the swelling. You should do the arm exercises while wearing the sleeve. Some doctors will perform surgery if the swelling continues over a long period of time.

Will all the pain, numbness, and tingling sensations eventually disappear?

Yes, they should. However, some women continue to have symptoms for many months after the operation has healed. Some patients say they have pain radiating from under the arm to the waist when they touch under the armpit. As with other operations, the symptoms are affected by the weather. If you have unusual sensations, discuss them with your doctor.

Will I get full muscle strength back in my arm?

That depends upon the operation which has been performed. In some radical mastectomies, you may be limited in the strength of certain motions and feel some permanent muscle weakness.

Are there some medical reasons why I should wear a prosthesis?

Yes, there are. The weight of the remaining breast, particularly for women with medium-to-large breasts, can cause shoulder, neck, and back pain. You may find that your posture will change, with the affected shoulder rising, if you do not have a prosthesis. The larger the remaining breast, the more vital the need, not only for appearance but also for weight. For your own well-being, emotional comfort, and self-confidence, you should plan to buy a prosthesis. In many cases, a well-fitted prosthetic device means the difference between prompt, cheerful, total recovery and long-term personal distress. You will need some device to make your clothing fit well.

Can I wear the prosthesis all the time?

Yes. Many patients wear it all the time, around the clock. Some patients start by wearing it a few hours a day and gradually increasing the number of hours of wear. Wearing the form to bed at night may help prevent a stiff neck and shoulder problems. Waterbeds have also been recommended by some, since they provide support and conform to the body.

I am ashamed to let my husband look at the scar. Is that an unusual feeling?

Unfortunately, we have heard that comment from many women. Several told us that they felt self-conscious about having their husbands or anyone else see the scar, that they did not expect the scar to be so ugly and disfiguring. That is one of the reasons why we suggested you look at the scar before you leave the hospital and talk with a nurse about it. The Reach to Recovery volunteer can also be of help in this area. If you can talk with your husband about your feelings, that is an important step forward. The American Cancer Society in many parts of the country runs "support groups" where patients can discuss problems with others who have the illness. The YWCAs also run a program called Encore which is a combination of exercise and discussion for women who have had mastectomies.

Will I have trouble sleeping?

Some women do have trouble sleeping on the side of the operation. Others say that they cannot wear their prosthesis to bed because the elastic in the bra is too tight (you can get a "sleeping brassiere" which is much softer and more comfortable to wear). Some women described the feeling as like being in a cast, saying it is difficult to sleep because it is hard to find a comfortable position. Others talk about the difficulty of lying flat on their backs because of the pulling sensation. Yet others experience very little difficulty with this problem.

When can I expect all the stiffness, heaviness, and tautness to be gone?

As with most surgery, you shouldn't expect it all to be gone in a month. You may have to exercise many more weeks before the stiffness eases up, and you may, as with other surgery, feel some recurrent stiffness and pulling. If by six weeks after you have had the operation, when you are fully healed with all the stitches out, you don't have the full range of motion, you should tell your doctor or nurse. They may order additional exercises.

When can I go back to doing my regular work?

Again, this depends upon the extent of your operation and your own personal condition. You should discuss this with your doctor before you go home from the hospital. Most doctors recommend early resumption of work, including household chores and office duties.

Can I continue with sports such as bowling, golf, tennis, skiing, and swimming?

You can certainly go back to them, but you should check with your doctor as to when you can take up active sports again. Swimming is very good exercise for breast patients, and there are many styles of bathing suits which you can use.

Where do I go to buy a prosthesis?

There are several places: corset shops, surgical supply houses, foundation departments of most large department stores, and some special outlets. Some American Cancer Society offices offer a variety of forms that a woman can examine (but are not for sale), in a noncommercial setting. The Reach to Recovery volunteer or the American Cancer Society office can give you material describing the various forms and a list of suggested outlets available. Most of the outlets have fitters who can help you. The large mail-order houses also have prostheses available.

When should I go to get a breast prosthesis?

Most doctors will tell you to wait until the scar is fully healed before you get fitted for a breast prosthesis (a form to replace the missing breast). Most patients can begin using a full prosthesis a month or six weeks after surgery. However, soft forms can be worn from the very beginning. For instance, at the very beginning you can use simple clean padding in your brassiere. The Reach to Recovery volunteer who visits you may provide you with a temporary Dacron-filled prosthesis to wear. Some patients tell us they use items such as cotton balls, lamb's-wool, handkerchiefs, sanitary napkins, or padded bras during the period between their operation and being fitted for a prosthesis. You should check with your doctor before wearing the permanent prosthesis.

How can I be sure I find the right prosthesis?

First of all, you should not shop for the prosthesis by yourself. It is much better if an involved person, such as your sister, mother, husband, or a good friend, goes along with you. Second, you should make sure you try on several different kinds and models so that you can be sure the one you finally buy is what you really want. Patients have complained that in some instances they have been faced with a hard-sell approach or have been shown only the most expensive models in shopping for prostheses. Make sure you shop around and try on different types and different brands. It is important to pay close attention to how it feels and how it fits—the form should match your other breast from the side, the bottom, and the front. The form should feel comfortable. Remember you will be wearing it every day for a long time to come.

Can I make my own prosthesis?

Some people do make their own prothesis. Some of the material put out by the American Cancer Society has instructions for making your own breast forms and night bras. Some small-breasted women or women who have had both breasts removed find that they can use homemade forms. However, in many cases, the homemade forms are too lightweight and tend to ride up. Again, you must be careful because you might end up with aches in your shoulders, backaches, and posture change if you wear a prothesis which is not of the proper weight for you.

What is a special mastectomy bra?

It is a bra with a built-in pocket to hold the form in place. It also has extra material under the arm and above the breast. The form is placed in the pocket of the bra, which holds it in place. You can bend, stretch, or stoop without jarring it out of place. Some patients have complained that the special mastectomy bras do not fit properly. Many patients have altered their own bras with pockets, and still others have had seamstresses make pockets for their bras. In some stores, fitters will sew pockets into your bras to hold the prosthesis.

What should I wear when I shop for the prosthesis?

You should bring along some figure-revealing clothes to see how natural the form will look—a sweater or one of your more revealing dresses. If you want to use your own bras, make sure you bring them along so they can be altered if needed.

What is meant by a cover on the form?

Some of the forms, both lightweight and heavy ones, have nylon or cloth covers. The covers are made of washable, fast-drying materials. The cover allows the forms to be pinned directly into regular brassieres for occasional use instead of in the specially made pocket. Some women prefer to wear the covers on the forms at all times. They like the way they feel. The tricot covers, especially, are easy to wash out every night and dry so that they can be worn the next day.

I have a depression under my arm left from the surgery. Is there any way to fill that? ·

There are "back" pads which can be worn under the form or along the side. These are sold with most prostheses and can fill in the depressions left by the surgery.

·**What are the different kinds of prostheses available?**

There are several different kinds of breast forms made by several companies. Generally they fall into these classifications:

- *Silicone-gel-filled:* Form usually made of silicone skin. Very soft and flexible with the look, feel, and weight of the natural breast. Worn with regular bra. Adjusts to body temperature. Filled with silicone gel, fluid, or sponge. Can leak (gel or fluid) if fingernail or pin pricks it. One company makes a special adhesive so form can be worn without bra if desired. OK for swimming. Most expensive. ($75–$200)
- *Liquid- or air-filled:* Form usually a plastic shell or a soft plastic form. Soft form has natural feel, look, and weight. Usually comes with covers. Depending on make can either be worn with regular or specially made bra. Air-filled has pocket that can be inflated to vary shape or size. Liquid-filled can leak if pricked. OK for swimming. ($40–$80)
- *Foam-rubber:* Lightweight (molded foam or foam chips) but can have weights added. Spongy feeling. May get stiff and yellow with wear. Good for leisure wear, swimming (needs waterproof cover). Especially useful with lounging bra for postoperative period. Some people like them for general wear. ($4–$20)
- *Polyester:* Lightweight and long-wearing. Soft pads with tricot filling. Good for sleepwear and postoperative wear. (About $10)
- *Inflatable:* Lightweight, both forms and bras. Best for women who have had both breasts removed. ($30–$70)

Ask the American Cancer Society or the Reach to Recovery volunteer for a complete up-to-date list of prostheses manufactured in the United States.

Can I get a breast form with a nipple?

Some forms are made with nipples. Others can be worn with nipples that are sold separately and can be easily attached.

Can I get a form in a dark skin color?

Some forms are made in both light and dark skin colors.

Are there any cosmetics to cover the scars I have after surgery? I find that the ordinary kinds just don't seem to work.

There is a special brand of cosmetics, Covermark, which is designed to blend into one's individual skin color. The cosmetics are waterproof and when carefully applied are particularly useful for swimming. Available from Lydia O'Leary, 575 Madison Avenue, New York, N.Y. 10022, and in many drug and department stores.

The tight elastic bothers me in my bra, but I like the way this particular one fits. Can I do anything about that?

Notion stores and girdle and corset shops sell bra extenders which can be used to make a bra more comfortable. They also sell shoulder strap pads which some women use to relieve discomfort on the shoulder strap area.

Can I have a prosthesis custom-made?

There are a few manufacturers who custom-make prostheses. The American Cancer Society can give you an up-to-date listing.

What does a prosthesis look like?

Usually it is flesh-colored. The prostheses are sized to match the remaining breast both in its shape and its weight. Normally, they are teardrop-shaped. The flat side goes against the wall of the chest and the tail end goes toward the armpit. One manufacturer makes a reversible one which can be used on either side.

Do the prostheses feel cold against your chest?

Most of them, when they are first put on, feel a little cold. But after they have been worn for a few minutes, they warm to body temperature and feel like a normal breast to the touch.

Will my insurance cover a prosthesis?

It depends on your insurance plan. Some health insurance (and Medicare) covers part or all of the cost of the first prosthesis. The doctor should write the prescription for the form. Breast forms and mastectomy bras may also be tax-deductible when medically prescribed. In most cases, only the first prosthesis is covered. A replacement form is not covered. Be sure to read your insurance policy, because some say you must buy the form within a specific period of time and buy a certain type. Keep all your receipts. Most prostheses are covered by warranty.

During the summertime, I perspire under the prosthesis. Can I do anything about that?

You can buy a sheepskin pad, which you wear facing the body, behind the form, to absorb perspiration. Some patients sometimes use facial tissue under the form during the summer.

Is anyone making special bathing suits for women with mastectomies to wear?

Many of the major bathing-suit companies make special bathing suits for mastectomy patients. You can usually get them through the same source where you got your prosthesis or in large department stores. Your local unit of the American Cancer Society can usually supply you with a list of available styles. There is also a mail-order house which carries these suits: Cameo Stores, Inc., Rockwell & Hartel Avenues, Philadelphia, Pa. 19111.

Is there anything that a family member or a friend can do to help a woman who has had a mastectomy adjust to the loss of her breast?

Patients who have gone through the experience tell us that several things have been helpful to them. Of course, different things are beneficial to different people.

- Many women find that talking about the loss of the breast is very helpful.

- A husband who tells his wife that he still loves her and needs her and will help her through these difficult days and makes her feel worthwhile is of great reassurance to the patient. It helps if the husband can also talk about the loss of the breast with his wife.
- Friends and family members who are willing to talk and who are not afraid to bring up the subject make it easier for conversation to begin.
- Nurses who encourage the patient to look at the scar and who listen to what she has to say are helpful.
- People who are willing to go with the patient to buy her prosthesis are helpful.

There is also help from the American Cancer Society—the Reach to Recovery program and the support groups for cancer patients are designed to help. In some towns and cities, the YMCAs run programs of exercise and support for recent breast patients.

I have had a breast removed. I felt that I had faced this fact very honestly and well and had accepted the mastectomy. Now a few weeks have gone by and I feel very depressed and cheated. Is this a normal reaction?

Patients react to a mastectomy in very different ways. Much of the reaction, it has been found, depends upon the expectations you have and how you approached the operation.

It is not unusual for women to have emotional distress. It may be a feeling of panic. Some women cry. Others say they don't feel like eating. Some can't sleep or concentrate. Still others can't talk about the operation to others. Many women have a "why did this have to happen to me" feeling. These are normal kinds of feelings for mastectomy patients.

It is not abnormal to be afraid of what the disease will mean to the rest of your life. If you are married, you may be worried about your husband's attitude and what he will think about your scar. If you are not married, you might worry about what you might face with a mate in the future. You may be concerned about how you can face people when you return home or to work. Discuss these concerns if you can.

Don't be concerned about when you have these feelings— some people have them directly after the operation, others not until a month or several months have gone by. Just understand they are normal reactions to losing an important part of your body and to the feeling of helplessness about it.

Most important, don't feel that you are strange because you have these feelings. It is normal to have them. Get some help. Sometimes you can talk with a member of your family or a good friend. Other people turn to the American Cancer Society or the Cancer Information Service to have someone to talk with. The American Cancer Society in some areas runs sessions where cancer patients can talk with each other. You may want to go back to the hospital and talk with the social worker or a nurse who was helpful to you during your admission. Or maybe your physician or your clergyman can help you.

How often should I see a doctor after my surgery?

It depends upon the follow-up treatment you will receive. If you are to receive radiation or chemotherapy, you will be referred by your surgeon to either a radiation oncologist or a medical oncologist (be sure to read Chapters 7 and 8 on these two treatment types). If you are to have no follow-up treatment, the surgeon will probably ask you to come back every three to six months for the first year, then every six months to a year.

What will the surgeon do during these follow-up visits?

The doctor will probably check your scar, the other breast, and the lymph nodes. He will tell you to make sure you are practicing breast self-examination on your other breast each month and make sure you know what you are looking for. He will answer any questions you might have about how you are feeling. At the annual visit, he will give you a physical examination, including a Pap smear. He will probably order blood tests, x-rays, a mammogram, and bone scans.

When is hormonal treatment used for breast cancer?

Hormonal treatment is one of several alternatives available to the doctor when breast cancer recurs. It is the use of hormones or endocrine therapy, either through the use of hormone drugs or the removal of one of the hormone-secreting organs, such as the ovaries, the adrenal glands, or the pituitary gland. The growth of cancer in the breast may depend on the presence of the hormones to which these tissues normally respond. Scientists feel that changing the normal hormonal environment may affect these cancers.

Is it true that only about one-third of the women can benefit from hormonal therapy?

No, it is not true. Women whose tumors contain estrogen receptors benefit from hormone treatment in about 60 percent of the cases. If the tumors do not contain receptors, less than a 10 percent response can be expected. The estrogen-receptor test is a means of predicting with a high level of accuracy which women will undergo a worthwhile remission as a result of this treatment.

What is an estrogen-receptor test and when is it done?

The doctor sends an adequate sample of the tumor to the laboratory to be measured for a chemical marking called an estrogen receptor. The test is done usually during the original breast operation or at the time of recurrence of the disease. It is best done before chemotherapy treatments are given to provide for accuracy. Not all hospitals have the facilities for performing this laboratory service, but its use is becoming more valuable in planning treatment for breast cancer patients.

Is radiation used in treating breast cancer?

Yes. Radiation is often advised after lumpectomy or segmental mastectomy as well as when the lymph nodes under the armpit are involved or when the tumor is located in the center of the breast. In some cases of Stage III breast cancer, radiation is used before operation. Various sequences of radiation, surgery, and chemotherapy are also being investigated.

Is it unusual to have chemotherapy treatment after a mastectomy?

No, it is not unusual. Chemotherapy treatment is used both as a preventive treatment for breast-cancer patients whose disease shows spread to one or more lymph nodes at the time of initial surgery and for breast-cancer patients with distant metastases. If chemotherapy has been recommended, ask for a consultation or a referral to a medical oncologist.

I am a breast-cancer patient taking chemotherapy. The doctor told me I must be on the drugs for a year. Does that mean my case is bad?

No, it does not indicate that, but it does mean that you are at a high risk for the cancer to spread because the disease was found in some of your lymph nodes. Chemotherapy as a preventive measure can be given for as long as 24 months. The length of the treatment time does not necessarily indicate the seriousness of your disease.

What chemotherapy drugs are usually used in treating breast-cancer patients?

There are many different combinations of drugs being used in treating breast cancer. Among the drugs used are chlorambucil, cyclophosphamide, melphalan, triethylenethiophosphoramide, methotrexate, 5-FU, Adriamycin, mitomycin, testosterone propionate, fluoxymesterone, testolactone, diethylstilbestrol, ethinyl estradiol, prednisone, vincristine and tamoxifen. Be sure to read Chapter 8 if you are to be treated with this method.

Is the use of immunotherapy new in the treatment of breast cancer?

There are several experimental trials being done using chemotherapy and immunotherapy in combination.

Can I have a baby after having had a mastectomy?

Before you make a decision about having a baby, be sure to discuss the ramifications of your cancer history with your doctor. Hormonal changes that accompany pregnancy can have an effect on cancer growth, and it is important for your doctor to evaluate your condition.

I would like to have breast reconstruction after my surgery for breast cancer. Can this be done?

You should ask your surgeon for a consultation with a plastic surgeon before the mastectomy if possible. The full extent of the reconstruction cannot be determined until after the incision has healed, but it is wise to have the consultation before the operation if possible. Depending on the individual, breast reconstruction is available to women who have had either a single or a double mastectomy. The results and the difficulty of the operation will vary with each individual case. Many women having mastectomies may be candidates for breast reconstruction if they and their surgeons know the facts about current techniques. In many cases, if arrangements are made before the operation, the plastic surgeon can be in the operating room at the time of the mastectomy.

Questions to Ask Your Doctor Before Breast Reconstruction

- How many breast reconstruction operations have you done? With what results?
- Do you have before and after pictures to show me?
- Can I talk with someone who has had the operation?
- Will you be present during the mastectomy?

Will the breast look as it did before the mastectomy?

You should not expect that it will. However, most patients are pleased with the results of the reconstruction. They say it makes them feel more like their old selves. Women who felt inhibited about undressing before their husbands lose the inhibition and say they feel more attractive. Although the new breast will not be a perfect replica of the old one, most women who have the reconstruction surgery can wear a normal bra or a bikini. The plastic surgeon will talk to you about your expectations. If they are not realistic, he may suggest that you not have it done.

What is involved in breast reconstruction?

Breast reconstruction means a second operation, and sometimes even two or more additional operations. The plastic surgeon implants a silicone-rubber envelope (usually a half-moon of silicone gel which has been specially molded) under the skin. Unlike silicone injections which have been used to enlarge breasts (and are now banned in many states), the silicone implant appears to be entirely safe. This implant forms a breast mound. If you have had a radical mastectomy, you may need additional operations to fill in the chest cavity. The plastic surgeon can take muscle tissue from another part of the body to rebuild the breast area.

Will I be able to have a nipple as part of the breast reconstruction?

If you wish to have one, it is usually possible. However, construction of the nipple and areola may require a second operation.

Are nipple reconstructions usually successful?

Nipple reconstruction is an amazing art. Nipples are reconstructed from tissue taken from either the inner thigh, the outer lip of the vagina, from the original nipple or from the nipple remaining in the other breast.

Is it true that reconstruction can hide a recurring cancer?

There is no proof that reconstructing the breast will hide a recurring cancer—or will make a dormant one become active. However, patients who are on chemotherapy may not be able to have reconstruction performed because of depressed white cell counts, which can increase the risk of infection.

Are more women having breast reconstruction performed?

Until recently, fewer than 1 percent of mastectomy patients in the United States had breast reconstruction. Now that there is more experience and improved techniques, many patients are electing to have breast reconstruction done either immediately or later.

When can breast reconstruction surgery be done?

It depends upon the kind of operation you have had and the extent of your cancer. If you have had a simple or modified radical mastectomy, you will probably have to wait for three months until the scar has healed, although some doctors say that patients with minimal disease can have reconstruction immediately following cancer surgery, or even at the same session. If you are having chemotherapy treatments, most doctors prefer to wait until you have completed the chemotherapy treatments. Most doctors wait another three months between the operation which creates the breast mound and the construction of the nipple.

I had my mastectomy more than ten years ago. Can I still have breast reconstruction?

There are women who have had successful reconstructions with mastectomies over 20 years old. The fact that you had a mastectomy many years ago does not disqualify you as a candidate for the operation. Nor does your age.

I have had radiation treatments. Can I still have a breast-reconstruction operation?

This will depend upon the condition of your skin. You need to have enough thick, soft, and loose skin, well nourished by blood vessels, to be able to hold up the implant. If your skin has been damaged by radiation treatments or if you need skin grafts, you may not be able to have the operation. You should discuss the question with a plastic surgeon, who can make the decision after examination.

My remaining breast is large. Can I have the reconstruction operation?

Yes. However, there is a limit to the size of the reconstructed breast. The limit is based on what the skin can support. Usually the surgeon will reduce the size of the remaining breast so that it will match the new breast. This operation is usually done at the same time as the operation to make the nipple. The operation to reduce the size of the remaining breast is called reduction mammoplasty.

Is it true that it is more difficult to have breast reconstruction if I have had radical surgery for my breast operation?

Yes, it is true that women who have had radical mastectomies require more extensive surgery to rebuild their breasts. This is because the chest cavity must be reconstructed as well as the breast itself. More operations must be performed in order to get a cosmetically good result. It is important, if you think you will want breast reconstruction, to discuss it with the surgeon beforehand. It may affect where he places the incision, since even the placement of the scar can make a difference in the reconstruction. Although the choice of the original operation is the cancer surgeon's, plastic surgeons recommend that breast-cancer surgeons leave as much skin and as little scar tissue as possible to facilitate reconstruction.

Are there any complications from the surgery for breast reconstruction?

You must remember that there is always the possibility of complications from any surgery. Even with the best surgeon there can be some complications. Sometimes, though rarely, an implant is rejected. You can try again and it may take the second time. Sometimes there is some hardening of the tissue around the implant. It is important to be sure that a qualified doctor is performing the plastic surgery.

How long does a breast reconstruction operation take to perform?

The reconstruction operation usually takes about 1½ hours. The operation for nipple graft also takes between 1 and 1½ hours. The stay in the hospital for the actual reconstruction is usually two or three days. More complicated surgery will require a longer stay.

Is general anesthesia used?

Usually, although some surgeons do the simpler reconstructions using local anesthesia.

What if my doctor does not think I should have breast reconstruction?

This depends upon his reasons. If his decision is based on health reasons, you should probably abide by his judgment. However, you could ask to have his reasoning confirmed by a second opinion. If he simply has given you the feeling that breast reconstruction for cosmetic reasons is frivolous or unnecessary, and you strongly want to have breast reconstruction, you should arrange to talk with a plastic surgeon about your case.

What kind of doctor should perform the plastic surgery?

A board-certified plastic surgeon should do the breast reconstruction. Be sure that he is experienced with the operation. Ask him how many he has done and what his results have been. Most doctors have before-and-after pictures they can show you.

Ask your doctor to recommend someone for the consultation or call a teaching hospital in your community. There is also a society of reconstructive surgeons: American Society of Plastic and Reconstructive Surgeons, 29 East Madison St., Suite 807, Chicago, Ill. 60602.

Is it possible for me to talk with someone else who has had the operation?

You should ask the plastic surgeon if he will allow you to talk with some of his patients. Some of them will have given him the permission to discuss it with other potential patients. There is also an organization in New York which will give you the chance to talk to a woman who has had the operation: AFTER, (Ask a Friend to Explain Reconstruction), 99 Park Avenue, New York, N.Y. 10016. The organization has a pamphlet which it will send to you on the subject.

How much does breast reconstruction cost?

The operations are expensive and depend upon the extent of the surgery as well as other factors. The operation alone can run as high as $5,000. Most of them range from $1,500 to $3,000. Almost all of the Blue Cross/Blue Shield plans and many of the private insurance plans now cover postmastectomy surgery. Some only cover the hospital costs, while others will also pay part or all of the plastic surgeon's costs. Be sure to know the cost and what your policy will cover before deciding on the operation.

Suggested Reading

COWLES, JANE. *Informed Consent.* New York: Coward, McCann and Geoghegan, 1976.

COPE, OLIVER, M.D. *The Breast: Its Problems—Benign and Malignant—and How to Deal with Them.* Boston, Mass.: Houghton Mifflin. $8.95.

KUSHNER, ROSE. *Breast Cancer: A Personal History and an Investigative Report.* New York: Harcourt Brace Jovanovich. $10.00. New edition (*Why Me*) also now available in paperback.

BLOCK, JEAN LIBMAN. *I Am Whole Again.* New York: Random House. $7.95. By a reconstruction patient.

chapter 12

Lung Cancer

Those Most Likely to Get Lung Cancer

- Age 50–64 and live in a city
- Have smoked one or more packs a day for 20 years or longer and/or began to smoke before age 20 and still smoking
- Smoke and work in an industrial plant with high-risk materials (such as asbestos)
- Have a persistent or violent smoker's cough
- Don't smoke but have had a violent cough for more than two weeks
- Have a nagging chest pain unrelated to cough
- Breathe with a wheezing sound
- Have noticed blood in sputum—even once
- Have had a change in color or volume of sputum

Symptoms of Lung Cancer

- A smoker's cough which has become persistent or violent
- A nonsmoker whose cough hangs on for more than two weeks
- A chest pain that is persistent and unrelated to a cough
- A wheezing sound in your breathing
- Bloodstained sputum
- Change in color or volume of sputum

- What are my chances for cure?
- Is the operation worth the pain and discomfort?
- Has the cancer spread outside the lungs?
- If I am not operated on, what other treatment do you suggest?
- Is my other lung in good enough condition so that I can still function fairly normally after the diseased lung is removed?
- How limited will I be in my activity?
- Will I need radiation therapy?
- Will you prescribe chemotherapy?
- How long will it be before I regain my strength?
- Do I have small-cell (or oat-cell) carcinoma?

What kind of doctor should I see if I have symptoms of lung cancer?

Usually the internist or general physician would refer you to a surgeon. It is important that he be a thoracic surgeon and one who specializes in lung diseases.

Is the National Cancer Institute supporting any studies on lung cancer?

The National Cancer Institute's clinical cooperative groups are presently studying new treatment methods for oat-cell and large-cell carcinoma, adenocarcinoma, and epidermoid cancers as well as some of the more unusual cancers. (See Chapter 23.)

What are the lungs?

The lungs are two spongy, pinkish-gray organs that take up much of the room inside the chest. They enfold the other organs of the chest such as the heart, the large blood vessels entering and leaving the heart, and the esophagus (tube carrying food from mouth to stomach). The left lung has two lobes or sections. It is smaller than the right lung because the heart takes up some of the space on the left side of the chest. The right lung has three lobes and is a little bigger than the left one.

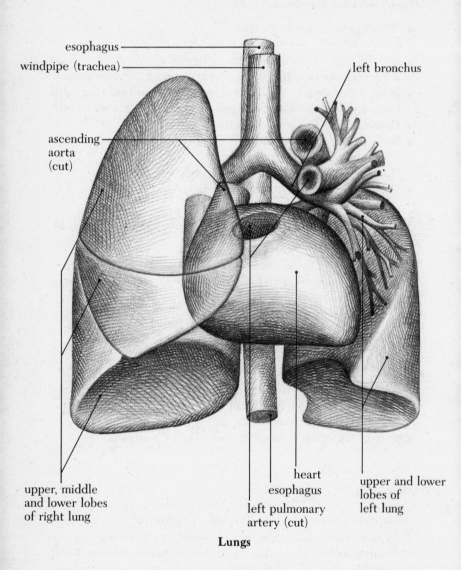

esophagus

windpipe (trachea)

left bronchus

ascending
aorta
(cut)

upper, middle
and lower lobes
of right lung

heart
esophagus

left pulmonary
artery (cut)

upper and lower
lobes of
left lung

Lungs

How does the air get into the lungs?

Air passes through the mouth or nose into the windpipe (trachea). The windpipe divides into two tubes called the left bronchus and the right bronchus. These large bronchi are about the size of a man's little finger. They divide into ever-smaller branched tubes like the branches of a tree and lead to the several lobes of the lungs. These air passages get smaller and smaller until they are only 1/100 inch across.

How do the lungs work?

The lungs bring needed oxygen into the body and expel carbon dioxide. The bloodstream brings the oxygen to the cells, which need it to carry out their work and stay alive. When we inhale, air enters the lungs through the bronchi. Cells of the lung are self-cleaning. Certain cells that line the bronchi produce mucus to wash out foreign materials. Other cells, which are equipped with tiny hairs, called cilia, sweep the mucus toward the throat. Impurities are carried away into the bloodstream or lymph system by other cells.

Where does lung cancer start?

Most lung cancers begin in the bronchi (the larger air tubes) or the bronchioles (the smaller tubes branching off the bronchi) in the moist mucous layer of the breathing tubes. Some cancer researchers think that 20 or more years may pass between the time someone is first exposed to a cancer-producing substance such as tobacco smoke and the time cancer actually develops.

Are there different kinds of lung cancer?

There are actually 13 different types of lung cancer. Nine of them are relatively rare. The four most common ones are epidermoid carcinoma (also known as squamous-cell carcinoma), adenocarcinoma, large-cell carcinoma, and small-cell carcinoma (also known as oat-cell carcinoma, which is usually treated differently from the other types). These four types make up over 90 percent of all lung cancers. They are named for the four different cell types found in the tumors when looked at under the microscope.

Tests For Lung Cancer

TEST	EXPLANATION
Physical exam and full health history	Important for doctor to know your health habits. Will listen to lungs to see if fluid has collected. Will check lymph nodes on neck to see if normal. Includes complete blood and liver-function tests.
Chest x-ray	A basic test. Detects tumors already about ½ inch in diameter. Can also show fluid or enlarged lymph nodes. X-ray useful in detecting changes in lung tissue. Should be part of regular checkup. Heavy smokers should have one every six months or on doctor's recommendation.
Sputum examination	Can detect abnormal cells in sputum. Sometimes used to tell what kind of cancer is present. Can sometimes detect cancer before large enough to appear on x-ray.
Bronchoscopy	Doctor looks into bronchial passages in search of tumor. Allows doctor to take cell samples. Performed under local anesthesia. Helps locate source of cancer cells found in sputum. Can use rigid or fiberoptic bronchoscope depending on location.
Tomogram	Three-dimensional x-ray used to detect location and size of lump. Shows one thin layer of lung at a time. May show cancer not seen in regular x-ray. Also called laminagram. CT scan is a type of tomogram.
Bronchogram	Specialized x-ray exam using radio-opaque dye to better define area.
Pulmonary-function test	Uses radioactive materials plus camera or computer to measure breathing and evaluate patient's ability to get oxygen into blood.
Biopsy	All-inclusive term. There are different methods of obtaining tissue, but tissue examination is essential part of determining presence of cancer, cell type, and degree of malignancy.
Mediastinoscopy	Method of getting diagnosis. Also necessary to tell whether lung cancer has spread to lymph nodes behind breastbone (mediastinum). Doctor passes instrument through small incision in neck, taking lymph nodes for biopsy.

TEST	EXPLANATION
Bone scan, liver scan, brain scan, bone-marrow biopsy	Also known as metastatic workup. Depending on results of other tests, one or more of these tests may be done. Scans are painless, routine outpatient diagnostic procedures, similar to x-rays. Tests help determine whether cancer has spread to bones, liver, and brain. Bone-marrow biopsy is done with needle on breastbone or hipbone.
Thoracentesis	Fluid examination used when there is fluid and other attempts to find cancer have failed. May be used to relieve pain or shortness of breath caused by fluid collection. Fluid is drawn by needle from space between lungs and chest wall and checked for cancer cells. Can be done in examining room or hospital.
Thoracoscopy	Relatively new test which helps pinpoint location of cancer. Done in operating room. Incision is made between two ribs, slender tubular instrument is inserted into lung cavity, lung is deflated, and instrument is used to examine entire surface of lung and chest wall for tumor. Tissue taken for examination. Lung reinflated.
Thoracotomy	Exploratory chest operation. Used as a diagnostic tool when other tests have failed to locate tumor. Question doctor carefully before submitting to this test to be certain that all other diagnostic tests available have been made. This is major surgery used to examine lung. If tumor is found, immediate testing is done and if cell type is favorable and there is no evidence of metastases outside lung (which normally should have been determined before this procedure was done), surgical removal of lung is usually performed at this time.

Are all kinds of lung cancer treated the same way?

No. There are different forms of treatment, depending on the cell type, on the extent of the disease, and on the way the disease responds to the treatment. Small-cell (oat-cell) carcinoma calls for a different form of treatment than do the other cell types.

What is oat-cell cancer and why it is treated differently?

Oat-cell or small-cell carcinoma was once considered the most lethal variety of lung cancer. However, major advances in treatment of this type of lung cancer have been made, with chemotherapy and radiotherapy. The tumor is highly sensitive to these treatments. If you have this type of cancer, you should either be treated at a major medical center or be certain that your doctor contacts someone at one of the cancer treatment centers who is using the new treatments.

Is lung cancer common?

Cancer of the lung is the commonest cancer among men in the United States and is on the increase among women. It is the third leading cancer killer. All cancers of the lung have a high degree of malignancy. When lung cancer is diagnosed in its earlier stages, of course, the chances of cure are much greater. Small epidermoid carcinomas, for example, can be cured in a large percentage of patients. The other carcinomas are more difficult to cure. The survival rate is better for those persons whose lung cancer is found before it spreads outside the lung. Each year approximately 100,000 new cases of lung cancer are diagnosed in the United States.

What is sarcoidosis?

Sarcoidosis, a disease characterized by noncancerous growths called granulomas, can be very difficult to diagnose, since it closely resembles some cancers or tuberculosis. It is not cancer. It most often affects the lungs but can also be found in the skin, liver, spleen, eyes, and bones. The course of the disease varies with the patient and the form of sarcoidosis. There are two forms of this disease. The acute type is characterized by an abrupt onset and sometimes sudden disappearance of symptoms. The chronic form has a slow, poorly defined beginning. Persons with relatively mild symptoms often do not need treatment. Drug treatment can relieve symptoms but will not prevent the granulomas from forming and appearing in other locations. Symptoms may include enlarged lymph nodes in the neck plus lung problems. Fever (especially a fever up to 101° daily), weight loss, and tiredness are also symptoms of sarcoidosis.

How does lung cancer spread?

Lung cancer usually begins as a tiny spot, most often on the inner lining of a bronchial tube. Lungs have a rich supply of blood and lymph vessels close to the cancer cells. If these cells get into the bloodstream or the lymph system, they can act as seeds and spread to other parts of the body. When this happens, it is called a metastasis. A metastasis (or "met," as it is sometimes called) is not a new kind of cancer, but is the lung cancer which has moved to another part of the body and begun to grow there. Therefore, even if it has spread to the bone, for example, it is not bone cancer but simply an extension or metastasis of the lung cancer. The metastasis looks and behaves in the same way as the original lung cancer, and therefore the same treatment which has been used to contain the lung tumor is likely to be successful in treating the metastasis.

How does the original lung tumor affect the lung?

There can be several effects on the process of breathing. As the tumor on the lining of a bronchus or bronchiole grows, it may interfere with the flow of air through the breathing tube and cause a wheeze or whistling noise as the air passes through the narrowed part of the bronchus. Or the tumor may cause a cough as it obstructs the upward movement of mucus. Sometimes it makes an already existing cough worse or, because it is bleeding, produces blood-streaked sputum (mucus and/or pus coughed up from the bronchial tube).

Are tumors of the lung ever found to be benign?

Benign tumors (adenomas) do occur—but they are rare. Prior to surgery they are difficult to distinguish from cancerous tumors and are therefore treated in the same manner.

Are most cases of lung cancer operable?

No. About 50 percent of all cases of lung cancer are inoperable.

What if the tumor has spread outside the lung? How does it affect other parts of the body?

Sometimes fluid accumulates in the space between the lungs and the ribs. This can cause chest pain and make it hard to breathe. A tumor growing between the two lungs may press on the esophagus and make it hard to swallow. It may affect the nerves that go to the voice box and make you hoarse. When it grows in one of the smallest bronchial tubes it may not have any effects that you notice.

When should I have a cough investigated to make certain it isn't something more serious?

It is wise to investigate the source of any cough that lasts for more than two or three weeks. This rule goes for the cough that hangs on after a chest cold or for the cough of chronic bronchitis—even though you have had it checked before. A cough, or a change in cough habit, is found in most lung-cancer patients at some time during the course of the disease. The tumor seems to act like a foreign body or obstruction within the lung and the cough represents the effort to expel it.

Are there any other symptoms I should be looking for?

Other signs which are fairly common in lung cancer are vague chest pains, a faint wheezing sound in breathing, or blood-streaked sputum. Chest pain is the second most common symptom. It is usually felt as a persistent ache unrelated to a cough and is commonly experienced on the side on which the tumor is located. Faint wheezing is fairly common at a relatively early stage. It is not necessarily constant. Blood-streaked sputum is a first symptom in a small percentage of cases. However, even small amounts of blood in the sputum—fine streaks, for instance—must be regarded seriously. Its appearance, even once, should always be reported to the doctor. Coughing up blood, either in flecks or streaks, occurs in over half the patients with lung cancer.

How much time does it take for symptoms of lung cancer to show up?

Lung cancer is fairly slow-growing and it ordinarily takes about 20 months from the time the tumor becomes visible on an x-ray to the appearance of the first symptom. And that symptom is usually a change in the character or severity of a chronic cough. Unfortunately, what happens all too often is that the patient usually waits two or three months before seeing a doctor—and then another three or four months go by before treatment is started, so that by the time the cancer is discovered, the disease has had a chance to spread.

Who are the people most likely to get lung cancer?

People most likely to develop lung cancer are males between 50 and 70 years old who have smoked almost all of their adult lives. And although lung cancer is about four times as common in men as in women, the incidence in women is increasing rapidly.

Do industrial pollutants cause lung cancer?

Studies being supported by the National Cancer Institute are beginning to show that occupations and environmental factors may play a role in the development of lung cancer. Persons who have been exposed frequently and for many years to irritating substances (such as asbestos, chromium compounds, radioactive ores, nickel, arsenic, and uranium) in the air they breathe in an industrial plant are thought to have a somewhat greater chance of developing lung cancer. A worker in these kinds of industries who smokes faces an even greater risk. If you are over 40, smoke two packs a day, and/or are in an occupation that is thought to be cancer-producing, you should have frequent medical checkups.

How do I know if I have been exposed to asbestos?

If you have worked for any length of time in a shipyard building or repairing ships, in a factory manufacturing asbestos materials, or as an insulation installer, a construction worker, or in automotive brake lining repair, you may have been exposed to asbestos on the job. The National Cancer Institute and other governmental agencies are informing workers and their families that job-related exposures to asbestos can result in certain diseases, particularly asbestosis and lung cancer.

What are the symptoms of the various asbestos-caused diseases?

Asbestosis is a chronic lung disease whose signs and symptoms result from permanent changes in lung tissue. The earliest and most prominent sign is shortness of breath after exertion.

Lung cancer has a cough or change in cough habit as its most common symptom. Chest pain is the second most common. Blood-streaked sputum, coughed up from the lungs, is the first symptom in a small number of cases.

Mesothelioma is a relatively rare cancer that affects the membrane lining the chest cavity (the pleura) or the membrane lining the abdominal cavity (peritoneum). The most common first symptoms are shortness of breath, pain in the wall of the chest which is aggravated by deep breathing, or abdominal pain which may vary from vague discomfort to severe spasms.

How can I find out if I have medical problems resulting from asbestos exposure?

If you have been exposed to asbestos on the job you should tell your doctor so he can watch for signs or symptoms of asbestos-related diseases. Tests for asbestosis include a physical exam with x-rays and lung-function tests. Tests for cancer, if suspected by your doctor, are more extensive and depend on your specific symptoms.

How does smoking affect the lungs?

Constant irritation of the bronchial lining by cigarette smoke causes the tiny hairs (cilia) that line the bronchial lining to disappear. Without these tiny hairs to sweep it into the throat in the cleansing action, the mucus remains trapped and "smoker's cough" often results. Continued smoking can cause the cells to form abnormal growth patterns and eventually to turn into cancer. Some recent studies indicate that lung cancer could be cut by as much as 80 percent if all smoking ceased. When a person stops smoking, the lungs begin to cleanse and repair themselves.

What kinds of tests does the doctor do when he is looking for lung cancer?

Usually the doctor starts by getting a health history, which gives him important clues to the most likely diagnosis. Then he will do a physical exam, looking, for example, for a hard lump in the neck which would suggest that cancer may have spread from some nearby part of the body to the lymph nodes of the neck. He will order complete blood counts and tests to check the functioning of your liver. A chest x-ray is a very basic test for lung cancer. If it is present, it usually shows up as a shadow on the x-ray. However, the smallest tumor which can be seen on an x-ray of the chest is about 1/2 inch in diameter. At this time metastasis may already have occurred. The doctor may see fluid that is collected in the space between the lung and the chest wall. This fluid, called pleural effusion, can be seen on the x-ray film. Pleural effusion is not always a sign of lung cancer. Usually when the cancer is in the very small bronchial tubes or in the air sacs in the outer portions of the lung, it is easy to see on the x-ray. Cancers in the larger bronchi are less easy to see, but they frequently cause a change in the adjacent lung tissue, and that can be located through the x-ray. The chest x-ray might also show enlarged lymph nodes that have filled with cancer cells even when the original tumor cannot be seen in the lung. When this happens, the doctor must continue to look for the original site of the cancer, using other diagnostic tools.

Is the chest x-ray ever used when the doctor has already made the diagnosis of cancer with other tools?

The initial x-ray will give the doctor a basis with which he can compare later x-rays, following the patient's progress and watching for changes in the lung tissue by comparing the early chest x-rays with later ones.

What other diagnostic tools does the doctor use to detect lung cancer?

There are several other diagnostic tools which can be used: They include sputum examination, bronchoscopy, tomogram, bronchogram, pulmonary-function test, biopsy, mediastinoscopy, bone scan, liver scan, brain scan, bone-marrow biopsy, thoracentesis, thoracoscopy, and thoractomy.

Isn't there a new test called sputum examination?

There are several new studies underway to try to find sensitive diagnostic tests which can be done easily, accurately, and inexpensively on a large number of people, since if lung cancer is found in its earliest stages, cure is possible in many cases. One such test that has already shown some success is sputum examination. The patient is asked to cough up some sputum (material coughed up from the lungs). The sputum is examined under a microscope to see if there are cancer cells present which have been shed from the inner lining of the breathing passages. Abnormal cells in the sputum can indicate a hidden cancer too small to be seen in x-ray photographs. The tumor is then located by such techniques as flexible fiberoptic bronchoscopy—this is an important part of the test because the sputum examination by itself does not tell the doctor where the tumor is located in the bronchial tree.

How is the sputum cytology test done?

You will be asked not to have anything to eat or drink except water or tea without milk. The nurse will give you a specimen jar which contains 50 percent alcohol to act as a fixative. You must cough very deeply and spit into the specimen jar. If you are unable to cough deeply enough the doctor will order a machine to assist in getting a good specimen.

What is a bronchoscopy?

A bronchoscopy is performed with the use of a rigid bronchoscope or a fiberoptic bronchoscope, depending on the location. The doctor using this instrument can look into the bronchial passages. The bronchoscope is a slender tube with a light at the far end which slides down the throat and into the bronchi.

Bronchoscopy sounds like a very uncomfortable procedure. Is it?

It doesn't need to be if you cooperate with your physician and the anesthesiologist. Local anesthesia is sprayed into the throat and bronchial tubes, making them feel numb. The bronchoscope is put into only one bronchus at a time, so you have no trouble breathing normally during the examination. You are relaxed and responsive to instructions and remain awake, although you will not remember much of the procedure afterward. Your head will be draped and your eyes covered. You will be asked to cough so that the doctor can obtain a good sample.

What does the doctor see during the bronchoscopy?

Looking through the bronchoscope, the doctor can illuminate the walls of the bronchi and examine the area. The development of new, flexible fiberoptic bronchoscopes means that the doctor can see around corners and into the inside of much smaller bronchial tubes. The flexibility of the instrument makes it possible for the doctor to take cell samples, using special attachments for biopsy, brushing, scraping, or washing.

How is that done?

Once the tumor is found, a small bit of liquid can be squirted through the bronchoscope onto the tumor and then withdrawn by suction. This liquid is then examined under the microscope for the presence of tumor cells, just as a sputum specimen might be. A slender cutting tool can be put through the bronchoscope. The doctor uses it to snip a small sample of tissue, which can then be examined under the microscope.

Are there any aftereffects of a bronchoscopy?

It is common for patients to cough up a small amount of blood after a specimen has been taken. This should be no cause for alarm. Some patients have a sore throat. Many people report no discomfort.

What is a tomogram? Is it related to a CT scan?

A tomogram or laminagram is a special chest x-ray, perfected within the last few years. If the regular chest x-ray shows a shadow in the lungs, tomograms can tell the physician more about the size, shape, or other characteristics of the lump. It is a series of pictures of various sections of lung tissue which when put together give a three-dimensional picture of abnormal lung growth. In cases of benign lumps, the tomogram tells the doctor enough about the tumor so he can make the diagnosis based on the tomogram pictures alone. If the tomogram suggests that the lump is cancerous, more tests will be needed to narrow down the diagnosis. Sometimes a newer type of tomogram also called a CT ("computerized tomography") scan proves to be helpful.

What is a bronchogram?

A bronchogram is another specialized x-ray examination which is sometimes used. A small amount of radiopaque dye is put into the bronchial tubes, and usually into the trachea after the area has been numbed. The patient is tilted into various positions to distribute the dye into the lungs and throughout the bronchi. X-rays are then taken.

What are pulmonary-function tests?

Pulmonary-function tests (also called lung-function tests) are given to measure your breathing and evaluate your ability to get oxygen into your blood. The tests measure the amount of air moving in and out of the lungs and indicate if there is an obstruction in the air passages. The tests give a baseline value of how well your lungs are presently functioning. The doctor will do these before the operation to be sure that your lungs are in good enough condition to keep you functioning even if a part of them is removed.

How are pulmonary-function tests done?

The test consists of various breathing exercises. It takes about one to two hours and will probably make you tired. You breathe pure oxygen. Then you have blood samples drawn. Cooperation is very important in this test and you must follow the instructions closely. The tests themselves are painless but time-consuming. In some places, radioactive materials and a camera or a computer are used in performing these tests.

Is a biopsy a necessary test?

A biopsy is an *essential* test. It means obtaining and examining a piece of tissue under the microscope. The tissue can be obtained in many different ways, as discussed above. You should remember that not all spots on the lungs are cancerous. As a matter of fact, according to the Mayo Clinic, an estimated 50–60 percent of lung biopsies are benign or noncancerous, depending on age. If lung cancer has spread to the lymph nodes in the neck or to other body tissues, a specimen of these might be taken for biopsy. When the pathologist studies a biopsy specimen under the microscope, he can identify the cell type of lung cancer along with its degree of malignancy.

What is a mediastinoscopy?

This is a minor surgical procedure that tells whether lung cancer has spread to the lymph nodes behind the breastbone in the area called the mediastinum. It is common for lung cancer to spread here first. The doctor passes an instrument through a small incision in the neck. You are anesthetized and asleep at the time. The nodes that are taken out are looked at by the pathologist. If they contain cancer, surgery may not be done. Radiation may be given instead to try to diminish or shrink the tumor tissue in the chest.

What is thoracentesis?

Fluid from the space between the lungs and the chest wall is removed by needle. A local anesthetic is applied to the skin where the needle will be inserted to minimize discomfort. Gentle suction draws the fluid through the needle into a syringe or bottle. There is then an examination of the fluid under the microscope to see if there are cancer cells. This test is usually used after other attempts to find cancer have failed. It can also be used to relieve pain or shortness of breath caused by the collection of fluid in the pleural space. This test can be done either in a hospital room or in an examining room.

What is a thorascopy?

This is a relatively new surgical procedure for diagnosing cancer in the lung. The patient is anesthetized and asleep in the operating room. A small incision is made between two ribs, and a slender tubular instrument is inserted into the space occupied by the lung. The instrument is much like a fiberoptic bronchoscope. When the instrument slips into the lung cavity, the lung is deflated and the thorascope can be used to examine the entire surface of the lung for tumor growth as well as the lining of the chest wall. Suspicious tissue is snipped, withdrawn through the thorascope, and given microscopic examination. The lung is reinflated at the end of the procedure. The lung not being examined remains expanded and able to function during the entire procedure.

This seems like a lot of tests. Are they all necessary?

Not all of the tests are done on all patients who are suspected of having lung cancer. However, it is important to have thorough testing and staging in lung cancer before any surgery is done. The time spent in doing diagnostic tests is time well spent. For example, if lung cancer has spread to the lymph nodes in the neck, to the opposite lung, or to other distant organs such as the liver or the brain, surgery alone will not cure it. Small-cell cancer of the lung is rarely cured by surgery. For it, other forms of treatment—chemotherapy and radiation—must be relied on. Operations for lung cancer (thoractomy with lobectomy or pneumonectomy) are major surgery and are usually not performed unless the patient stands a reasonable chance for cure.

Why would the doctor decide to give me radiation before he operates?

In some cases, depending on the size and the location of the tumor, radiation is given to shrink the size of the tumor. This can be done either in conjunction with the operation or in place of the operation, depending on the circumstances of the case.

Is radiation therapy sometimes used after surgery?

Yes. It can be used this way. About a month after the operation, when the chest tissues have had an opportunity to heal, radiation treatment may be started. Radiation is given to that part of the chest where metastases were found or seemed likely to occur. For more information on x-ray therapy, see Chapter 7.

Can x-ray therapy be given to the other lung if one has been removed?

Since radiotherapy to the lung can cause scar tissue to form, making it difficult for the lung to function, radiotherapy is usually not given to the opposite lung.

How does the doctor determine the stage of lung cancer when it is found?

The staging will include three sets of letters and numbers. The first two grade the tumor size, the second two indicate the nodal involvement, and the third pair relate to whether or not the tumor has metastasized. The general categories of staging and more information on how it is done can be found in Chapter 3.

The General Stages of Lung Cancer

STAGE	OTHER CLASSIFICATIONS	EXPLANATION
Occult:	TX N0 M0	This indicates secretions containing malignant cells but without other evidence of tumor or metastasis.
Stage I:	TIS M0 N0 T1 N0 M0 T1 N1 M0 T2 N0 M0	Carcinoma in situ or noninvasive cancer. This stage also includes tumors nearly 3 centimeters in size or less which have metastasized only to the lymph nodes or a tumor which may be larger but shows no signs of metastasis.
Stage II:	T2 N1 M0	A tumor larger than 3 centimeters with only a small amount of nearby lymph-node involvement.
Stage III:	T3 with any N or M N2 with any T or M M1 with any T or N	Any tumor more extensive than above or any tumor with metastasis to the lymph nodes in the mediastinum or any tumor with distant metastasis.

What treatment is most often recommended for the various stages?

- Stages I and II: Lobectomy or pneumonectomy with removal of suspected nodes. Postoperative radiation sometimes used.

- Stage III: Radiation therapy to primary and mediastinal nodes. Chemotherapy used, especially for the oat-cell variety.

Is surgery usually used for lung cancer?

Yes, in most cases. The doctor will usually operate if he feels that the entire tumor can be removed or if the operation will remove a portion of the tumor and will help the patient live with the disease better. If the cancer affects only one lobe it will be removed. If it affects both lobes on the left side or all three lobes on the right side, the whole lung on the involved side may be taken out. If the lymph nodes involved are around the main bronchus and the large blood vessels of the lungs or in the center of the chest, it might be possible to remove all of the malignancy as long as only one lung contains the cancer. The use of surgery and the operation which will be performed depend upon many factors.

What happens if the cancer has spread to the chest wall?

Again it depends upon the amount and location of the spread. It is possible to treat with surgery if the cancer has grown directly from the lung into a small area of the chest wall. Then the involved part of the chest wall is taken out along with the lung, and skin and muscle are used to cover the part of the wall which has been removed.

When is surgery not used?

Surgery usually is not the treatment—or not the only treatment— for lung cancer in which the tumor has grown directly into one or more of the important structures in the chest, such as the heart, the esophagus, large blood vessels, or windpipe, or if it has spread to the lymph nodes in the neck, to the opposite lung, or to other organs far from the lung, such as the liver, kidneys, or brain. When this happens, radiation and chemotherapy, used alone, in combination, or with surgery, are used, depending upon the location and the extent of the disease.

What if I decide I don't want my lung removed?

If your general health is good and it seems that the cancer is confined to one lobe or one lung, the doctor will probably recommend removal of the entire tumor. If all the cancer is removed, statistics show there is an excellent chance for recovery. Radiation following surgery is not usually necessary in cases where the entire cancer is removed. If surgery is not recommended, radiation therapy can be used. However, radiation therapy may not be as successful a treatment as surgery. New combination programs employing chemotherapy, as well as radiation and/or immunotherapy, are being tested. Chemotherapy has been found to be successful in treatment of lung cancer of the small-cell (oat-cell) variety.

What is a coin lesion?

This is a term sometimes used to refer to a small tumor of the lung which is confined to the lung without extension to adjacent structures. It is often found as the result of a routine chest x-ray. A coin lesion is considered to be potentially curable.

Where does lung cancer spread to most often?

Unfortunately, distant metastases can spread to virtually any organ of the body—liver, skeleton, and other lung, for instance. One of the most common sites for metastases is the brain. Radiation of the sites is usually used for treatment in these cases.

What are the various types of lung operations called?

The three most common types of lung operations are thoractomy, lobectomy, and pneumonectomy.

What is a thoracotomy?

This is a major operation used as a diagnostic tool when other diagnostic tests have failed to locate the tumor or to clarify the nature or extent of the tumor. The operation is performed in the operating room under anesthesia. It involves opening up the chest on one side and examining the lungs and nearby areas, such as lymph nodes. To perform the procedure, the doctor removes a rib or goes between two ribs, just below the shoulder blade. His cut follows the curve of the ribs, going from the back just under the shoulder blade around to the front of the chest. He spreads the ribs apart so he can see and work in the area of the lung. If a tumor is found, an immediate examination of it is made by the pathologist. If his report shows that the cell type of the tumor is favorable for operating, the surgical removal—lobectomy or pneumonectomy—is usually performed immediately.

What is a lobectomy?

A lobectomy involves the surgical removal of one lobe of the lung. The procedure for operating is similar to a thoractomy.

What is a pneumonectomy?

A pneumonectomy is the removal of the entire lung. Again, this is a major operation done in an operating room with the patient under anesthesia and follows the same procedure as the thoractomy.

Does the surgeon ever change his mind and not remove the lung?

If the surgeon finds that the cancer has spread too far for him to remove it all or is in an area where removal is impossible, he may leave the lung intact and close the incision. Then radiation and chemotherapy will be used to help shrink the tumor growth.

Will the surgeon ever remove the lung even though the cancer cannot be totally removed?

It depends on many conditions. If, for example, the tumor is causing serious bleeding and the patient is coughing up blood or if there is an infection with abscess formation, it may be necessary to remove the lung. X-ray therapy and chemotherapy will then be used to help reduce the remaining cancer.

How does the patient breathe during lung operations?

Special equipment is used to assist breathing. The other lung continues to breathe while the surgeon is working on the diseased lung.

After a lung operation, what happens to the space that's left in the chest?

Like empty closets, the space manages to get filled up. Body fluid and scar tissue take up most of the room. Structures from the opposite side shift toward the side of the operation. The other lung expands a little. At the beginning there may be a feeling of one-sidedness or emptiness on the side of the operation.

Where are the incisions made for a lung operation?

They are made beneath and behind the shoulder blade paralleling the ribs and will not be visible unless the back is exposed, as in a bathing suit.

How long do most lung-cancer operations take to perform?

Approximately two to four hours.

When can I get out of bed?

You will be up in from one to three days, depending upon the extent of the operation and your physical condition.

Will breathing be painful?

Breathing may be painful for about a week after the operation.

Is the incision painful?

Most people experience no pain. However, some find that scars are sensitive for several months.

Can a patient breathe and live normally after the removal of one or two lobes of the lung? After the entire lung is removed?

A patient can breathe and live normally after the removal of one or two lobes of the lung, except that there might be a slight restriction placed on strenuous physical exercise. Those with an entire lung removed tend to get short of breath when they exert themselves. But at rest, they breathe normally. Therefore, it is necessary to restrict their activity somewhat.

How long a hospital stay is necessary on the average?

Most doctors will send their patients home—barring complications—in about 10 to 14 days.

Why am I asked to cough after the operation?

Though it sounds cruel and though your entire insides hurt, coughing is necessary to dislodge secretions in the lungs. The nurse will explain just how it is done and will show you how to support the incision. Coughing is one of the most effective ways of keeping the lungs free of secretions and of avoiding complications. With any respiratory surgery done under general anesthesia, the area becomes dry and mucous plugs form at the lung bases. Coughing helps dislodge the mucus and helps prevent pneumonia.

Why are arm and leg exercises necessary following the operation?

Since the thoractomy incision usually runs under one arm, there may be a tendency to favor that arm and hold it close to the body. To prevent the arm and shoulder from getting tight, you can exercise it by bringing the affected arm up slowly in front of the body to shoulder height and extending it out to the side to shoulder height. Simple leg exercises should be performed while in bed to help prevent phlebitis. You will probably be wearing elastic stockings to help decrease the possibility of phlebitis.

What should I know about the chest-drainage equipment?

The tube is there to permit drainage of any air or fluid that accumulates during surgery and will usually remain in place after surgery for two to four days. The first few days the tube will drain bloody fluid. This is normal. Each day, the amount of drainage will decrease and the color will get lighter. The tube is sutured to the skin and will not come out during deep breathing or coughing. In fact, you will be encouraged to get up, to take deep breaths, and to cough. This will help the lung to expand and will force out the air and fluid that has accumulated in the lung area. The only caution you must take is not to allow the tube to kink up or to fold over, since this can cause pressure to build up in the chest, resulting in pain or shortness of breath. It will probably not hurt when the tube is taken out.

Why does it hurt when I lift my arms or take a deep breath?

Sometimes this happens after lung surgery and is due to the surgery. Your nurse or doctor will instruct you in breathing deeply—you will be encouraged to breathe each time to the point of pain. Amazingly enough, the pain on breathing will go away more quickly if you breathe deeply than if you try to prevent the lung pain by shallow breathing.

Will I be needing intravenous fluids?

Probably, for at least 24 hours after the operation.

Can I catch lung cancer by kissing someone who has it?

There is no indication that cancer can be "caught" by kissing a person. There is also no evidence to suggest that living in the same household with a cancer patient, sharing his or her possessions, or being physically intimate over a long period of time will increase a person's chances of getting cancer. You should not be afraid that you will "catch" cancer.

I have recently had an operation in which one lung was removed. I am very depressed and tired. I can't even climb the stairs without being short of breath. Does that mean that my cancer is worse?

No. Many patients complain of fatigue after a lung operation. Remember that the body needs to repair itself after any operation—and surgery in which a lung is removed is a major operation. Take time and rest and do not worry. When your body gets adjusted to having only one lung, you will be able to climb stairs more easily. Try not to get depressed over it.

Suggested Reading

Cox, Barbara G. *Living with Lung Cancer.* Rochester, Minn.: Mayo Foundation, 1977. Order from Schmidt Printing, Inc., 1416 Valley High Drive N.W., Rochester, Minn. 55601. $2.55.

chapter 13

Skin Cancers

Those Most Likely to Get Skin Cancer

- Light-skinned persons living in the southern part of the country
- Persons who have had excessive exposure to the sun without protection, such as farmers, seamen, ranchers, etc.
- Persons over 40 years of age, males more often than females
- Persons with fair complexion whose skin sunburns rather than tans
- Relatives of persons with basal-cell skin cancer
- Persons who have had excessive exposure to x-rays

Symptoms of Skin Cancer

- Any lesion which forms a scab, rescabs and fails to heal
- A scaly skin thickening which develops in a small area, usually on face, neck, or hands
- A molelike growth that increases in size, becomes ulcerated, and may bleed easily
- A pearly or waxy growth
- Any sore, blister, patch, pimple, or other blemish that does not show signs of healing within two to three weeks.

Tests for Skin Cancer

- Excisional biopsy for lesions of less than 2 centimeters
- Incisional biopsy for larger lesions
- If doctor suspects melanoma, electrocautery biopsy or electro-excision should *never* be performed. If there is any question, ask for a second pathologist's opinion.

What do I need to remember?

- Skin cancer is the most common kind of cancer, is the most easily diagnosed and treated, and is the most curable.
- Ninety-five percent of skin-cancer patients are free of their disease following medically approved treatment (usually surgery).
- Any sore, blister, patch, pimple, or other skin blemish that does not heal in two to three weeks should be seen by a doctor.

Questions to Ask Your Doctor About Skin Cancer

- What kind of skin cancer do I have?
- What kind of treatment will you give me? Why?
- What are the alternatives?
- Will I need a skin graft?
- Who will do it?
- How extensive will it be?

What kind of doctor should I see if I have symptoms of skin cancer?

You should see your own family doctor or a dermatologist. If you have malignant melanoma, a surgeon specializing in cancer treatment or an oncologist should be handling your case. If you need reconstructive work done as a result of some kind of skin cancer, a plastic surgeon, dermatologist, otolaryngologist, or maxillofacial surgeon would be the doctor of choice.

Skin Cancer

Type	Symptoms	Treatment	Remarks
Basal-cell	Raised lump. Center sometimes a crusted sore. Skin covering it looks tense and shiny, sometimes pearly. Usually found on head or neck. Sometimes on face, nose, or upper lip. Rarely found on trunk or body.	Surgery, radiation, heat, freezing, chemotherapy drugs, immunotherapy	Most common form of skin cancer. Found in lowest skin layer. Grows more slowly. Does not metastasize. Rarely spreads. Tends to run in families. Most common in men over 50.
Squamous-cell	Usually looks similar to basal-cell cancer. Lump raised from skin surface. Sometimes looks like wart. Usually scaly without center ulcer. Found on neck, face, near lower lip, ear, on hands.	Same as basal-cell	Next most common form but seen much less frequently than basal-cell. More likely to spread than basal-cell. Can metastasize. Generally seen in persons over 60.
Malignant melanoma	Mole which changes in size or appearance. Red, white, or blue specks appear in long-standing moles. Moles that bleed, become darker in color, or have tiny dark spots appearing in skin around them.	Surgery, chemotherapy, radiation	Relatively rare. Much more serious than basal-cell and squamous-cell. Be sure to have qualified cancer specialist. Difficult to diagnose and treat.
Mycosis fungoides (not a true skin cancer, but manifested first in skin tumors)	Reddish, plaquelike tumors of scaly, thickened skin. Itchy.	Chemotherapy drugs, radiation therapy	Thought to be related to Hodgkin disease. Lymph-node involvement.

Is the National Cancer Institute supporting any studies on skin cancer?

The National Cancer Institute's Clinical Cooperative Groups are presently studying new treatment methods for malignant melanoma and mycosis fungoides, two types of skin cancer (see Chapter 23).

What is the skin?

The skin is one of the largest organs in the body. It has two main layers with several sublayers. The main top layer is called the epidermis, and the main underlying layer of connective tissue is called the dermis. The two skin layers together with specialized structures (such as nerves, hair, nails, and various types of glands) protect the body from injury, receive sensory impulses, excrete waste products, and regulate body temperature. The skin in performing these functions is constantly exposed to the sun, wind, industrial elements, and other harsh external and internal stresses.

What results from these exposures?

What usually results are benign abnormalities. However, sometimes the results are malignant. When they are malignant, they develop as two main kinds of skin cancer, which are distinguished by the cell type: basal-cell cancer and squamous-cell cancer.

Is it true that skin cancer is the most common cancer?

Yes. Skin cancer is the most common form of cancer. Fortunately, it is also one of the easiest to diagnose and to find at an early stage. It is estimated that 45–50 percent of all persons living to age 65 will have had at least one skin cancer.

Is skin cancer curable?

Yes. Today, 95 percent of skin-cancer patients are free of their disease following medically approved treatment. If patients were to seek medical attention early enough, it is possible that the cure rate could be even higher—98 percent or even 100 percent. And most skin cancer can be treated either in an outpatient clinic or in a doctor's office.

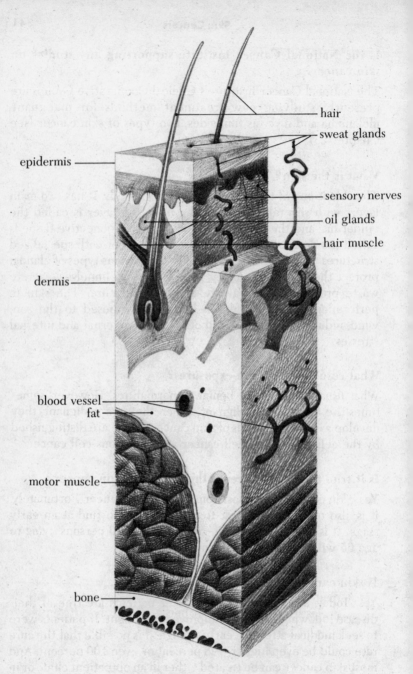

hair

sweat glands

epidermis

sensory nerves

oil glands

hair muscle

dermis

blood vessel

fat

motor muscle

bone

Cross-section of skin (enlarged)

342

Do the rays from sunlamps cause skin cancer?

Many sunlamps produce ultraviolet radiation that, like ultraviolet rays from the sun, can cause eye injuries, skin burns, and possibly even cancer. In addition, some sunlamps also give out ultraviolet rays of a short wavelength that can be dangerous to the cell structure of your body. Most of the time, the cells repair the damage. But sometimes this results in changes in cell character called mutations. Some mutations may be cancerous. The FDA is developing a performance standard for sunlamps, because they are potentially hazardous. The standard would require that sunlamps prominently display warning labels and that they have timers that shut them off automatically.

Do black people get skin cancer?

Most skin cancer is directly related to overexposure to the sun's damaging ultraviolet rays, and while black people do indeed develop skin cancer, they do so much less often than people with lighter skin. The pigmentation in their skin, a substance called melanin, protects them. Very fair people are most susceptible to skin cancer.

I've heard that arsenic causes skin cancer. Is that true?

Arsenic in the form of Fowler's solution was used to treat problems like asthma and psoriasis some 20 years ago. Doctors are reporting that some people who used arsenic for prolonged periods have developed skin cancer.

Are there different kinds of skin cancer?

Yes, there are two basic common kinds of skin cancer—basal-cell cancer and squamous-cell cancer. The overwhelming proportion of skin cancers are basal-cell cancer. Squamous-cell cancers are next most common but are seen much less frequently than basal-cell cancers. There are two other conditions which are quite uncommon, but which also appear on the skin. They are malignant melanoma and mycosis fungoides. These are not strictly classified as skin cancer because they are not confined to the skin, but they will be discussed later in this chapter.

What is basal-cell cancer?

Basal cells are spherical and are found in the lowest layer of the epidermis. The cancer involving these cells is the most common kind of skin cancer. You usually notice a lump that is about ¼ to ½ inch across. The edge of the lump is raised; sometimes the center is depressed and is an open sore. The skin covering it looks tense and shiny, even pearly. The lump enlarges at the point where it began. When it ulcerates in the middle, it becomes covered with a scab or crust. Basal-cell cancer grows slowly and rarely metastasizes, but if not treated for a long time, this slow-growing cancer penetrates the layers of tissue below the skin's surface and involves the bone.

Where is basal-cell cancer usually found on the body?

About 90 percent of these cancers are found on the neck and head. Many times they are found on the face, around the nose or upper lip. They are not usually found on the trunk. Basal-cell cancer rarely spreads to the lymph nodes, so usually a simple removal assures a permanent cure. Since basal-cell cancer rarely metastasizes, it is the most curable skin cancer.

What is squamous-cell cancer?

Most of the epidermis is composed of squamous cells, which are flat. Squamous-cell cancer is less common than basal-cell but it is more serious, because it is more likely to spread to the lymph nodes and it metastasizes more often. Squamous-cell cancer grows more rapidly than does basal-cell cancer. As with basal-cell, you usually first notice it when the lump is about ¼ to ½ inch across. The lump is raised from the skin surface slightly, sometimes looking like a wart. It doesn't have the shiny surface of the basal-cell cancer. Instead it is usually scaly without a central pit or ulcer. Squamous-cell cancer metastasizes but usually not until the primary cancer has been present for a long time.

Can you really tell the difference between the two kinds by looking at them?

A skilled dermatologist or a doctor experienced in detecting skin cancer may be able to tell the difference by looking at them. However, sometimes they look like benign growths and further tests are needed to determine whether they are cancerous.

What are the major things I should be checking?

You might notice a pimple or a small sore that hasn't healed or disappeared but instead is gradually growing bigger. Or you may have had a skin lesion for many years which has started to grow or become irritated. As noted before, any pale, waxy, pearly-looking lump which eventually becomes an open sore or red, scaly, sharply outlined patches should be seen by a doctor.

Moles which change in appearance or size are especially important to watch. Go to the doctor at once if any red, white, or particularly blue specks appear in a long-standing mole. Moles that are a uniform bluish-black, bluish-gray, or of uneven surface also should be looked at by a doctor. If the mole begins to bleed, becomes darker in color, or has other tiny dark spots appearing in the skin around it, it may have become a malignant melanoma—a condition which will be discussed later in this chapter. You should remember that any sore, blister, patch, pimple, or other skin blemish that does not heal in two to three weeks should be seen by a doctor.

Can skin cancer spread to other parts of the body?

Yes, skin cancer is still cancer, and although it grows slowly and usually doesn't metastasize, if it does spread to the structures beneath it, it may be necessary to do extensive and sometimes disfiguring surgery. As with all cancer, the best safeguard against it is early treatment.

What are precancers?

An abnormal skin condition that tends to become cancerous at a later date is referred to as precancer. The most common are senile or actinic (sun-ray) keratosis and hyperkeratosis. Since they tend to become malignant, these precancerous conditions should be checked regularly.

What is keratosis?

Keratosis is a scaly skin thickening which develops in a small area, usually on the face, neck or hands. It usually develops in older persons whose skin has been exposed for many years to the ultraviolet rays of the sun. In older persons it is referred to as senile or actinic keratosis, and this variety frequently occurs on the unexposed parts of the body such as the chest, back, or arms.

There are several varieties, some are benign, some may become cancerous and should be checked by the doctor regularly.

What is leukoplakia?

This is a condition, resembling keratosis, which occurs as a white thickening on the lip or tongue or in the mouth. It frequently occurs in heavy pipe smokers and tobacco chewers.

What is hyperkeratosis?

This is a precancerous condition that appears as a scaly patch or small scab of the skin in a sharply limited, usually small area. Hyperkeratoses are usually caused by exposure to direct strong sunlight and to hot drying wind. They are nearly always found on the face, neck, and hands.

What is Bowen's disease? Is it a kind of skin cancer?

Yes. Bowen's disease is a rare form of skin cancer. It often occurs in several primary sites. The growth is reddish-pink, raised with scaling. It usually occurs on the unexposed areas of the skin. Some doctors regard it as a precancerous condition. Sometimes it is associated with internal malignancies.

What is sweat-gland cancer?

It is a very rare kind of cancer that may metastasize to the lymph nodes or to distant sites. It can originate from any gland but usually occurs near the anus, eyelids, ears, armpits, and scrotum.

What is xeroderma?

Xeroderma is an inherited condition. It is thought to be a precancerous disease. The skin is irregularly pigmented and scaly and later becomes thin, ulcerated, and scarred. It is strongly sensitized to sunlight, and cancer occurs on the areas which have been exposed to it, even briefly.

What is a lipoma?

Lipomas are not cancerous. They are soft, fatty tumors that lie directly beneath the skin. They are the most common tumor in the body. They can be small like a pea or as big as a grapefruit. You can find them almost anywhere on the body. Usually they are underneath the skin of the trunk or the neck or on the arms and legs. They feel soft and move freely under the skin. They are usually not firmly attached to surrounding structures. If they are somewhere where you can see them or if they show signs of growth, the doctor might remove them for cosmetic reasons. Removal is usually done in the hospital. However, they are usually not removed. They do not cause pain and rarely become cancerous. If they do become malignant, they will show rapid growth and the feel of the tissue will change.

Do warts ever turn into cancer?

No. Warts do not turn into cancer.

What are hemangiomas?

Hemangiomas are usually nonmalignant. They are blood-vessel tumors of the skin. They may appear at any time from birth to old age on any part of the body. They look like red spots on the skin and can be anywhere from the size of a pinhead to the size of a nickel. Sometimes they bleed if they are in an area which gets irritated, such as a man's face. Most of them are harmless and do not grow. They very rarely become malignant. Doctors usually do not remove them unless they are unsightly.

What is a ganglion?

A ganglion is not a cancer. It is a thin-walled cyst which appears in the tendons or joints. It is filled with a colorless, jellylike substance. Ganglions are usually seen on the inside wrists of children and young adults.

What is a sebaceous cyst?

Sebaceous cysts, or wens, are thin-walled sacs which contain a soft cheeselike material. The openings of the glands which secrete oils into the skin (sebaceous glands) get clogged and the cysts develop. They can be the size of a nut or get as big as a plum. Usually you find them on the scalp, on the upper back, behind the ear, or on the neck and face.

Do sebaceous cysts turn into cancer?

These cysts rarely turn into cancer. Those which are stable in size usually are left alone unless they are located in areas where there is constant or repeated irritation. When cysts increase in size over a period of weeks or months, they are usually removed. Sometimes they become infected and are treated with warm wet packs or antibiotics or, if needed, with incision and drainage. These cysts can be removed in the doctor's office or in the hospital.

What is a fibroma?

Skin fibromas very rarely form cancer. They are small, hard lumps about the size of a cherry pit. They are quite common and sometimes are referred to as fibrous tumors. They are not usually removed.

Are there any other skin conditions which are not cancerous?

Yes, there are several others. Seborrheic keratoses (raised, warty-looking, appear to be stuck onto the skin's surface, easy to scrape off with a fingernail), skin tags (papilloma—little outpatchings of skin), syringomas (benign tumor caused by an enlarged sweat gland), histiocytomas (solitary, well-rounded firm nodule), senile lentigo (liver spots), and sebaceous hyperplasia (shiny, yellow, waxy-oily tumors) are skin conditions that are almost always benign and rarely turn into cancer.

Can a tattoo cause skin cancer?

No, a tattoo usually does not cause cancer. However, if there is itching or bubbling around the edges, it should be checked by a doctor.

How can I tell whether or not a growth is cancerous?

You cannot. You should bring any skin change to the attention of your doctor. Only a physician can determine the nature of an abnormal skin growth—whether it is benign, precancerous, or malignant.

Can a doctor tell just by looking whether or not a growth is cancerous?

An experienced doctor can tell when a growth looks suspicious and will order a biopsy to make a definite diagnosis. The doctor will take out the entire lesion if it is small, or if it is large he will take a small wedge of it for the biopsy. As with all cancers, the only way the doctor can be sure whether or not a growth is malignant is on the basis of a biopsy, in which the cells are examined under the microscope.

How does skin cancer spread?

Basal-cell and squamous-cell cancer typically spreads by sending out tentacles through the surrounding tissues. Although these kinds of skin cancer may be destructive locally, they seldom metastasize or spread to bones, lungs, or other organs.

Should all growths on the skin be removed?

No, most growths on the skin need not be removed. They should be seen by a doctor if:
- They show a change, such as increase in size.
- They are painful.
- They become infected.
- They bleed.
- They are being irritated by something such as a bra strap, a belt, shaving, etc.

Should all skin growths which are cancerous be removed?

Yes. They should be treated with some kind of therapy.

Are any tests other than a biopsy needed for skin cancer?

It depends on what the biopsy shows. If the biopsy shows squamous-cell cancer, a chest x-ray is usually taken, particularly if the growth is large. Although metastases are rare, if they do occur, they are likely to be in the lung. Also if the biopsy shows squamous-cell cancer the physician is likely to check the lymph nodes in the area.

How are skin tumors classified?

The following designations are used:
- TIS: Preinvasive carcinoma
- T0:   No primary tumor present
- T1:   Tumor 2 centimeters or less in its largest dimension, no perceptible depth
- T2:   Tumor more than 2 centimeters but not more than 5 centimeters in its largest dimension or with minimal infiltration of the dermis, irrespective of size

How are skin tumors classified? (continued)

- T3:   Tumor more than 5 centimeters in its largest dimension or with deep infiltration of the dermis regardless of size
- T4:   Tumor involving other structures such as cartilage, muscle, or bone

Sometimes N or M classifications are added if there is nodal involvement or metastases. More information on staging can be found in Chapter 3.

How is skin cancer treated?

There are several ways of treating skin cancer. The most common ones are surgery and radiation therapy. However, heat, freezing, chemotherapy, and immunotherapy are all being used in some instances.

What factors determine the treatment used?

The treatment depends upon many things: the type of growth, its location, its size, the rate of growth, the degree of extension and metastasis, and whether or not it is a recurring growth. The doctor must also take into account the physical condition of the patient and how the person might respond to the various treatments. The treatment chosen should be the one which will give the best results both medically and cosmetically. The patient's preference should be taken into consideration.

When are surgery and radiation therapy used?

A small growth which is easily accessible is usually removed completely by surgery in the doctor's office. If the growth is large or is in a place where the surgery might leave a disfiguring scar, the procedure would be different. A biopsy would be done by removing a piece of the growth and having it checked microscopically to make sure it is cancer. If it is, there are several alternatives. Surgery would generally be used if it would leave a smaller and less visible scar. Radiation would be the treatment in areas where it gives better cosmetic results. For example, in an area such as the eyelids, where surgery would involve additional reconstructive work, radiation or one or more of the other treatments might be recommended.

When is a curette used?

A curette is a surgical instrument used to take out some lesions. Many of the skin tumors are scraped off the skin either with a scalpel blade or a curette—a stainless-steel hand tool. The open bottom has sharp edges which pry away a raised lesion.

When are heat or freezing used?

Electrocautery and the use of electric needles are sometimes used on small cancers. This treatment is usually performed in the office and healing takes place in a week or two. Cryosurgery is showing some promising results—the cancer is subjected to subzero temperatures without damage to underlying vital structures such as cartilage.

How does an electric needle work?

Sometimes the doctor uses an electric needle to take out the growth. He holds a stylus whose point is giving out raw cutting electricity. The amount of electricity is regulated with a foot pedal. Sometimes this treatment is called desiccation, which means "drying up."

When are chemotherapeutic drugs and immunotherapy used?

Chemotherapeutic drugs such as 5-FU in the form of ointment have been effective for both cancers and precancers of the skin. Chemotherapy and immunotherapy are used to treat melanoma and mycosis fungoides when these tumors have spread or to prevent spread.

Are the different treatments ever combined? Are the treatments for skin cancer usually repeated over a long period of time?

Sometimes one treatment is sufficient. In other circumstances, repeated treatments are necessary. In some cases, a combination of methods may be used. Again, it depends upon the individual case.

Does skin cancer recur?

Yes. Skin cancer is one of the most common recurrent cancers. A person with skin cancer has a 50–60 percent chance of having a second cancer, usually another skin cancer. Therefore, patients should have followup visits two to four times a year.

Are operations for removal of skin cancer, especially around the eyes and the mouth, disfiguring?

No, they need not be. Usually some kind of skin graft or other plastic surgery is done so that a person with these skin cancers on the face need not worry about disfigurement.

What is malignant melanoma?

Malignant melanoma is a rare form of skin cancer. It is dangerous because, unlike the other skin cancers, it metastasizes early and spreads quickly. It is one of the more uncontrollable cancers. Sometimes malignant melanoma is called black cancer because as a rule the lesion is black or dark-brown. The cell involved is the melanocyte, which is a melanin-producing cell located in the basal layer of the epidermis or in the portion of the skin just below.

What are the symptoms of malignant melanoma?

Malignant melanoma usually begins with a flat or slightly elevated brown spot that is somewhere between ¼ to 1 inch across. It looks like the moles which you have in other places on your body. Some begin in a preexisting mole. It is very important to remember that any mole that shows signs of change—moles which suddenly start growing or bleeding, moles which become darker or lighter in color, moles which have darker spots in the skin around them, moles that have red, white, or particularly blue specks in them, moles that are uniform bluish-black or bluish-gray or have an uneven surface—should be examined by a doctor. Although most moles are benign, if any of these changes occur in a mole that you have had for years, you should immediately go to the doctor.

Should moles which do not show any change be removed?

No. Moles (or nevi as the doctors usually call them) are very common in various places on the body. It is estimated that most people have from 15 to 50 of them on the body. Since melanoma is relatively rare—about 1 to 2 percent of all human cancers—the odds that any one mole will become malignant melanoma are less than one in several million. It would be impractical to recommend removal of all moles.

Are there any places on the body where moles should be removed?

Moles on the palms of the hands, the soles of the feet, or the genitalia are more apt to turn into malignant melanoma than are moles elsewhere. In addition, if you have a mole in a location that is likely to be repeatedly irritated, such as where a brassiere strap rubs, or where it might be nicked in shaving, it is wise to have it removed. You can have this done in a doctor's office or in an outpatient clinic in the hospital. Usually it will be examined under the microscope just to make certain it is not cancerous.

I am pregnant. The moles on my body are getting darker. Should I be worried about that?

No. Moles on a woman's body may become darker than usual during pregnancy. This is normal and not a sign of melanoma, but you should mention it to your obstetrician.

Is it true that a hair growing from a mole means that the mole is not malignant?

Most doctors agree that the presence of hair suggests that a mole is not malignant, but this is not a hard-and-fast rule. As with any other mole, any change in the color, size, or shape should be regarded as a symptom that should be investigated by the doctor.

Where do melanomas usually occur?

Melanomas can start anywhere there is pigment, but about 80 percent of them start from the skin. Other sites of origin are the eye, intestines, and salivary glands. Skin lesions are commonest on the lower extremity, frequently occur on the head and neck, and occur less often on the trunk.

Who usually gets melanoma?

About 70 to 80 percent of malignant melanoma of the skin occurs in light-complexioned, sandy-haired, freckled individuals. It is most commonly seen in persons between 30 and 60 years old and is about evenly distributed between men and women. It is very rare in black persons.

Where does malignant melanoma metastasize?

Malignant melanoma can metastasize to any part of the body but most commonly to the lungs, liver, and brain. The cells in malignant melanoma show a tendency to metastasize early, traveling through the lymph system and/or the blood system. The commonest route of spread is to the regional lymph nodes.

What kind of doctor will be used to treat melanomas?

Melanomas are usually found by dermatologists, who usually perform the biopsy, which is then read by a pathologist. If the lesion is found to be malignant, further treatment should be carried out by a specialist—either a surgeon who specializes in cancer or an oncologist.

Is there more than one kind of malignant melanoma?

There are three fairly distinct forms of primary (original-site) melanoma. They are superficial spreading melanoma, nodular melanoma, and lentigo maligna melanoma. Superficial spreading melanoma and nodular melanoma start from a preexisting mole or as a new growth. Lentigo maligna (also known as Hutchinson's melanotic freckle) is a relatively rare tissue abnormality which tends to occur in areas of the body exposed to the sun in light-skinned individuals.

What will the doctor do to a mole which has shown some change?

The doctor will arrange to have it removed for examination under the microscope. If it is small, he will take out the whole mole. If it is large, a partial biopsy will be done. It is generally considered wise for the doctor to take out the entire mole if possible, although there is no strong scientific evidence that a partial biopsy is harmful to the patient.

Is it easy for the pathologist to tell whether or not the mole is malignant melanoma?

Diagnosis of this kind calls for an experienced pathologist, since malignant melanoma is a very difficult cancer to diagnose correctly. If there is any doubt at all about the diagnosis, the slides should be reviewed by several pathologists before any decision about treatment is made.

After biopsy, what other tests are needed before treating malignant melanoma?

Usually, before any treatment is begun, a complete evaluation is undergone by patients with malignant melanoma. This usually includes a complete physical, documentation of the size and location of any tumor present, the site of primary origin, a history of past and current symptoms, complete blood count, a survey of blood chemistry, and a chest x-ray. In addition, if needed, a bone-marrow aspiration and biopsy, x-rays of the skull and lumbar spine, liver and spleen scans, an electroencephalogram and brain scan, and a stool examination for the presence of occult blood are done.

The General Stages of Malignant Melanoma

STAGE	OTHER CLASSIFICATIONS	EXPLANATION
Stage I	Any T or N0 Any T N0 M0	Localized to area or site of origin
Stage II	Any Ta, Tb N0 or N1 M0	Spread confined to regional lymph nodes
Stage III	Any T, Ta or Tb, any N, M1 or M2 Any T, Ta or Tb, N1 or N2, and M	Disseminated spread to lymph nodes, multiple cutaneous and/or subcutaneous sites or organs

What is the treatment for malignant melanoma?

The treatment for malignant melanoma depends upon the location, extent, and stage of the disease. If the microscopic examination shows that the mole is a malignant melanoma, then further surgery is usually done. The doctor will remove some of the normal-appearing skin around the mole. Sometimes the nearby lymph glands are also removed.

Is chemotherapy ever used for malignant melanoma?

Sometimes single-drug or combination chemotherapy is used, usually in combination with surgery or immunotherapy. If a limited treatment of a single part or organ of the body is needed, chemotherapy in isolation perfusion (introducing the drug to an isolated part of the circulatory system) may be the treatment.

Is radiation treatment ever used for malignant melanoma?

Although surgery is generally considered the treatment of choice for malignant melanoma, radiation therapy is sometimes used for treatment, especially for those patients who cannot have an operation for some reason. Radiotherapy is used in certain eye tumors and is frequently used to control localized pain.

What is the role of immunotherapy in malignant melanoma?

There is a great amount of research now going on in the use of immunotherapy as an adjuvant therapy for malignant melanoma. Clinical trials are being conducted with immunostimulants such as BCG.

Will reconstructive surgery be needed in a person with malignant melanoma?

It depends upon the location and the extent of the operation. Patients with facial and neck areas involved usually need cosmetic surgery, either skin grafts or other plastic surgery.

What is a skin graft?

A portion of healthy skin is taken from one area of your body (called the donor site) and moved to another area (called the recipient site). In skin cancer, such grafts cover the areas that have been left bare by the surgical removal of portions of the skin. The skin is usually taken from the back or thigh or other part of the body and is stitched to the injured part. The graft is nourished by small arteries from the tissue surrounding the injured area.

Are there different ways of doing skin grafts?

There are several different ways:
- *Pinch grafts:* Small pieces, usually about ¼ inch in diameter, are taken from the uppermost layer of the skin and spaced in the area missing the skin. The small pieces grow in the new location and spread out to cover the bare area. This method is used usually in very small areas such as the eyelid.

- *Split-thickness grafts:* These are sheets of skin, sometimes measuring several inches in diameter, taken from the uppermost layer of flat surfaces such as the back, the thigh, or the stomach. This method is used when a larger area needs to be covered. Stitches are taken around the edges of the grafts and compression bandages are put on top.
- *Full-thickness grafts:* These contain all the layers of the skin but not the fat tissue which lies underneath. They are used in areas subject to friction or in weight-bearing areas. The grafts are cut so that they will exactly cover the bare area.
- *Pedicle grafts:* One portion of the skin remains attached to the donor site while the rest is transferred to a recipient site. These are used to cover defects on the face when a wide area of skin has been removed along with the tumor or to cover a finger or hand with new skin.

Are skin-graft operations dangerous?

No. The doctor must be sure that both the donor site and the recipient site are free from infection. The graft must be evenly applied and held in place snugly.

Is it painful to have a skin graft?

No. There is usually only a little pain and a burning sensation in the area from which the skin has been taken and no pain at the site where it is applied.

What is used to cover the skin graft when it is done?

Firm bandages are used to keep the graft snugly applied to the area. The dressing is not changed for one or two weeks until the grafted skin is living and growing in its new location.

Does the grafted skin look like the normal skin?

This depends upon where the graft is taken from. Sometimes it might be a different color and texture. The graft will develop sensation after a few months. The new skin can get sunburned but often it does not get as dark as the surrounding skin. The new skin will grow hair only if it grew hair in its original location.

What kind of doctor would do a skin graft?

It depends upon the size and the type of grafting which needs to be done. Facial procedures are done by dermatologists, otolaryngologists, maxillofacial surgeons and plastic surgeons.

Are there some precautions that can be taken to help protect against skin cancer?

Avoid repeated overexposure to the sun, especially between 10 a.m. and 2 p.m. when most of the sun's total ultraviolet radiation reaches the earth's surface. Repeated sunburns accumulate damage to the skin that eventually can develop into skin cancer. Use a sunscreen preparation to absorb ultraviolet rays or use a sunblock preparation that will deflect ultraviolet rays. Tan gradually. If you are not able to tan, don't risk sunburning. When you play outdoors—tennis, baseball, sailing—use sunblock preparation and avoid the midday sun. Wear protective clothing, such as long-sleeved shirts and wide-brimmed hats, especially if you work outdoors. If you're a farmer, put a canopy on your tractor. If there is a history of skin cancer in your family and you have skin similar to those members, be more cautious when outdoors.

Are some sunscreens better than others?

Look for sunscreens which contain benzophenone or para-aminobenzoic acid, usually abbreviated "PABA." You should apply sunscreens evenly and reapply them often when you are outside, especially after swimming and when playing tennis.

What is the difference between a sunscreen and a sunblock?

Sunscreens selectively screen out redness-producing rays. Sunblocks screen out everything. If you are the kind of person who cannot tolerate any exposure at all, the best sunblock for you is zinc-oxide paste. You can buy this over the counter. If you need even more protection, use a sunscreen with PABA plus a titanium-dioxide paste. Your druggist can make this up for you.

I hear that when you are taking some kinds of medicine you get a worse sunburn. Is that true?

Yes, it is true. There are some substances that are photosensitizing—that is, when you are taking them you can get a bad sunburn from relatively little exposure. Among them are birth-control pills, thiazide diuretics (prescribed for high blood pressure), oral hypoglycemics (antidiabetic drugs), and Thorazine (tranquilizer). Also watch out for saccharin, halogenated salicylanilides (the active ingredient in deodorant soap), oil of bergamot (used in most perfumes), and essences of lemon and lime (in many aftershave lotions and bath soaps). Persons taking some of the chemotherapeutic drugs or who have had radiation must be careful to protect their skins from sunburn.

I borrowed suntan lotion from a person who has skin cancer. Can I catch cancer from using the suntan lotion?

No. Cancer is not an illness which you can catch from someone else. Although the exact cause of many cancers is unknown, after many tests and studies, the results show that cancer is not contagious in humans. Skin cancer is most often caused by overexposure to the sun. Using suntan lotions, swimming in pools where patients swim or kissing a cancer patient in no way increases the risks of contracting cancer.

What is mycosis fungoides?

Mycosis fungoides is an uncommon chronic type of malignancy which can last for many years. In its early stages it usually affects the skin and may stay confined to one area for years. Eventually the lymph nodes and internal organs may become involved.

Is mycosis fungoides some kind of fungus?

The disease was named several centuries ago when it was thought that the disease was due to some kind of a fungus. It has long been recognized that it is a disease primarily affecting the reticuloendothelial system—cells scattered throughout the body which destroy other cells, bacteria, and fragments of foreign materials, form antibodies, and regulate the immune reaction and the formation of blood cells.

Is mycosis fungoides a form of leukemia?

Because it may arise simultaneously in many different areas of the skin, mycosis fungoides is thought to be related to Hodgkin disease and leukemia, two other systemic cancers which affect the lymph and blood systems. However, mycosis fungoides has a tendency to remain confined to the skin for long periods of time, unlike Hodgkin disease and leukemia, which spread rapidly if untreated.

What are the stages of mycosis fungoides?

There are three stages of the disease. The first is called the promycotic stage. Reddish, plaquelike tumors of scaly, thickened skin develop. They itch and have a tendency to spread and ulcerate. The plaques, which may resemble eczema or psoriasis, may be found almost anywhere—on the back, arms, stomach, face, or scalp. This stage can persist for several years or longer without distinctive biopsy changes which would enable a positive diagnosis to be made.

The second stage is the infiltration stage. The skin becomes infiltrated with an overgrowth of the reticuloendothelial cells of several kinds. This allows a microscopic diagnosis to be made.

In the third stage, large tumors develop on the skin. They may become ulcerated, painful, and odoriferous.

How is mycosis fungoides treated?

In the first stage, treatment is directed to relieving the itching. Soothing baths, antihistamines, and topical steroid creams are sometimes used. As the tumors become more advanced, radiation therapy may be the treatment. Nitrogen mustard may be used topically. Chemotherapy may be prescribed as the disease progresses. Sometimes radiation treatment is added to the chemotherapy.

chapter 14

Adult Leukemia and Lymphoma

What is leukemia?

Leukemia is a cancer of the blood-forming tissues characterized primarily by uncontrolled multiplication and accumulation of abnormal white blood cells.

What causes leukemia?

The cause of leukemia is not known. Certain specific factors, such as excessive exposure to radiation and possibly to certain chemicals, such as benzene, have been identified as maybe having some connection to the onset of leukemia. Certain viruses are known to cause leukemia in animals, but this has not been proved so in humans.

Isn't leukemia a children's disease?

Though it is thought of by many people as a disease that only strikes children, leukemia actually affects more adults than children. More than half of all leukemias occur in persons over 60 years of age. ALL is the type of leukemia that appears most often in children and young adults. (For information on ALL, see Chapter 20.)

Adult Leukemia

TYPE	OTHER NAMES USED IN REFERRING TO THIS TYPE	AGE	SYMPTOMS	TREATMENTS
CLL	Chronic lymphocytic	Usually appears in later life—60–70. More males than females.	Usually none. Often discovered on routine examination. Blood tests reveal elevated white cell blood count, lowered or normal red cell and platelet count. Enlarged lymph glands, spleen or liver.	Often no treatment necessary. Steroids such as prednisone or chlorambucil may be prescribed. Some types considered to be inactive or progressing slowly and can be held in check for long periods of time.
CML	Chronic granulocytic Chronic myelogenous Chronic myelocytic	Seldom occurs before age 25; usually 40–60.	Spleen enlargement, fatigue, sweating, early satiety, heat intolerance, easy bruising. Bone marrow shows excess of granulocytes. Philadelphia chromosome identified in bone marrow.	Chemotherapy to suppress excessive production of granulocytes; x-ray therapy to spleen; splenectomy. Must be followed closely since it can accelerate and become unresponsive to treatment.
AML	Acute myelocytic (AMoL) Acute myeloblastic Acute myelogenous Acute granulocytic Myelomonocytic (AMML)	Seen at any age, but primarily in 20–55 age group.	Low-grade fever, fatigue and pallor, bleeding and bruising, bone and joint pain. Many myeloblasts, low platelet count. Infection that persists despite antibiotics.	Chemotherapy. Other supportive treatments including red-cell or white-blood-cell platelet transfusion, immunotherapy, antibiotics used depending on condition.
ALL	Acute lymphocytic Lymphoid	Found in children and young adults, occasionally older age groups.	See Chapter 20	

Is the outlook for adult leukemics more hopeful today?

Yes. Prior to the development of chemotherapy, the majority of patients who developed adult leukemia showed a rapid and progressive downhill course. More than 20 percent of patients died within two weeks and 80 percent within two months. The management of the disease with chemotherapy has made it possible to control the activity of the leukemic cells and, in some cases, to reverse the malignant process.

What kind of doctor should I see if I have symptoms of leukemia, Hodgkin disease, or non-Hodgkin lymphoma?

Your internist or family physician will usually refer you to an oncologist if he finds evidence of these diseases. A hemopathologist should be consulted to properly stage the disease if classification is difficult. If you have lymphoma and the necessary x-ray equipment or radiotherapeutic expertise is not available in your community, you should be referred to the nearest major medical center for high-precision radiotherapy.

What studies is the National Cancer Institute supporting on leukemia?

The National Cancer Institute's clinical cooperative groups presently have studies in the following categories: acute leukemia (general), acute lymphocytic leukemia, acute non-lymphocytic leukemia, chronic nonlymphocytic leukemia, chronic lymphocytic leukemia, extramedullary leukemia, and leukemia (general).

Questions to Ask Your Doctor If You Have Leukemia

- Exactly what type of leukemia do I have?
- Is it chronic or acute?
- Exactly which cells are affected?
- Can you explain my blood counts to me? What would you consider normal for me?
- Was my type of leukemia difficult to diagnose?
- Has the diagnosis been checked by another hematologist?
- What kind of treatment are you planning for me?

- How often will you want to see me?
- What is the usual prognosis for this kind of leukemia?
- Is there a leukemia specialist in the area?

Are the terms "acute" and "chronic" leukemia accurate?

No. Until the 1950s there was a clear distinction between acute and chronic leukemias. The acute leukemias were characterized by a short and severe course of illness, the chronic leukemias by a much slower progression of the disease. Survival time for patients with acute leukemia was measured in weeks or months, and for patients with chronic leukemia in years. Today, because of the new therapies which are prolonging the lives of patients with the acute leukemias, the distinctions, in terms of survival implications, are no longer as clear as they once were.

How are leukemias classified?

Presently, leukemias are classified in two categories—acute (or poorly differentiated) and chronic (or well differentiated).
  Acute leukemia includes:
- Myelogenous (AML)
  - Myelomonocytic (AMML)
  - Monocytic (AMoL)
  - Erythroid
- Lymphoid (ALL)
- Unclassifiable
  Chronic leukemia includes:
- Myelogenous (CML)
- Lymphoid (CLL)

I find all the different names of leukemia confusing—can you help me get them straight?

Basically, there are three types of adult leukemia. The confusing thing is that each type is known by a variety of names—and with changing techniques, the names no longer reflect the true nature of the disease. The chart at the start of the chapter lists the different types and different names by which leukemias may be known. We will refer to them by the initials CLL, CML, and AML to help make the designations less confusing.

What are the most common types of adult leukemias?

The two most common types among adults are CLL and AML. CML is more rarely seen.

Can you tell me more about blood to help me understand leukemia?

Blood is made up of cells and fluid. The three major types of cells in the blood are red blood cells, known as erythrocytes, white blood cells, known as leukocytes, and platelets, known as thrombocytes. All of these cells are produced in the bone marrow. After the red blood cells, white blood cells, and platelets are made, they remain inside the marrow until they mature and become adult cells. After maturing, the adult cells slowly leak into the blood vessels and become part of the blood. The bones which produce red blood cells include the ribs, the breastbone, the wide top portion of the hipbone, and the spinal vertebrae.

What is the function of red blood cells?

Red blood cells act as a transportation system. They carry oxygen from the lungs to the other cells of the body and bring back waste products or carbon dioxide. If there are too few red blood cells, anemia results and the body cannot get enough oxygen to do its work.

What do white blood cells do?

White blood cells defend your body against illness. They capture, destroy, and remove germs. They prevent infection. White cells are made in the bone marrow and the spleen. If you have too few white blood cells, you are more likely to develop an infection and less able to fight an infection. There are several kinds of white blood cells. Granulocytes fight infections by engulfing bacteria. Lymphocytes play a role in producing antibodies. Leukocytes is a general term used to include all white cells.

What is the role of the platelets?

Platelets work by clotting your blood after an injury or cut. They act as "stoppers" which keep the blood from leaking out. If you have too few platelets, your blood clots more slowly and bleeding may be prolonged following an injury.

What are the symptoms of leukemia?

In some varieties of leukemia, there are no symptoms—and leukemia is found during the course of a routine physical examination, pointing up the need for physical examinations on a regularly scheduled basis. As with all other cancers, the earlier the illness is diagnosed, the better the chances of a cure. Fatigue, fever, weight loss, bone pain, easy bruising, or abdominal discomfort may indicate the presence of leukemia. In CML some patients will experience excessive sweating and heat intolerance.

Is leukemia difficult to diagnose?

While leukemia is usually not difficult to diagnose, certain preleukemic states and poorly defined types of leukemia may make it difficult for the doctor to classify the illness. The various classifications have been modified and renamed as greater understanding about leukemia has come about through the medical advances in the last ten years. A blood picture resembling leukemia may appear with some infections such as mononucleosis, tuberculosis, and whooping cough.

What kind of treatment is used in arresting leukemia?

Specific treatment varies depending on the type of leukemia diagnosed—so do not try to compare your treatment with that of another leukemia patient, since a great many factors enter into the type of treatment you will receive. Most acute leukemias (ALL and AML) are being treated with the administration of two or more drugs. CML is most commonly treated with oral doses of busulfan. X-ray therapy is sometimes used as a secondary treatment—and may be repeated. CLL may be left untreated until there is evidence of further progression of the illness. Overtreatment in this case is believed to be more dangerous than undertreatment. Chlorambucil and steroid therapy are sometimes used for CLL.

Are the leukemias really different diseases?

Each of the three adult leukemias, though related, has its own set of symptoms, treatments, and problems. The two chronic leukemias—CML and CLL—are quite different from each other.

CML usually affects younger people (age 40—60) than does CLL (60—70). CML requires early treatment, CLL often requires no treatment. AML occurs at all ages but most commonly after 40. The chronic leukemias rarely occur before the age of 30. ALL is a disease of children and young adults. There are numerous other leukemias in which other cell types predominate, such as eosinophils, basophils, reticulum cells, monoblasts and mono- cytes, plasma cells, and a variety of poorly identified stem cells, as well as lymphosarcoma and erythroleukemia. For these reasons it is important to know precisely what type of leukemia you are dealing with. Don't make the mistake of comparing treatments and blood counts with other leukemia patients, since there are so many variables in both symptoms and treatments.

What is the usual course of AML?

AML sometimes begins as an apparently infectious process, with abrupt onset, high fever, and secondary infection of mouth, throat, or lungs. Joint pains may be present. Or the patient may complain of progressive weakness and pallor. AML is seen at all ages, with a somewhat higher proportion of patients in the 20—55 age range. Primitive white blood cells in the bone marrow accumulate rapidly and invade many tissues—and can be rapidly fatal if left untreated. Improvement in the treatment of AML has resulted from better combinations of drugs used and from better supportive care, especially the use of white blood cell transfu- sions. Immunotherapy is also being studied and some reports indicate that it may be helpful.

Who usually gets CLL?

This is a disease usually of later life and many patients are safely observed without treatment for many years. Since it often appears late in life, death is often unrelated to it.

How is CML treated?

This leukemia occurs at any age but chiefly in the 20-to-50 age group. It is more often seen in males. Unlike CLL, once the initial diagnosis is made, treatment usually begins immediately. It can be controlled by chemotherapy for varying periods. It is extremely important for patients with CML to stay in touch with their doctors so that blood counts can be taken regularly and analyzed. Treatment can maintain the patient in almost normal health and activity, but the disease can take an "acute" course called a blast crisis. Persistent anemia, hemorrhage, fever, exhaustion, and secondary infections are common. X-ray therapy or radiophosphorus is sometimes used if the spleen continues to enlarge.

Is it usual for patients with CML to feel extremely well in the early stages?

Yes. The usual course of the illness is for early treatment to be successful and for the patient to feel extremely well. However, because of the way this type of leukemia progresses, patients must remain under constant care of the doctor. Do not be fooled into thinking that because of your feeling of well-being you can stop your visits to the doctor. This is foolhardy, since the disease can accelerate and become unresponsive to treatment unless closely followed.

Just to give me some handle on what the doctor is talking about, what is the meaning of some of the tests he does?

The table explains the terminology and some of the average values that the doctor uses as indicators. It is important to remember that averages mean that "normal" varies a great deal from person to person. The average ranges given here are broad. More important is *your* change from what is normal for you. If you wish to know, ask your doctor exactly what your counts are and how they relate to your case.

Why all the emphasis on blood tests?

When you have leukemia, blood tests become a part of your life. Since leukemia means that there is an abnormality in the production of blood, the blood counts tell the doctor about the state of your disease. His blood checks help him determine how you are progressing.

Blood Tests For Leukemia

TEST	MEANING	AVERAGE COUNT
WBC	White blood cell count	Averages 5,000–10,000 for adults
Differential count	Percent of white cells in peripheral blood	Based on 100 cell count
Hematocrit	Percentage volume of red cells to total blood	Average for men: 42–46 Average for women: 38–42
Hemoglobin	Amount of oxygen-carrying protein in known volume of peripheral blood	Male: 13–16 Gm/100 ml Female 12–15 Gm/100 ml
Platelets	Also called thrombocytes. Microscopic estimate of number of platelets per cubic millimeter. Indicates blood-clotting condition.	Normal range 150,000–300,000 for most laboratories.
Granulocytes	Those white blood cells that have ability to fight infection.	Average between 2,000–4,000. Below 500 indicates body's ability to fight infection is limited.
Erythrocytes	Red cells. Carry oxygen from lung to other areas of body.	Average red cell count is 4.5–5 million.
Reticulocytes or "retic"	Count of young new red cells being manufactured	0.5–1.5 percent of red cells
Blasts	Abnormal cells found in marrow of blood	Less than 5 percent in normal marrow
Leukocytes	A general term used to include all white blood cells.	Normal 5,000–10,000

What are petechiae?

These are little spots on the skin due to tiny hemorrhages. The spots may form a red or brown rash. They are a result of a low platelet count and decreased clotting function. They should be reported to the doctor.

What is thrombocytopenia?

It is a decreased number of platelets (those substances that along with plasma help blood to clot). There are different causes of thrombocytopenia. Leukemia is one of them.

Is the white blood cell count always high in leukemia?

No. The white blood cell count may be high or low. The more reliable diagnostic indicator is the proportion of immature or leukemic white cells present.

What happens when the platelet count is low?

If there are too few platelets, your blood clots more slowly and bleeding may be prolonged following an injury. Blood may "leak" out of the small blood vessels near the skin and cause spots called petechiae. Extra care should be taken to avoid bleeding. Avoid situations where you might be injured. Use an electric razor rather than a blade for shaving. Use toothette swabs instead of a toothbrush for cleaning your teeth. Do not take aspirin at this time because aspirin may increase your tendency to bleed. If you cut yourself or have to have an injection or shot while your platelet count is low, make sure pressure is applied for five or ten minutes to stop the bleeding.

What is a remission?

A remission is the goal of therapy for acute leukemia. It means that the abnormal immature blood cells have disappeared from your bone marrow and bloodstream, allowing normal red blood cells, white blood cells, and platelets to form. Remissions can last for any length of time—from a few days to years. Remission, however, is not considered a cure. Rather, it is a healthy state brought about by treatment. A patient in remission can go about living his or her normal life, though it will be necessary for the doctor to continue to follow progress with regular blood and bone-marrow testing.

What does bone-marrow depression mean?

This refers to the inability of the bone marrow to produce a sufficient number of blood cells—often the result of treatment with medication for leukemia or other kinds of cancer.

What is the meaning of induction therapy?

Induction therapy is the initial aggressive course of chemotherapy which is designed to wipe out abnormal cells and allow the regrowth of normal cells. At the time of this initial treatment, the patient is extremely susceptible to infection, since normal cells which fight infection are destroyed along with the abnormal cells. Two or three courses of therapy may be necessary before a complete remission is obtained.

What is maintenance therapy?

It is an effort to keep the patient in remission, prevent the reappearance of leukemic cells, and maintain a normal bone-marrow and blood picture.

What is consolidation therapy?

This is the treatment given after remission has been obtained in an attempt to prolong the duration of remission. It is a slightly less intensive course of chemotherapy given after the initial induction has been achieved. It is used in hope of improving the results of maintenance therapy.

How is a bone-marrow aspiration done?

The bone-marrow test may be done on the breastbone or hipbone. The breastbone test is done with the patient lying on his or her back. The patient usually lies on the stomach when it is done on the hipbone. The area is numbed with a shot of Xylocaine and a tiny opening is made in the skin. The doctor will use a special two-part needle made up of a hollow tube with another solid tube fitted into it. When this has been inserted into the bone marrow, the solid tube is removed and an empty suction tube is attached to the opening of the needle. The doctor will pull some of the marrow out by pulling back on the plunger. You are likely to feel pressure but it will hurt for just a few seconds. If the first attempt is not successful, the doctor will repeat the process. Sometimes it is difficult to obtain a bone-marrow specimen and the doctor will try again. Sometimes when aspiration will not give adequate information, a bone-marrow biopsy may be needed.

What is involved in a bone-marrow biopsy?

A similar type of needle is used as for the bone-marrow aspiration. The hollow needle is pressed farther into the bone so that it can pick up a piece of whole marrow and take it out so that a biopsy can be performed. Bone-marrow biopsies are usually taken from the hipbone.

How long does it take to do a bone-marrow test?

The whole procedure only takes five or ten minutes, and complications are rare. You will be able to feel the needle but the pain is minimal.

What is a bone-marrow trephine?

This is a less commonly used procedure than the bone-marrow aspiration or biopsy and involves taking a tiny piece of whole bone for examination. A larger needle than that used for an ordinary bone-marrow test is usually used for this purpose.

When the doctor does my bone-marrow test, he refers to spicules. What does that mean?

Spicules are bits of bone marrow with fat in them, which give a representative sample of marrow cells. Without spicules, it is impossible to make an accurate diagnosis of the bone-marrow cells.

Does leukemia change the bones?

No. It does not change the shape or strength of the bones but it does interfere with the work of the bone marrow. The red blood cells, along with the platelets and certain of the white blood cells, are formed primarily in the bone marrow and are then released into the bloodstream as they become mature.

The doctor talks about "blast" or "leukemic" cells. What does that mean?

Blasts or leukemic cells are immature white blood cells.

What complications are most common in leukemia patients?

Anemia (low red cell count), thrombocytopenia (low platelet count), and infections are complications of the illness. You may have none, any, or all of these in your course of treatment—but it is important to be aware of them and report them to your doctor as soon as they occur. Your doctor will also be checking for bone pain, kidney problems, gonadal involvement, and central-nervous-system involvement.

Is it unusual for leukemia patients to stop passing urine?

If you have trouble passing urine, be sure to let your doctor know. When cells are dividing often or when the treatments are causing them to die in large numbers, it is more difficult for your body to dispose of wastes. The doctor will usually ask you to drink lots of fluid and to take pills (allopurinol) if you have this problem.

What is plasmapheresis?

This is a process which makes it possible to get large numbers of platelets for transfusion by the use of a continuous-flow centrifuge which removes both platelets and plasma from the whole blood and returns red blood cells to the donor in a single operation. This technique permits donors to give platelets as often as twice in a single week for periods up to three months. Formerly, the limit was once in six to eight weeks. Since transfusions of blood platelets are often effective in preventing or stopping hemorrhage, this advance is an important one for leukemia patients. Plasmapheresis enables a single adult donor to provide the major portion of the platelets required by a patient with leukemia.

Can this method be used for other types of blood cells?

Granulocytes can also be obtained by using a continuous-flow centrifuge. Leukopheresis is the donation of white blood cells through the same process.

What is the role of transfusions in treating leukemia?

Often different types of blood transfusions are used during treatment (particularly with patients who have AML) to help prevent infections and hemorrhaging. White blood cells, red blood cells, and platelets can all be transfused. It has been found, for example, that patients who are given transfusions of leukocytes and platelets early in their treatment may have fewer infections and less hemorrhaging. Since patients can become resistant to platelets from persons of different platelet types, platelets can be closely matched, if necessary, to the patient's own platelets through the same tissue-typing methods that are used in kidney and heart transplants.

What do the doctors mean when they talk about DAT, POMP, COAP, DOAP, etc.?

These abbreviations are shorthand to describe the various combinations of chemotherapy drugs which are used in treating the various kinds of cancer, usually derived from the initials of the drugs being used. For instance, DAT refers to the combination of daunorubicin (D), ara-C (A), and thioguanine (T). POMP refers to the combination of 6-mercaptopurine (P), Oncovin (O), methotrexate (M), and prednisone (P). COAP is the combination of Cytoxan (C), Oncovin (O), ara-C (A) and prednisone (P).

What is the relationship of leukemia cells to the central nervous system?

Even after a remission has been achieved, studies of spinal fluid may reveal the presence of leukemic cells in the central nervous system of some patients. The fact that some leukemic cells have found a sanctuary in the central nervous system makes them a threat to the patient. Due to the properties of the capillary walls that prevent certain substances from passing from the blood to the central nervous system, these leukemic cells are not killed by the chemotherapeutic drugs. Radiation therapy and drugs administered directly into the spinal fluid are being used to help prevent and control central-nervous-system leukemia. This is more common with ALL than with other types of leukemia.

What is a bone-marrow transplant?

Bone-marrow transplantation is a recent approach to the treatment of acute leukemia and lymphoma. The state of the art is in the early stages, and the preparation for a transplant is complicated. This treatment is available only in a few of the large cancer centers at the present time.

When is a bone-marrow transplant used?

It may be used in some cases of three types of diseases—aplastic anemia (when patients do not have enough red cells to carry oxygen, enough white cells to fight bacteria, or enough platelets to help clotting), in some types of acute leukemia, and for some lymphomas. Donor bone marrow is transplanted to reseed the nonfunctioning bone marrow with new cells capable of replacing the entire blood system.

Can anyone undergo a bone-marrow transplantation?

No. This is used only for specific cases, and only with patients who have a donor with the same red blood cell and white blood cell types. This is usually a brother or sister or other person whose blood samples match those of the patient. Once a match is determined, the patient receives preparative drug and/or x-ray therapy necessary for the body to accept the grafted bone marrow. In the case of leukemia, the patient will also receive drug therapy to destroy the cancerous cells.

How is the bone marrow given to the patient?

The bone marrow itself is given to the patient in the same way as a blood transfusion. The preparation of the donor is more complicated. Testing may be done over the period of about a week. If there is a "match" and a bone-marrow transfusion is decided upon, the donor must be prepared to be in the vicinity of the hospital for about three weeks.

How is the bone marrow taken from the donor?

The bone marrow is removed from the donor with a special needle. The procedure is the same as that used for a bone-marrow test which is routinely done on leukemia and lymphoma patients. Marrow is obtained from multiple punctures, mainly in the hipbone.

Is the procedure painful for the donor?

The procedure is performed in the operating room with the donor under general anesthesia. The donor will feel nothing during the procedure. The procedure will leave tiny punctures on the donor's hip which heal over quickly and leave no scars. The donor may feel a bit of soreness in the area for a day or two after the procedure.

Does bone marrow normally replace itself?

Yes. The marrow taken from the donor is only a small portion of the donor's healthy marrow and replaces itself within a few days.

What is a splenectomy?

This operation involves the removal of the spleen. It is sometimes used in the treatment of leukemia, especially CML, or in lymphomas when the spleen enlarges and is responsible for destroying large numbers of normal blood cells.

Spleen removal is performed under general anesthesia. The incision is usually made in the upper left abdomen and is about 8 inches long. Once removed, the spleen does not grow back, but since its normal functions are taken over by other body tissues, the absence of the spleen does not interfere with normal living. Cancer of the spleen is rare, but when it does occur a splenectomy is the usual treatment.

Is immunotherapy used in the treatment of leukemia?

Some research is being done in this area, but results are still early and uncertain. Once the patient is in remission, immunotherapy is sometimes used to strengthen the body's ability to recognize and destroy cancer cells. (See information in Chapter 9.)

Persons Most Likely to Get Hodgkin Disease and Non-Hodgkin Lymphoma

Hodgkin disease: Mostly persons under 45 years of age, more males than females, peak age 20–25.
Non-Hodgkin lymphomas: Peak age 55–70, very few under 40.

Symptoms of Hodgkin Disease and Non-Hodgkin Lymphoma

- An enlarged lymph node, in the neck, armpit, or groin
- Pain in abdomen, back or legs
- Persistent fatigue
- Fever
- Loss of weight
- Night sweats
- Itching
- Nausea and vomiting
- Pain in enlarged lymph nodes after alcohol ingestion

Tests for Hodgkin Disease and Non-Hodgkin Lymphoma

- Complete history with special attention to unexplained fever, night sweats, or weight loss of more than 10 percent in prior six months
- Physical examination with particular attention to lymph nodes, liver, spleen, and bone tenderness
- Chest x-ray and/or whole-lung tomography
- Blood and urine tests
- Bone-marrow tests
- Lymphangiography
- Intravenous pyelogram (IVP)
- Inferior venacavagram (IVC)

Depending on condition, these may also be needed:

- Liver, spleen, and bone scans
- Staging laparotomy (except for some non-Hodgkin or Stage IV lymphomas)
- Splenectomy
- Liver biopsy
- Skin tests

Careful and complete testing is of the essence before any treatment is given—so be patient. The initial treatment determines the course of the disease, so tests must be done in depth to assure the most effective treatment. (Of course, the extent of testing is determined by the age and state of health of the patient. In those whose age and medical problems limit therapy, less aggressive testing procedures are done.)

Questions to Ask Your Doctor If You Have Hodgkin Disease or Non-Hodgkin Lymphoma

- What have you found that makes you think I have Hodgkin disease or non-Hodgkin lymphoma?
- Is the disease confined to one area or more than one area?
- Can my case be discussed with someone at one of the cancer centers?
- Will I need a laparotomy to diagnose my case accurately?
- Will my spleen need to be removed?
- Are you absolutely certain about the extent of the disease?
- Has a hemopathologist checked the pathology?

- I want to be certain that the diagnosis has been confirmed by someone else.
- Did the pathologist find Reed-Sternberg cells?
- Can you explain what cell type is involved and how my disease has been staged?
- What plans do you have for my treatment, and what alternatives do I have?
- How many cases like mine have you treated?

For female patients of childbearing age (or younger):

- Can I plan on being married and having children?
- If I am pregnant, will the pregnancy need to be terminated?
- Would you advise me not to have any more children?
- What effect would pregnancy have on me and the child?
- How long would I have to wait before I can think about becoming pregnant?

For young male patients:

- How will this affect my ability to father children?
- What can be done to avoid sterility?

What studies is the National Cancer Institute supporting on lymphomas?

The National Cancer Institute's clinical cooperative groups presently have studies in all types of lymphoma including Hodgkin disease and non-Hodgkin lymphoma.

What is malignant lymphoma?

The lymphomas are characterized by abnormal growth of cells making up the lymphatic tissue. They differ and are categorized according to which cells are affected. This group of diseases is sometimes referred to as Hodgkin and non-Hodgkin lymphomas or malignant lymphomas and includes a wide variety of related illnesses. In the past, many of these diseases were categorized by terminology which is no longer in use—such as lymphosarcoma, lymphogranuloma, giant follicle lymphoma, renticuloendothelial sarcoma, macrofollicular lymphoma, and reticulum cell sarcoma—and newer classifications based upon better understanding of the disease are now used. All lymphomas have certain similarities, including the approach to diagnosis and treatment, so questions in this chapter referring to lymphomas cover both Hodgkin and non-Hodgkin diseases.

What is the role of the lymph system in the body?

The lymph system is made up of nodes and thin-walled tubelike veins along which the nodes lie. Its job is to help fight diseases and infection, and it serves as part of the body's drainage system. Lymph nodes are usually very small and soft but become enlarged when there is an infection or disease present, such as mononucleosis or strep throat. Lymph glands are found throughout the body—behind the ears, in the groin, behind the knee, in front of the elbow, under the armpit, at the angle of the jaw, deep inside the abdominal cavity, at the junction of the right and left bronchi, and in many other areas. Lymphatic tissues include the tonsils, adenoids, and spleen. The lymph system is a sensitive indicator of illness in the body.

How is lymphoma diagnosed?

It is usually diagnosed by biopsy of a lymph node and the examination under the microscope by a hematopathologist.

How are lymphomas treated?

The treatment depends on where in the body the disease is found. Lymphomas differ from many other cancers in that they are not treated by surgery. However, lymphoma can be successfully treated by chemotherapy and/or radiation.

What is lymphangiography or a lymphangiogram?

A lymphangiogram is a test which shows where malignant lymph nodes are located in the abdomen. This is done by injecting a special dye into the lymph vessels of the foot. The lymphatic system carries the dye to all lymph nodes. When the x-rays are taken, the dye outlines the lymphatic system. It shows the size of various lymph nodes, their shape, and even their internal structure. This allows the doctor to identify abnormal nodes. The patterns of lymph flow that show up on the x-rays are also important, because lymph does not pass easily through the nodes that are filled with cancerous cells and abnormal patterns of lymph flow develop. From this x-ray, the doctor is able to identify involved nodes and to choose several lymph nodes to remove and examine. Because the dye remains in the lymph vessels for long periods of time after a lymphangiogram, x-rays can be taken during and after therapy to monitor the effects of treatment on the cancer.

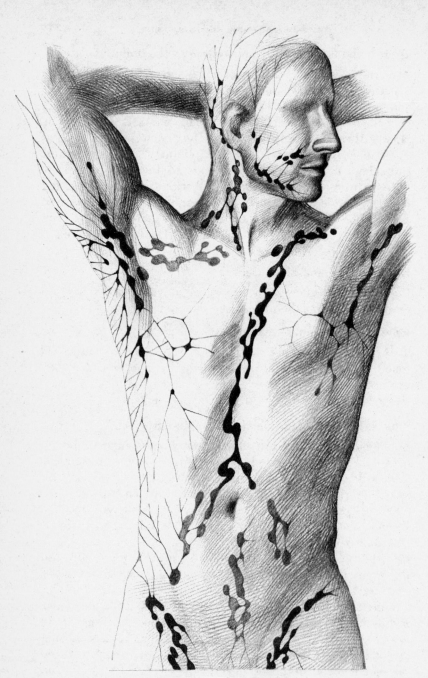

Lymph system

380

When is a laparatomy used to diagnose lymphoma?

Some doctors feel that for patients with early stages of Hodgkin disease, an accurate diagnosis is important enough to warrant a routine laparotomy (a surgical operation to explore the entire abdomen)—except in cases where the patient's age or health makes this a problem. This procedure enables the doctor to determine the extent of the disease and if it has spread to the abdomen. In most non-Hodgkin cases, laparatomy is not recommended for diagnostic purposes, since other clinical methods can be used to determine the extent of the disease accurately enough to stage the disease properly.

Why is staging so important?

The nature and extent of your first treatment influences and can severely limit future treatment. Therefore, it is important for the doctor to stage your condition correctly before beginning treatment. The staging procedure—during which time all the necessary tests are completed—may take from one to three weeks. While that seems like a long time to postpone treatment, it is important because it allows the doctor to have complete information before the treatment is started.

What definitions do doctors use in classifying lymphomas?

Doctors use a variety of terms to classify lymphomas in an attempt to describe the cell where the lymphoma originates as well as to indicate certain microscopic features of the cells. So much progress has been made in the study of lymphomas in the past ten years that new terminology is constantly being invented and old terminology updated. Some of the latest classifications include, for Hodgkin disease, lymphocyte predominance (LP), nodular sclerosis (NS), mixed cellularity (MC), and lymphocyte depletion (LD). For non-Hodgkin disease, cells are classified as either nodular or diffuse in four categories: poorly differentiated lymphocytic, mixed cell, histocytic, or well-differentiated lymphocytic. These classifications have replaced the use of such terminology as large-cell lymphosarcoma, reticulum-cell sarcoma, lymphoblastic lymphosarcoma, small-cell lymphosarcoma, giant follicular lymphoma and lymphocytic lymphosarcoma. All of this terminology makes it extremely confusing for a patient who is trying to understand the nature of his disease, but if you ask the doctor, he should be able to clarify for you exactly what is involved in your disease process.

Is pregnancy a problem for a woman with lymphoma?

Although pregnancy has no effect on the course of the illness, women with lymphoma should consult with their physicians about family planning. Treatment cannot be given during pregnancy, since drugs can harmfully affect the fetus. Family planning is an important issue because it is difficult to predict when treatment may be needed. Men should also discuss the possible effects of changes in sperm due to drugs and radiation therapy. Some work has been done in the field of repositioning ovaries to sites that can be shielded when x-ray therapy is performed. The disease itself does not seem to have an adverse effect on fertility, the course of pregnancy, labor, or the baby. The treatment and its side effects, however, must be taken into consideration in making a judgment. If at all possible, a waiting period of two years after remission is advised before becoming pregnant.

How does Hodgkin disease differ from non-Hodgkin disease?

All are classified as lymphomas. Hodgkin disease is distinguished from the other lymphomas by the presence of a particular abnormal cell, called the Reed-Sternberg cell, in the patient's lymph nodes. (Reed-Sternberg cells may be found also in patients with infectious mononucleosis.) Hodgkin disease usually appears first in one group of lymph nodes—often in the neck—but it may also involve many lymph nodes as well as the spleen, the liver, the bone marrow, and other organs. The diagnosis is usually made through the biopsy of a lymph node.

What is the most usual symptom of Hodgkin disease?

The most common first sign is a swollen lymph gland, usually in the neck. Many doctors believe that Hodgkin disease begins in one area of the lymph system and, if left unchecked, spreads throughout the system and later to other tissues and organs. Unexplained weight loss and unexplained fever and night sweats should all be reported to the doctor. An enlarged spleen or liver may be present in some instances. Skin rashes, itching, and weakness may occur. Anemia and reduced ability to fight infection may develop.

If I have an enlarged lymph node should I see a doctor immediately?

Lymph glands may be enlarged as a result of infections or other illnesses such as mononucleosis or rheumatoid arthritis—but any lymph gland in the neck, armpit, or groin that remains enlarged for three weeks or longer should be checked by your doctor.

Is itching a common symptom for those with Hodgkin disease?

Itching—or pruritus, as it is sometimes referred to by the medical profession—is not unusual. It usually disappears with treatment of the disease, and some relief may be possible with antihistamines. It may reappear at a later time and should be reported to the physician if it occurs. This symptom is one of the most distressing and most difficult to cope with for many patients.

Is fever often a symptom of Hodgkin disease?

A low-grade fever is not uncommon, though some patients may be unaware of it unless they experience night sweats. A pattern of high fever alternating with normal or subnormal temperature may also be seen.

Are there any other symptoms?

Some patients report that an alcoholic drink can induce pain in enlarged lymph nodes, sometimes accompanied by nausea and vomiting. This symptom occurs in less than 5 percent of all patients.

What causes Hodgkin disease?

Though there is a great deal known about Hodgkin disease, its actual cause remains a mystery. Some researchers suspect that it may be caused by a virus, but direct proof is lacking. Neither does there seem to be a hereditary factor involved, although there are instances where more than one person in the family has had Hodgkin disease. More males than females are listed with Hodgkin disease, but the proportion of females affected has recently shown a definite increase. Two age groups appear to be most frequently involved—those in the 20–35 age group and those over 50.

What are Reed-Sternberg cells?

These are abnormal cells necessary to make a diagnosis of Hodgkin disease. Seen under the microscope, these cells and their cellular surroundings confirm a diagnosis of Hodgkin disease. They are named for the two scientists who first identified them. Reed-Sternberg cells alone are not sufficient for diagnosis of Hodgkin disease, since similar cells have been described in mononucleosis and other diseases.

Why is it important to have Hodgkin disease properly classified before treatment is started?

A complete evaluation before the start of treatment is necessary because the nature and extent of previous treatment influences and can severely limit future treatment.

Why is the spleen sometimes removed in Hodgkin disease?

If a laparotomy is performed to aid diagnosis, the spleen is usually removed at the time of surgery. This is done so that it can be examined for disease and because x-ray treatment of the spleen usually would be indicated if it were not removed. Since the spleen lies over the left kidney and part of the lung and stomach, x-ray treatment would affect these organs. Therefore, removal of the spleen helps prevent potential injury to other organs.

How is Hodgkin disease staged?

Hodgkin disease is classified into four stages, depending on the extent of the disease. Stages I and II denote involvement of one or more lymph-node regions on the same side of the diaphragm. Stage III includes disease limited to the lymph nodes, but on both sides of the diaphragm. Involvement of the spleen or other localized involvement of an extralymphatic organ or site or both are also classified as Stage III. Biopsy-proven involvement of the liver or bone marrow is defined as Stage IV disease. When involvement is found in the other extralymphatic tissues, such as the lung, pleura, or bone, individual judgment is made, depending on whether the disease is localized or multiple—meaning that it could be classified at any stage depending on whether it is confined to one or more regions. Involvement of only one organ, such as the stomach or bowel, in other words, does not signal Stage IV disease, but rather Stage I, E (extranodal).

Stage B refers to patients who also have fever, night sweats, or weight loss. Therefore, a patient might be Stage IIIA, without these symptoms, or Stage IIIB, with one of these symptoms.

Because of these distinctions, which have a bearing on treatment, it is extremely important that the disease be properly researched before treatment begins.

What is the usual treatment for Hodgkin disease?

Treatment depends upon the stage the disease is in when the patient is diagnosed. Latest scientific evidence indicates that the patient with early-stage previously untreated Hodgkin disease has the best chance of cure if he is treated with high-precision radiation therapy. Take note that if the up-to-date radiation equipment or radiotherapeutic expertise is not available in your community, you should be referred to the nearest major medical center for this treatment. The use of small radiotherapy units, operating at treatment distances of 80 centimeters or less, results in a patchwork of small treatment fields which invite frequent technical errors. In cases where the disease is more widespread, combination chemotherapy can be added to the treatment. Patients with Stage IIIB or IV disease usually require combination chemotherapy, with moderate-dose radiotherapy either in a "split-course" approach or at the end of multiple drug cycles, when complete remission has been attained. More than 60 percent of patients with Stage I or II disease treated with radiation therapy are free of disease ten years after diagnosis. Similar results are now being obtained with patients with Stage III or IV disease treated with combination chemotherapy and irradiation.

What treatment is available to a patient who relapses after the first series of treatments?

This depends, first of all, upon what treatment was previously used. If treatment was with radiotherapy only, chemotherapy supplemented with judicious radiotherapy can be used. Those who develop relapse more than 12 months after completion of their last combination chemotherapy cycle usually do well on another course of the same drugs; those relapsing earlier are best treated with one of the newer combinations of chemotherapy. The available options make it possible for the patient to feel optimistic about the ability of his or her doctors to keep the disease in check with proper treatment.

Is Hodgkin disease responsive to treatment?

Yes. This tumor responds dramatically to treatment, even with patients in whom the disease has spread. Even in cases which are not curable and recur after initially successful treatment, control for long periods of time is often possible.

What is the outlook for patients with Hodgkin disease?

Excellent. Within the last ten years, tremendous progress has been made and, with proper treatment, Hodgkin disease can be controlled for long periods of time. Even conservative doctors are talking about patients who have been cured of Hodgkin disease. Following radiation and/or chemotherapy treatments, ten-year disease-free remissions are not uncommon, even in cases which were discovered in Stage III or IV.

What tests are usually required to diagnose non-Hodgkin lymphoma?

Routine tests, including complete blood count and liver- and renal-function tests, are needed. Bone-marrow biopsy and intravenous pyelogram, as well as some of the more complicated tests used in diagnosing Hodgkin disease, may be required.

What symptoms usually accompany non-Hodgkin lymphoma?

A history of a lump or other mass, recurrent infections, or an episode of herpes zoster (shingles), as well as unexplained anemia or bleeding, are sometimes symptoms of lymphoma. Sometimes this disease starts with a tumor in the adenoids, tonsils, or nose and throat area or as a lesion of the lung or nervous system. Careful evaluation of these symptoms must be made by the doctor and further tests conducted so that the extent of the disease can be fully evaluated.

How do doctors stage non-Hodgkin lymphoma?

The staging procedure is similar to the procedure used in staging Hodgkin disease. Stages I and II denote involvement of one or more lymph-node regions, respectively, on the same side of the diaphragm. Stage III includes disease limited to the lymph nodes, but on both sides of the diaphragm. If the spleen is involved, an "S" designation is added to Stage III. Stage IV indicates lymph-node plus other visceral involvement such as the marrow or the liver. Involvement of only one organ, such as the stomach or bowel, is classified as Stage I, with an "E" added to this classification to denote extranodal involvement.

What treatment is prescribed for non-Hodgkin lymphoma?

Though few patients have Stage I or II non-Hodgkin disease, the most common treatment for these stages is with supervoltage cobalt-60 radiation, sometimes followed by chemotherapy. For those with Stage III and Stage IV disease, chemotherapy, usually a multi-drug series, is recommended, sometimes with radiotherapy. In elderly patients or those in poor health, less aggressive therapy is usually prescribed.

What is the outlook for patients with lymphomas other than Hodgkin disease?

These cover a wide variety of conditions, and the stage in which they are discovered and the age of the patient naturally have a great deal of bearing on the outcome. Progress in the management of non-Hodgkin lymphoma has not been as dramatic as in the control and cure of Hodgkin disease, but good results are being reported. Treatments which have been successful in Hodgkin disease are being applied to the other lymphomas, but well-controlled studies have not yet resolved the ideal number of drugs or their schedule of administration. The natural history of these diseases varies considerably and some types (nodular well-differentiated or poorly differentiated lymphocytic) progress very slowly, sometimes for years.

What is myeloma?

This is a type of cancer in which abnormal plasma cells destroy normal bone tissue, causing the bones to become extremely fragile. It is often referred to as multiple myeloma, and in Europe is known as Kahler's disease.

Who usually gets multiple myeloma?

Multiple myeloma is most often seen in adults between the ages of 50 and 70. Statistics show that more men than women have multiple myeloma.

What are the symptoms?

The main symptom is bone pain, which seems to worsen at night. Back pain is often present. Bone fractures may occur. Abnormal bleeding, difficulty in urination, and susceptibility to infections are all possible symptoms.

How does the doctor diagnose multiple myeloma?

X-rays may show destroyed patches of bone. Blood and urine tests can detect certain abnormal proteins which suggest the presence of the disease. (The term "Bence-Jones protein" is used in connection with multiple myeloma to identify a specific protein excretion which is used in diagnosing the condition.) A small-needle aspiration of bone marrow, made under local anesthesia, is needed to make a final diagnosis.

Are most myeloma patients anemic?

Since the bone marrow is producing fewer oxygen-carrying red blood cells and disease-fighting white blood cells, myeloma patients are often anemic and susceptible to infections such as pneumonia. As the plasma cells act against the bone tissue, calcium is released sometimes in amounts exceeding the kidney's capacity to dispose of it. The patient may become weak, nauseated, and disoriented.

Is exercise important to the myeloma patient?

Yes. Since immobilization can aggravate the imbalance of calcium, exercise and adequate fluid intake are important. Every effort is made to provide pain relief through radiation and chemotherapy so that the patient will be able to be ambulatory.

What treatments are prescribed for multiple myeloma?

Treatment depends upon the extent of the disease. If limited to one area, x-ray therapy can control the disease for long periods of time and is helpful in relieving pain. Combination chemotherapy has been found to be effective in shrinking plasma-cell tumors, improving the sense of well-being, and reducing bone pain. Several studies by the National Cancer Institute's clinical cooperative groups are in progress to determine the most effective combinations of chemotherapy for this disease. (See Chapter 23.)

Is Sjögren's syndrome a form of cancer?

Sjögren's syndrome is a combination of symptoms associated with inflammation of the cornea and conjunctiva of the eye, enlargement of the parotid glands in the neck, and dryness of the mouth due to lack of normal secretions. The syndrome itself is not a form of cancer, but in some cases lymphoma later develops, and it is believed that there may be an association between the two diseases.

What is polycythemia vera?

The disease is characterized by an increase in the mass of red blood cells and the total blood volume and in some cases, the disease can over a period of many years become truly malignant with the development of AML leukemia. There can be a later transition to enlargement of such organs as the spleen and liver and progressive anemia.

The symptoms of aplastic anemia make it sound like cancer. Is it?

No, although the National Cancer Institute is supporting several clinical studies of the disease, it is not classified as cancer. Its main symptom is a reduction below normal in the number of red cells present in the blood. It is a serious condition that occurs when the bone marrow fails to make adequate numbers of red blood cells, white blood cells, and platelets. This type of anemia generally does not respond to specific therapy, and many patients die as a result—but it may remit spontaneously without treatment. The clinical studies include investigations of bone marrow transplantations. (See Chapter 23.)

chapter 15

Gastrointestinal Cancers— Colon-Rectal, Bladder, Kidney, Stomach, Liver, Pancreas

Symptoms of Gastrointestinal Cancer

- Signs of blood in stool or urine (this is always a warning—must see doctor immediately)
- Change in bowel habits, increased use of laxatives, change in stool size
- Sense of incomplete evacuation
- Gas pains or cramps
- Constant indigestion or heartburn
- Abdominal pain or distended feeling
- Burning sensation when urinating
- Need for frequent urination
- Vomiting
- Feeling of lump or mass in abdomen

Those Most Likely to Get Gastrointestinal Cancer

- Age 50–74
- Personal or family history of rectal polyps
- History of ulcerative colitis
- History of stomach cancer among close relatives
- History of chronic liver disease (hepatitis)
- Diet heavy in smoked, pickled, or salted foods

Tests for Gastrointestinal Cancer

- Health history and physical exam
- Digital rectal examination
- Endoscopy, proctosigmoidoscopy, or colonoscopy
- Barium enema, barium swallow (GI series)
- Occult blood test (hemocult, stool guaiac test)
- Intravenous pyelogram (to assess kidney and bladder function)
- Hematologic studies
- Blood-chemistry studies
- Cytology
- Liver biopsy (if there is suspicion of liver metastases)

Questions to Ask the Doctor Before an Operation

- Where exactly is the cancer located?
- Do you have any evidence that the cancer has spread?
- Who will be performing the surgery? How often does he do this operation?
- What kind of anesthesia will be used?
- Is there a patient who has had the operation who could talk with me about it?
- Will I need to have an opening outside the body?
- If the answer to the preceding question is yes: Will I be able to continue to work? Can you show me exactly where the opening will be? Will the opening be permanent or is there a chance that it would be reconnected? Can I try on the appliance so that I can be sure that the opening will be comfortable?
- Will the operation change my eating habits?
- Will I still be able to have sexual relations?
- Will I be scheduled for radiation therapy? (If yes, be sure to read Chapter 7.)
- Will I be scheduled for chemotherapy? (If yes, be sure to read Chapter 8.)
- Can immunotherapy be used in my case?

Abdominal Cancer

Type	Symptoms	Diagnostic Tests	Treatment
Colon-rectal	Rectal bleeding, blood in stool, jet-black stool, change in bowel habits, alternating constipation/diarrhea, crampy abdominal pain, weakness, loss of weight, loss of appetite	Digital exam, sigmoidoscopy or proctosigmoidoscopy, barium enema, colonoscopy, CEA	Surgery (can range from snipping of polyps in doctor's office to colostomy or ileostomy); chemotherapy and/or radiation therapy is being tested on an investigational basis.
Bladder	Bloody urine, change in bladder habits, increase in urination, retention of urine, incontinence	Cystoscopy, cystogram, intravenous pyelogram, cytology	Electrosurgery, surgery, radiation, radioisotopes, chemotherapy
Kidney	Back or side pain, blood in urine, abdominal mass, fever, weight loss	Intravenous pyelogram, blood studies, urinalysis, renal arteriography, scans	Surgery, radiation, chemotherapy, immunotherapy
Stomach	Indigestion, dark stools, vomiting, weight loss, early fullness	Barium x-rays, gastroscopy, cytology (gastric washing), CEA	Surgery, chemotherapy, radiation therapy
Liver	Discomfort in upper abdomen on right side (more acute with deep breathing), hard lump, pain in right shoulder, jaundice	Needle biopsy, radiography, angiography, tomograms, liver scans	Surgery, regional chemotherapy
Pancreas	Jaundice, itching of skin, abdominal pain and discomfort, nausea, diarrhea, belching, feeling of fullness, intolerance of fatty foods, weight loss, loss of energy and strength, clay-colored stools	Barium x-rays, liver-function tests, angiography, ultrasound, CEA, CT scan	Surgery, chemotherapy, radiation therapy

What kind of doctor should I see if I have symptoms of gastrointestinal cancer?

The specialists who deal in this area include gastroenterologists (who treat diseases of the GI tract from mouth to anus, including the stomach, liver, pancreas and intestines), endocrinologists (who treat diseases of the organs which secrete hormones in the bloodstream, such as pancreas), nephrologists (who treat diseases of kidneys), proctologists (who treat colon and rectal conditions), and urologists' (surgeons who treat the urinary system).

Is the National Cancer Institute supporting any studies on gastrointestinal cancer?

Yes, the National Cancer Institute's clinical cooperative groups are presently conducting studies on colon-rectal, bladder, stomach, pancreas, and kidney cancers as well as on general genitourinary tumors. (See Chapter 23.)

What is the colon?

The colon, or large intestine, is the final 5 to 7 feet of the intestinal tract. It starts at the right lower part of the abdomen and, defying the laws of gravity, continues upward on the right side of the abdomen, close to the liver under the ribs (this section is known as the ascending colon). It makes a left turn and crosses to the left portion of the abdomen (this 2-to-2½ foot portion is known as the transverse colon). The next portion heads down the left side of the abdomen to the pelvis (called the descending colon). The final section, which is S-shaped (the sigmoid colon), and the final 8 or 10 inches located in the pelvis behind the urinary bladder are known as the rectum, with the final 2 inches being referred to as the anal region. The colon joins the small intestines to the rectum. The colon and rectum form the lower end of the digestive tract.

What kind of tumors develop in the colon?

There are two kinds, primarily—benign growths such as adenomas or polyps, and malignant growths, which are cancer.

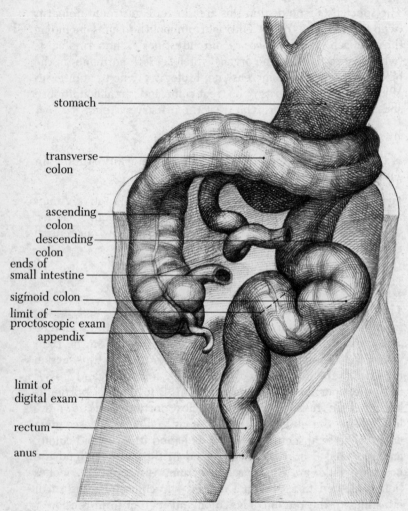

stomach

transverse
colon

ascending
colon

descending
colon

ends of
small intestine

sigmoid colon

limit of
proctoscopic exam

appendix

limit of
digital exam

rectum

anus

Colon-rectal area

What is a polyp?

A polyp is simply a growth originating from the mucous membranes of the colon (polyps also occur in the bladder, uterus, nose, etc.). They are very common, occurring in 10 to 15 percent of all adults. Usually they cause few symptoms and are most often found during routine intestinal examinations. Cure, through removal, entails little surgical risk. If cancer is found in the polyp, the area surrounding it is removed. Painless rectal bleeding is the most frequent symptom of a polyp. Because some polyps have a tendency to become cancerous, their removal is recommended by many doctors.

How does the doctor remove a polyp?

This depends on where the polyp is located. If it is within 8 inches of the rectal opening, it can be removed with a sigmoidoscope through the rectum—either burned off or clipped and removed through the rectum. With improved techniques of colonoscopy almost any polyp with a "stalk" can be removed through a colonoscope. Some will still require surgery if they are large or flat. The incision is made at the area of the polyp, the colon is opened, and the polyp is removed. The polyp will be carefully examined to make sure that it is not cancerous. If cancer is found, the segment of the bowel where it grew must be removed.

What is a sigmoidoscope?

This is an instrument which enables the doctor to view about 12 inches of the intestinal tract through the rectum. This is the area where polyps and cancers are most usually found. Small polyps can be removed with this instrument in the doctor's office with general or local anesthetics. It also allows a small portion of tissue to be extracted from the wall of the colon for laboratory testing. The procedure using the sigmoidoscope is called a sigmoidoscopy or proctosigmoidoscopy and should be included by your doctor as part of your annual physical exam if you are over 40 years of age or earlier if you have had a family history of colon cancer.

What causes tumors to form in the colon?

The causes are unknown, but it is suspected that heredity as well as diet and poor bowel habits may play a role in some cancers of the colon. Conditions such as polyps, ulcerative colitis, and colitis also may be causes. Periodic checkups with a rectal examination make it possible for tumors to be discovered before they become dangerous.

What is involved when the doctor does a digital rectal examination?

With a gloved finger, the doctor will probe the rectum for lesions. This examination will detect the presence of any masses in the lowest 4 inches of the rectum. Any stool on the gloved finger may be tested for blood.

How do I prepare for a proctosigmoidoscopy?

Usually the doctor will instruct you to have a tap-water enema the night before or the morning of the examination. The conventional instrument he uses is a sigmoidoscope which allows him to view the last 12 inches of the colon. Some doctors prefer a flexible colonoscope which allows him to view higher into the colon. If bleeding, obstruction, or diarrhea is present, the doctor will suggest a less vigorous bowel cleansing.

Is a proctosigmoidoscopy dangerous?

No. Complications from this examination are rare—but an inexperienced doctor could perforate the bowel, causing serious problems. This procedure is best done by a proctologist or a gastroenterologist or someone else who is experienced in doing the procedure.

What is the stool-guaiac test?

The guaiac (pronounced *gwi-yak*) test (also called occult stool test or Hemocult) is a simple, inexpensive method of testing stools for traces of blood. Usually stool samples are taken of three consecutive bowel movements so that if there is intermittent bleeding, this can be discovered. To increase the accuracy of the stool analysis, the doctor may ask you to start a meat-free, high-fiber diet 48 hours before the collection of the first stool specimen and continuing through the next three days. Vitamin C and aspirin should be avoided during this time to ensure that the test is accurate. A simple, easy-to-use home kit has been designed so that the patient merely needs to put a small amount of feces on a slide and mail it in according to instructions.

Do hemorrhoids (piles) usually turn into cancer?

No. However, hemorrhoids may exist along with cancer. Any rectal bleeding should be followed by an examination by the doctor to determine its cause. Do not assume that all bleeding is caused by hemorrhoids, because one of the symptoms of cancer of the colon or rectum is bright-red blood in the stools.

What are some of the symptoms of a tumor in the rectum or colon?

Rectal bleeding, red blood in the stool, jet-black stools, a change in bowel habits or the size of the stool, alternating constipation and diarrhea, crampy abdominal pains, weakness, loss of weight, and loss of appetite. Sometimes you will see a streak of blood in the stool only once. It is important that any sign be checked by a doctor.

If tumors are found, must they always be removed?

Yes. Most doctors agree that even benign tumors (adenomas or polyps) should be removed because they may eventually develop into cancer.

How serious is the operation?

The operation varies depending on the location, kind, and size of the tumor. Polyps near the rectum can often be removed through the rectum without anesthesia in a surgeon's office, as an outpatient in a hospital, or during an overnight hospital stay. For any benign tumor, the procedure is simple removal of the tumor at its base. If the tumor is cancerous, the tumor as well as a generous portion of the colon above and below is removed.

What kind of operation is necessary for cancerous growths in the colon or rectum?

Again, this depends on the kind, size, and location of the tumor. In all cases, the surgeon must remove the entire tumor. If enough normal colon remains, he will rejoin the healthy pieces so that the patient can function in a normal manner. When this is not possible, then an artificial opening, called a stoma, is made on the abdominal wall.

What is this operation called?

This surgery is a colostomy. Whether permanent or temporary, a colostomy can be performed in any portion of the colon, and it takes the name of the segment where it is located. Following colostomy, bowel movements are received in a pouch placed over the opening.

Are all colostomies permanent?

No, many of them are temporary—that is, after a certain period of time, in a second operation, the colon is rejoined and the hole in the abdomen is closed up. These operations are often referred to as two-stage procedures. The first operation is a temporary colostomy. The second is an operation to rejoin the colon and close the colostomy. The number of patients who require colostomies has been reduced, thanks to new surgical techniques and materials. Often the doctor is able to perform a one-stage operation, bringing together the healthy sections of the colon after the tumor has been removed.

When is a permanent colostomy necessary?

Permanent colostomies are usually necessary when the growth is in the region of the lower portion of the colon and rectum— anywhere from the anus opening up to 6 inches above the rectum. In this case, the entire anus, rectum, and lower colon are removed and the upper portion of the colon is brought out onto the abdominal wall in the form of a permanent colostomy.

What are temporary colostomies called?

There are several different kinds, each of which requires two-stage operations: double-barrel colostomy, transverse-loop colostomy and cecostomy. Each of these requires the temporary use of an appliance outside the body to collect body wastes. Each, however, can later be repaired by the surgeon so that the colon is rejoined and the use of an appliance is no longer necessary.

Is a colostomy always due to cancer?

No. There are about twenty other diseases and conditions which lead to the need for this operation.

What is an ileostomy?

The ileum is a portion of the small intestine. When disease

necessitates its removal, an ileostomy is created. This is usually, but not always, a permanent arrangement, depending upon whether the rectum remains healthy or must be removed as well.

What is the difference between a colostomy and an ileostomy?

A person with a colostomy usually has had a portion of the colon and the rectum removed. A person with ileostomy usually has had the entire colon plus a portion of the small intestine removed as well. The word "ostomy" means a surgical procedure that creates a stoma (an artificial opening). A person who has had this kind of surgery is known as an ostomate.

What happens to bowel movements if the colon and rectum are removed?

You will need to have a permanent abdominal opening (colostomy) through which the bowels will be evacuated.

What is a total colectomy?

This is when the surgeon removes the entire large intestine and rectum.

The General Stages of Colon-Rectal Cancer		
STAGE	OTHER CLASSIFICATIONS	EXPLANATION
Stage 0	TIS, N0, M0	Carcinoma in situ as demonstrated by biopsy.
Stage I	T0, 1 N0, M0 T0, 1 NX, M0 T2, N0, M0 T2, NX, M0	Tumor has not extended beyond bowel wall. No evidence of regional or distant metastases.
Stage II	T3-5, N0 M0 T3-5, NX, M0	Tumor has extended beyond the bowel wall but has no metastasis either regional or distant.
Stage III	Any T, N1, M0	Tumor has spread beyond the bowel or rectal wall with regional metastasis but not distant metastasis.
Stage IV	Any T, any N, M1	Tumor has spread beyond the bowel or rectal wall and has distant metastasis. Can also have regional metastasis.

What is a stoma?

A stoma is an opening or hole. When a colostomy is performed the end of the small or large intestine is brought through the abdominal wall. It is fastened at the skin level so that it cannot slip back. The diameter may vary from ½ inch to 3 inches or more. This is called a stoma.

That sounds uncomfortable. Is it?

A well-cared-for, healthy stoma is comfortable and painless and does not interfere with physical activity. However, much of the success with which a patient is able to handle the stoma is determined by the way in which the surgery is carried out.

How can I be sure that mine will be a stoma that is easily manageable?

That is a hard question—but a very important one. First of all, make certain that your surgeon is someone who specializes in this particular type of operation. Some surgeons undertake these operations without the benefit of repeated experience, and though they provide a stoma which is surgically correct, the stoma may not be functional from the patient's point of view. So, be warned. Ask the doctor how often he has performed this surgery. Ask if he examines the ostomy each time the patient visits him. Ask him what kind of long-term routine supervision he is prepared to give you or can suggest for you. You might even ask him if he has a patient who has had this operation who would be willing to talk with you. Be absolutely certain that he has located a suitable site for the stoma before you are on the operating table. He will undoubtedly ask you to stand, sit, and lie down as he notes your body so he can determine the best site for stoma placement. Stomas situated in scars, in the navel, or where you wear your belt (particularly if you are a man) can be quite unmanageable. Proximity to bony prominences, or the waistline, or interference by rolls of fat—all can interfere with the use of ostomy appliances. These problems cause soiling and often make it difficult for the patient to make a good recovery. So be sure the doctor discusses with you the actual location of the opening. The type of ostomy you have determines where the stoma will be to some extent and the nature of the discharge you will have. Ask the doctor to show you on a diagram what portion of your colon he will remove and where the stoma will be.

What preparations are necessary before surgery of the colon?

Usually the patient is required to enter the hospital several days before surgery. Medication with antibiotic drugs and low-residue or liquid diets will be prescribed. Blood transfusions may be necessary if you are anemic, as well as vitamin, mineral, and glucose feedings by vein. If there is an obstruction, an attempt may be made to overcome it by passing a tube into the small intestine.

What kind of anesthesia is used?

General anesthesia is usually preferred. Spinal is sometimes used.

How long do I have to stay in the hospital for a colostomy?

The time varies according to the type of surgery. A simple operation for the removal of polyps through the rectum may require only one or two days of hospitalization. A tumor removed through the abdomen may require 10 to 14 days in the hospital. Complications, as with any surgery, can extend this time period. In the case of operations which are done in several stages, the patient may have to plan on several hospitalizations, each requiring a varying amount of time—from ten days to several weeks—in the hospital.

How does a colostomy affect my general health?

You will probably be healthier than ever. The problem area has been removed and the intestine that remains is perfectly able to take care of the absorption of food elements.

Can the body function without a large portion of the intestines?

A person has about 20 feet of small intestine and 5 feet of large intestine (the large intestine is larger in diameter than the small intestine, thus its name). He can live quite well without a portion of his small intestine and without his entire large intestine (colon). Most digestion actually takes place before food reaches the colon. The colon's function is to absorb the water from the already digested material and to transport waste through its length and store it until it is ready to be expelled from the body. The remaining portions of the colon learn to assume some of the water-absorption role of the intestine that was removed. Even though to a layman the removal of a portion of the small intestine or even all of the colon and rectum sounds as though it would make it impossible for the body to function, the fact is that after successful surgery the body adjusts to the loss of the large or small intestine and rectum with very little effect. The patient will usually be able to eat what he likes and function in exactly the same way—usually feeling better than he did before.

The thought of living with a permanent bowel opening is repulsive to me.

Better techniques and methods of caring for colostomies have really made care a routine and fairly simple matter. It will become a part of your regular routine. Many patients who at first thought they would not be able to care for their stomas are after a short time able to live a perfectly normal life. Hundreds of thousands of people are doing this and are in no way disabled.

Will I have to worry about my diet?

No special diet is needed. Your body will tell you which foods are best for you. You should be careful about eating highly laxative foods or foods which are "gassy"—such as beans, nuts, onions, cabbage. Just be sure you eat a complete and well-balanced diet.

Will I have the colostomy bag on when I come down from my operation?

Usually, patients who have had ileostomies will return from surgery with a temporary ostomy bag in place. A patient who has had a colostomy will not have fecal drainage until he begins to eat again a few days or a week after the operation. He will return from surgery with dressings but with no ostomy bag. When fecal matter begins to be expelled, a temporary colostomy bag will be applied. Because this is a temporary appliance, it may not work as well as the permanent one. Furthermore, the process is more complicated because you have so recently had the operation. Don't be dismayed by the whole procedure. It will become a simple, routine matter for you when you return home. Thousands of people from every walk of life have had colostomies and are able to attend to their businesses and their homes, marry, have babies, play golf or tennis, swim, dance, go to the movies—in other words, live perfectly normal lives.

How long will it take me to get adjusted to the bag and using it?

A lot depends on your attitude. There will be mental as well as physical adjustments for you to make. It is not an easy adjustment, but a positive attitude helps a great deal. Usually, after a few months' time, you will be accustomed to the routine and it will be a regular part of your daily life. The sooner you accept the fact that your stoma is a part of you, the sooner this adjustment will take place.

Will having an ostomy affect my having sexual relations?

It depends upon a lot of factors—your sex, the extent of the surgery, your attitude, and your age, to mention a few. This is a topic you should discuss with your doctor before you have the operation. There are also three good booklets which are published by the United Ostomy Association, Inc. (1111 Wilshire Boulevard, Los Angeles, Calif. 90017; telephone 213-481-2811): "Sex, Courtship and the Single Ostomate," "Sex and the Male Ostomate," and "Sex, Pregnancy and the Female Ostomate."

Can I get any other information on ostomies?

The United Ostomy Association is a very remarkable and active organization. Its entire reason for being in existence is to help people like you who have had ostomies. You can check your local telephone-directory yellow pages under "Associations" or "Social Service Organizations," for a local chapter of the United Ostomy Association, or call the American Cancer Society in your area and ask them where the nearest chapter is located. If you are not able to locate a local ostomy group, write to the United Ostomy Association (address given in the preceding answer). The association has helpful literature about caring for your ostomy and information on the manufacturers of equipment which you will find most helpful. The American Cancer Society also has literature on this subject and often sponsors ostomy group meetings. Be sure to avail yourself of this help.

Will Medicare pay for my colostomy supplies?

Medicare will pay for colostomy equipment and other prosthetic devices to replace internal organs if you have taken the supplemental benefits under medical insurance, Part B.

Is chemotherapy or radiation therapy ever used in treating colon-rectal cancer?

There are some studies now being carried out in which chemotherapy or radiation and chemotherapy are being used in treating colon-rectal cancer. Usually these treatments are used following surgery.

What is the function of the bladder?

The urinary bladder is the reservoir for the urine. It is located in the front part of the pelvic cavity. It is elastic and increases in size as the urine accumulates. It is the seat of many disorders, including bladder stones, tumors, infections (or cystitis), obstruction, and paralysis.

What are the symptoms of bladder cancer?

Bloody urine is often a first sign, although bloody urine can also be the sign of many other urinary problems. The color can range from a smoky shade to deep red. There is usually no accompanying pain, and the amount of blood does not usually relate to the size of the tumor. Any sign of blood in the urine, even if it happens only once, is a warning to see your doctor immediately so that whatever condition is present can be treated. Bloody urine can also be a sign of conditions such as tumors, infections, or bladder stones. Other symptoms of bladder cancer include a change in bladder habits with an increase in the frequency of urination and, rarely, retention of urine or incontinence.

Who is most likely to get bladder cancer?

Bladder cancer occurs most frequently in persons between 50 and 70 years of age. Four of every five patients are men. There are two main types of cancer of the bladder—papillary and transitional-cell carcinoma. Less frequently found are squamous-cell carcinoma and adenocarcinoma.

What is papillary cancer of the bladder?

This is the most common type and the most easily cured. It starts on the bladder wall but grows into the bladder cavity and remains attached to the bladder wall by a mushroomlike stem. This type of tumor may be single or multiple, pea-sized or large enough to occupy the entire bladder. The tumor cells appear to be almost normal.

Are most bladder tumors found to be cancerous?

No. Many bladder tumors are found to be benign. However, benign tumors may become malignant. The doctor can often detect the change of a lesion by doing a cystoscopy. When seen with the cystoscope, the growths may appear to be like a series of warts, with the larger ones taking on a cauliflower appearance.

Is bladder cancer likely to metastasize to other parts of the body?

Fortunately most bladder cancers are slow-growing and do not tend to spread to other parts of the body as do other cancers. Metastases usually are found first in the pelvic lymph nodes and usually remain localized there for a long time. Early detection and removal is the easiest and surest cure, since bladder cancer can spread to the lung, bones, and liver.

Is it unusual for bladder tumors to recur?

There is a great tendency for bladder tumors to recur either in the same location or in some other part of the bladder. Most of these growths are noncancerous, and many that are malignant are slow-growing. Most recurrences can be treated easily and successfully.

How is a diagnosis of bladder cancer made?

A urologist usually performs an examination with a cystoscope, which allows him to inspect the lining of the urinary bladder. If any suspicious-looking areas or growth are observed, a piece of tissue is removed for microscopic examination without major surgery. The examination involves little time or discomfort. Cystograms, made after filling the bladder with an opaque solution, give further information about the size of the tumor and the width of its base. Intravenous pyelograms can be done to

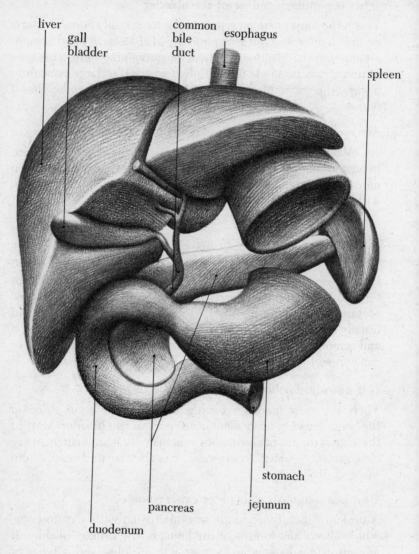

liver

gall
bladder

common
bile
duct

esophagus

spleen

duodenum

pancreas

jejunum

stomach

Front view, major internal organs

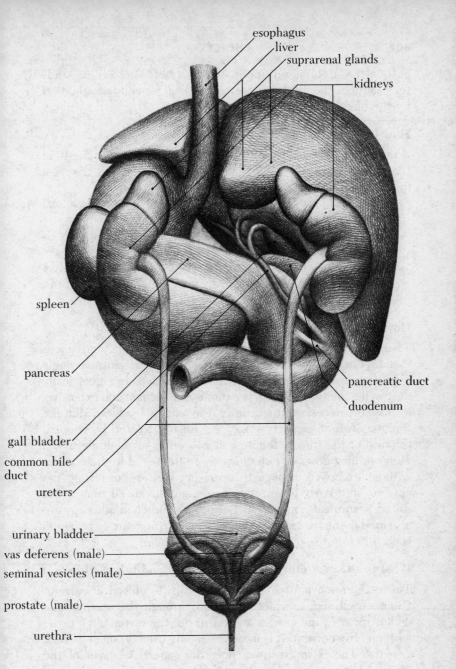

esophagus
liver
suprarenal glands
kidneys

spleen

pancreas

pancreatic duct

duodenum

gall bladder

common bile
duct

ureters

urinary bladder
vas deferens (male)
seminal vesicles (male)

prostate (male)

urethra

Rear view, major internal organs

outline the ureters and upper urinary tract. Microscopic study (cytology) of the urine for presence of cancer cells sloughed off by the bladder is routine.

How is cancer of the bladder staged?

A number of different methods are used. However, the depth of the penetration of the tumor into the bladder wall is the most important factor in determining treatment.

- *TIS, Ta, T1 and T2:* These designations indicate minimal penetration.
- *T3, T3a, T3b:* Deep penetration of bladder or muscle is indicated.
- *T4, T4a, T4b:* Indicates that the tumor is fixed to the pelvic wall and/or infiltrates the abdominal wall, prostate, uterus, vagina, or muscle.

How is bladder cancer treated?

There are so many different types and stages of bladder cancer that therapy varies widely among individual patients. A single papillary tumor may be successfully treated by electrically destroying the tissue. When the tumor is malignant and extensive, it may be necessary to remove the entire bladder. Multiple tumors, even at an early stage, are usually treated by surgical removal of the tumors themselves as well as surrounding tissue. Tumor-killing doses of radiation can be delivered to the bladder without excessive damage to overlying tissues, permitting the cure of both early localized cancers and advanced tumors not suited to surgical removal. Radioisotopes and chemotherapy are also used in the treatment of bladder cancer. Sometimes radiation is used before the operation in bladder cancer.

What is a transurethral resection (TUR) and fulguration?

This is the removal of a bladder growth with electrical current. Using a cystoscope, which is passed through the urethra, the doctor removes the growth and burns out the surrounding tissue with electric current. It is most commonly used on small, benign growths. This is successful if only the superficial layer of the bladder has been invaded. After this treatment your doctor will ask you to return every three to four months because new tumors have been known to grow in the same vicinity in about one-quarter of all cases. If no recurrences are found after a year, the intervals between examinations may be lengthened gradually.

What surgical procedures are used if the cancer is large and invasive?

Depending on where the cancer is located and how far it has advanced, the doctor will perform either a segmental resection or a cystectomy.

What is involved in a segmental resection?

A segmental resection is usually recommended if the tumor is localized in one area of the bladder with an adequate margin of tissue that can be removed from around the tumor. This operation is performed through a lower-abdominal incision and, when complete, the patient is left with a portion of the bladder and therefore can maintain urinary control. When this is not possible, then a cystectomy is necessary.

What is a cystectomy?

The operation for removal of the bladder is called a cystectomy. In order to remove all the tissue containing the cancer safely and completely, it is sometimes necessary also to operate on other nearby parts of the body. In women, this may mean the removal of the ovaries, fallopian tubes, and uterus, as well as a portion of the vagina which contains the urethra. In men, the prostate and seminal vesicles may also be removed. If the tumor is near the opening of the bladder neck or involves areas of the bladder lining, the urethra may also be removed. A cystectomy is a major operation, but with modern surgical techniques and anesthetics, it can be carried out successfully.

Is radiation sometimes used before surgery?

Preoperative radiotherapy has been found to produce partial or even complete destruction of tumors of the bladder and is often used before a cystectomy is performed.

How long will I remain in the hospital after my cystectomy?

Usually the recovery period lasts two or three weeks.

What anesthesia is used for bladder operation?

Usually spinal anesthesia is used. General anesthesia may also be recommended.

Where is the incision?

The incision begins in the midline, above the navel, and extends to the level of the pubic bone.

How long does the operation take?

This is a complicated operation which takes from five to six hours to perform.

What special preparations are made before surgery?

Usually, you are admitted to the hospital three to five days before the scheduled surgery. Daily enemas and laxatives will be given to you. In addition, you may be given antibiotics to reduce the amount of bacteria in your system. A special diet and vitamin supplements will be ordered for you. Your doctor or nurse may ask you to test a sample appliance to ensure that the area chosen for your stoma is on the flattest possible surface and provides maximum comfort for your various normal activities.

How is urine stored and emptied when one has had a cystectomy?

The most common method used is the ileal conduit or ileal loop bladder operation. A portion of the small intestine is used to carry the urine from the ureters to the outside of the body. An appliance is placed over the opening (stoma) to collect the urine. This technique has proved most satisfactory, since it maintains kidney function and is easy for the patient to manage.

Does this mean I'll have to wear a bag outside my body to collect the urine?

Yes. Though this is a large change in life-style, most patients find that they can adjust to the change once they understand that the existence of a stoma on the abdomen and a collection device over it need not be limiting or disabling. Hundreds of patients of all ages have had to face this adjustment and have found that they can handle it and resume normal activities.

Is there some way I can have a say in where the opening is placed?

Your doctor will usually discuss this with you, since the site should be determined before the operation. Generally it is located either in the right lower or upper abdomen. It should be placed where, when the collection appliance is attached, movements such as sitting, standing, twisting, and bending will not pull the appliance loose. It should not be located near an old scar or attached near rolls of fat. This should all be discussed with your doctor before the operation.

Will I be rigged to a urine-collection device when I leave the operating room?

The temporary appliance will be placed over your stoma in the recovery room. This appliance will be connected to a continuous drainage bag that will be emptied of urine by one of the nurses or nurses' aides. For the first few days someone else will take care of you and your stoma. As you gain strength you will be taught how to do this yourself. It is important that you learn to care for your appliance and have confidence in it before you leave the hospital.

Is there any way I can try the appliance out before the operation?

Yes. The nurse can help you try out the appliance. She can apply it and put water in the pouch to simulate the weight of the urine. You can dress yourself and try doing some of your normal activities. This trial is a good way to eliminate your own anxieties about wearing the appliance. Keep in mind that there are many different types of appliances and many different solutions. You may need to try several before you find one that suits you. The United Ostomy Association (1111 Wilshire Boulevard, Los Angeles, Calif. 90017; tel. 213-481-2811) publishes several helpful booklets listed earlier in this chapter in the section on colon-rectal cancer.

How long will the appliance stay in place?

Usually five to ten days. It should be changed only when it begins to leak or becomes uncomfortable.

How often should it be emptied?

About every two hours.

What happens to the appliance during sleep?

Usually during sleep the appliance is connected to drainage tubing attached to a bottle placed on the floor beside the bed. Running the tubing under the leg allows greater freedom of movement. Most patients find they can sleep in any position once they are accustomed to wearing their appliances.

Does the urine look the same as before?

It does not look exactly the same as urine from the bladder, since the conduit through which it passes is made from a segment of the small intestine, which secretes mucus. This mucous membrane is sensitive, and urination can cause mucus as well as slight amounts of blood to appear in the urine. Check with your doctor if there are changes in the consistency or color of the urine or a decrease in the amount of drainage.

Should I get a spare appliance?

Yes. It is a good idea to have one to wear and one to keep ready for use. This ensures that the one to be applied will be well dried and aired. You'll find you need a new appliance about every six months.

Can I bathe and shower as usual?

Yes. You can bathe and shower with or without the appliance. If the stoma seems irritated, remove the appliance and soak yourself in the tub of warm water.

How long will the stomach tube remain in place?

This tube, placed through your nose and into your stomach to drain the gastric juices and prevent accumulation of air and fluid in your stomach, usually remains in place after surgery for five to seven days, until your bowels have regained normal activity. This will allow your stomach and bowels to rest and give the connection time to heal.

How does a cystectomy affect a man's ability to function sexually?

It depends upon the extent of the operation. Sometimes there is permanent loss of sexual function, with the penis losing its ability to become erect, so impotence results. You should discuss this point with your doctor before he performs the operation so that you will know how extensive the surgery will be.

Are women still able to function sexually?

Sexual activity may be possible but it could be impaired if a portion of the vagina is removed. Again, this is a topic which you should discuss with your doctor before the operation is performed.

Is it usual for a patient to be depressed after this kind of operation?

It is not unusual to feel depressed. As a result of the depression, the patient's attention span may be short, and he or she may have difficulty in concentrating and be irritable. It is important for the family and friends to realize that this is a temporary but normal feeling. An inability to cope with the new way the body functions may reinforce the thought that the person may never be able to cope with anything again. The depression is usually short-lived and subsides when the patient finds that family and friends accept him or her and that he or she can return to a normal way of life.

What is the function of the kidneys?

There are two kidneys, one on each side of the back portion of the abdomen, located rather high in the loin. Their function is to filter waste products from the blood, returning to the circulating blood those substances that are necessary for normal chemical balance. The central portion of each kidney is hollow and receives the body fluids. The urine leaves the kidney and passes down its ureter—a long tubular structure—which connects with the bladder.

What are the symptoms of kidney tumors?

Four symptoms can warn the patient of the possibility of kidney tumors: persistent pain in the area over the kidneys, either in the back or along the side of the body; blood in the urine; a feeling of a lump or mass in the kidney region; and fever or weight loss.

Are all kidney tumors cancerous?

No. Many are benign. The benign growths often are filled with fluid and can be classified as cysts. They vary in size. However, malignancy cannot always be determined without surgery.

How is cancer of the kidney diagnosed?

The doctor will usually assess kidney and bladder function with an intravenous pyelogram. Blood studies will be made to reveal the presence of anemia. Urinalysis, renal arteriography, and scans are sometimes recommended. Because cancer of the kidney is difficult to diagnose it has been labeled the "internist's tumor."

How is cancer of the kidney staged?

Tumors of the kidney are classified as follows:
- *T1*: Small tumor, minimum distortion and deformity
- *T2*: Large tumor with deformity and/or enlargement of kidney and/or collecting system
- *T3a*: Tumor involving tissues around kidney
- *T3c*: Tumor involving renal vein and infradiaphragmatic vena cava
- *T4a*: Tumor invasion of neighboring structures such as muscle or bowel
- *T4b*: Tumor involving supradiaphragmatic vena cava

What symptoms are indicative of tumors of the ureter?

Usually blood in the urine, pain in the flank, and finally obstruction to the flow of urine to the bladder. This is an uncommon form of cancer and usually necessitates the removal of the kidney on the same side as the affected ureter.

Can one live normally if a kidney is removed?

Fortunately, people can live perfectly normal lives with only one healthy kidney.

What is kidney removal called?

The medical term is "nephrectomy," and it is considered a major operation.

Are nephrectomies done only for cancer?

No.

What kind of incision is made for this operation?

The incision extends from the loin, just below the last rib and above the hipbone, around onto the abdomen.

What anesthesia is usually used?

General anesthesia is usually used for this operation.

Are other treatments besides surgery ever used for cancer of the kidney?

Recently some doctors have been using a course of preoperative radiotherapy for several weeks followed by surgery. It has been found that sometimes an apparently inoperable tumor can be made operable. Postoperative radiotherapy, chemotherapy, and immunotherapy are being used in some hospitals. However, removal of the kidney is the most common approach.

Where is the stomach located?

The stomach is a pouchlike organ which makes up a relatively small part of the intestinal tract. It lies below the diaphragm in the left upper part of the abdomen, crossing over to the right below the liver. The stomach hangs comparatively free in the abdominal cavity and moves with breathing.

What symptoms indicate the possibility of stomach cancer?

Unfortunately, the symptoms of stomach cancer are often vague and nonspecific. The most common symptom of stomach cancer is indigestion. This may consist of a sense of discomfort or mild pain, fullness or bloating, burping, slight nausea, heartburn, or loss of appetite. Of course these are signs which we find easy to ignore, but if they persist—even intermittently—for a period of two weeks, your doctor should be consulted. Later signs might include blood in the stools or vomiting, rapid weight loss, and severe pain. These symptoms may also indicate the presence of an ulcer.

How is the diagnosis made?

A careful history and physical and rectal examination come first. Laboratory tests such as red and white blood cell count and analysis of the acidity of stomach contents will be ordered. The most important of all diagnostic methods is the x-ray examination, with the radiologist observing the flow of barium under the fluoroscope with x-rays of various areas of the stomach taken from different angles with the patient in various positions. Gastroscopy, in which a flexible instrument is passed into the stomach for viewing, along with a newer diagnostic procedure known as exfoliate cytology, is sometimes used. Cytology allows the examination through a microscope of cells shed by the lining of the stomach. In order to collect the cells, a gastric washing is done. An abrasive brush or balloon is introduced into the stomach and the stomach lining is gently scraped. The material collected is studied by a pathologist to determine if malignant cells are present.

How is cancer of the stomach usually treated?

The usual treatment for cancer of the stomach is prompt surgical removal of the malignant tumor. The operation usually involves the removal of a part or all of the stomach, depending on the location of the malignancy. Sometimes parts of other abdominal organs, such as spleen and pancreas, are removed if they are in the area of the tumor and are believed to be affected.

Is any other treatment recommended?

It depends upon the location and extent of the tumor. Sometimes chemotherapy is used following surgery. Some experimental work is being done with implantation of radioactive sources into the malignant stomach tumor to give relief from pain in patients whose cancers are inoperable. Stomach cancers usually are considered resistant to x-rays since a radiation dose safe for the surrounding normal tissues is not strong enough to destroy the cancer.

Do doctors sometimes suspect cancer of the stomach and find a benign tumor?

Yes. Preoperative x-ray examinations cannot always distinguish a malignant tumor from a harmless benign tumor. Furthermore, x-rays occasionally will give the appearance of a tumor but an ulcer may be discovered at surgery.

Is the same operation performed for ulcer of the stomach and stomach cancer?

This depends on the extent of the stomach cancer. The same procedure—removal of the stomach—is usually performed for either condition.

Do stomach ulcers lead to stomach cancer?

This is a question over which there has been much speculation. Most doctors feel that the danger of stomach ulcers rests not so much in the possibility that an ulcer may lead to malignancy, but rather that it may be cancerous even while being treated as an ulcer.

What is the difference in the usual treatment between a stomach ulcer and a duodenal ulcer?

A duodenal ulcer can be treated conservatively for long periods of time without the fear of cancer. A stomach ulcer must be followed closely. A patient is usually put on a strict diet, given appropriate medication, and subjected to further x-ray examination every two to four weeks. If a clean x-ray picture does not result from this treatment within a few weeks, an exploratory operation is usually performed to determine whether there is a malignancy.

How can a person live without a stomach?

Quite successfully. Sometimes, only a section of the stomach is removed. However, when necessary, the entire stomach is removed. The patient is required to eat smaller, more frequent meals—perhaps half as much food at each meal as previously. The patient learns to eat more often and more slowly and adjusts to this way of life quite easily.

What must be done to prepare for stomach surgery?

Patients are usually admitted to the hospital two to five days before the scheduled operation. They are put on a liquid diet and the stomach is washed out with a stomach tube once or twice daily. Often intravenous medications, vitamins, and blood transfusions are given prior to the operation.

Can the doctor tell immediately if there is a malignancy?

It is usually necessary to wait several days for the pathological examination of the stomach to determine if cancer is present.

The General Stages of Cancer of the Stomach

STAGE	OTHER CLASSIFICATIONS	EXPLANATION
Stage I	T1, N0, M0	Tumor is confined to the lining and connective tissue of the stomach. There is no regional or distant metastasis.
Stage II	T2, N0, M0 T3, N0, M0	Tumor involves the stomach wall but has not penetrated through it. There are no regional or distant metastases.
Stage III	T 1-3, N1 M0 T 1-3, N2, M0 T 1-3, N3, M0	Tumor has penetrated the stomach wall and invaded nearby structures. There is no distant metastasis. There may be regional metastasis.
Stage IV	T1-3, N3, M0 T4, N03, M0 T1-4 or TX or N03 or NX, M1	The tumor has penetrated the stomach wall and invaded nearby structures with regional and distant metastases.

Is the postoperative period for a stomach operation uncomfortable?

There is likely to be discomfort caused by the use of stomach tubes, intravenous feedings, and injections. Food and drink is usually withheld for two to four days. For at least the first three to four months, small, frequent feedings are recommended. The patient can then gradually return to a normal diet of bland foods. Spicy foods and alcohol should be avoided. The doctor may prescribe the addition of iron and liver extract to the diet.

What is the dumping syndrome?

Following gastrectomy, some patients develop what is known as the "dumping syndrome"—weakness, dizziness, sweating, nausea, vomiting, palpitation—which occurs when the remnant of the stomach empties itself of food too quickly. This can usually be controlled by frequent small feedings and by a high-protein diet with the addition of dry foods and fluids between feedings.

How long is the convalescence period following extensive stomach surgery?

The patient will usually be able to return to normal activity after about two months.

What does the liver do?

The liver performs more complex functions than any other organ of the body except the brain. It breaks down worn-out red blood cells and converts them into bile. It produces proteins essential to proper blood clotting. It regulates the level of many hormones. It stores sugar and regulates the amount which circulates in the blood. It controls the metabolism of cholesterol. It stores Vitamins A, D, E, and K. In fact, the functions of the liver are so many and varied that it is almost impossible to test them all in the clinical laboratory.

Where is the liver located?

It fills the upper right side of the diaphragm and is protected on both the right and left sides by the rib cage.

Can one function without a liver?

No, it is not possible to function without any liver. However, one can live normally with as little as 15 to 20 percent of the normal liver. The liver's powers of recuperation are truly amazing.

Can cysts on the liver be removed?

Yes, most cysts can be successfully removed.

Are all tumors of the liver cancerous?

Tumors of the liver may be malignant or benign. Cancer of the liver itself is rare—the cancer usually has started elsewhere and spread to the liver. Benign tumors are usually small, produce no symptoms, and may be discovered only during the course of another operation. Such tumors are usually not removed. Suspected malignant cancer of the liver alerts the doctor to the possibility of cancer elsewhere in the body. Cancers of the lung, breast, or gastrointestinal system can spread to the liver.

Is cancer of the liver and cancer which has spread to the liver treated in the same way?

No. They are two very different problems. Cancer of the breast which has spread to the liver is treated in the same way as breast cancer with metastases would be treated. Liver cancer—that is, cancer which has started in the liver and not metastasized there from some other organ—is treated as liver cancer. Many people whose cancer has spread to the liver from some other place think they also have liver cancer. This is not true.

What symptoms alert the doctor to the possibility of liver problems?

Vague discomfort in the upper abdomen on the right side, which becomes more acute with deep breathing, is one possible symptom. Sometimes an enlarged liver can be felt as a hard lump just below the rib cage on the right side. If the tumor is located under the diaphragm, pain can sometimes be felt around the right shoulder blade. Jaundice, which produces a yellowish look to the skin, may develop.

Will cirrhosis of the liver turn to cancer?

No. Cirrhosis of the liver will often be found in patients who have cancer of the liver. However, only about 4 percent of the patients who have cirrhosis of the liver later develop cancer. In cirrhosis of the liver, the liver may be badly scarred or swollen. Cirrhosis of the liver may be the result of a severe case of hepatitis, or may be caused by heavy drinking or by drugs such as carbon tetrachloride (cleaning fluid), chlorpromazine (a tranquilizer), or isoniazid (a tuberculosis drug). Damage leads to an obstruction of the liver, which prevents the normal rate of flow of blood through the liver. Surgery can help by lessening the quantity of blood delivered through the liver. Relief of the blood load often permits the liver to recover its normal function.

How is cancer of the liver diagnosed?

A needle biopsy is sometimes used to determine whether the liver is cancerous. A careful history and physical examination, radiography, endoscopy, angiography, tomograms, biochemical tests of the liver, liver scans—all can be employed in making a diagnosis.

Will the doctor attempt to remove the primary growth if he finds metastases to the liver?

Usually not. Extensive surgery may be too debilitating when metastases have spread to other parts of the body.

What treatment is possible if a cancer is found in the liver?

If cancer is confined to a segment or a lobe, surgical removal may be indicated.

What other forms of treatment may be recommended?

Regional chemotherapy—that is, chemicals introduced directly into the arteries which are supplying the tumor—is sometimes used successfully to deprive the tumor-bearing area of oxygen and some of its nutrient supply.

What is the pancreas?

It is a pulpy, flat gland about 5 inches long by a few inches high which lies far back on the rear wall of the upper abdominal cavity. The part it plays in the body is a vital and specialized one. It manufactures digestive juices which are passed through the pancreatic duct into the intestine for digestion of proteins, fats, and carbohydrates. Insulin, which is essential for the utilization of sugar, is manufactured in the pancreas and deposited directly into the bloodstream. A duct, called the pancreatic duct, runs through the entire length of the pancreas. The pancreas is often referred to as having a head, a body, and a tail. The head fits into the curve of the duodenum on the right, close to the common bile duct, and the tail curves up toward the spleen. At the head of the pancreas there is often a branching of the main pancreatic duct. These ducts are responsible for collecting the digestive juices manufactured by the gland and depositing them through their openings into the small intestine.

What are the symptoms of cancer of the pancreas?

A variety of symptoms that can also be the signals of diseases other than cancer of the pancreas, as well as the hidden location of the pancreas, combine to make cancer difficult to diagnose. For this reason, pancreatic cancer is often far advanced before it is detected. Cancer in the head of the pancreas, because it involves the common bile duct, usually causes jaundice, and often there is intense itching of the skin. There may be some abdominal pain and discomfort, nausea, diarrhea, belching, a feeling of fullness, and intolerance of fatty foods. Weight loss, loss of appetite, and loss of strength or energy may be other symptoms. The color of the bowel movement may be affected, being foamy, clay-colored, or, more rarely, silvery in color. All of these symptoms might also be present when there are cysts or benign tumors in the pancreas. Another set of symptoms can present themselves in cases where the tumor is located in the body portion of the pancreas. Severe back pain may be present as the result of the size of the tumor. The pain may worsen after eating or when lying down and be slightly relieved when bending forward or sitting. The disease is so difficult to diagnose that the majority of patients are treated for three to six months for other causes before actual diagnosis of the pancreatic cancer is made.

What tests will the doctor need?

The doctor will usually order barium x-rays, liver-function studies, and angiography to determine more clearly where the tumor is located.

Can cysts in the pancreas turn into cancer?

Rarely will a cyst in the pancreas become cancerous. Usually, cysts can be removed successfully with a good chance of recovery. If allowed to remain they can continue to grow and cause serious problems in pancreatic activity. It is important to remember that all cysts, tumors, or inflammations of the pancreas do not indicate the presence of cancer.

Can the doctor tell whether or not the condition of the pancreas is cancerous before he operates?

Usually he cannot. Benign tumors and growths often grow in the pancreas, causing the cells that produce insulin to overproduce, causing symptoms that include intense hunger, trembling, fainting, confusion, or convulsions. The operation to remove a cyst is a low-risk one. However, if the presence of cancerous cells is found, it may be necessary to operate so as to bypass the obstruction or to remove the entire gland. Then it becomes a complicated operation.

How does the doctor decide if there is cancer in the pancreas?

The only certain way at the moment is through a biopsy— which in this case requires a laparotomy. However, many experimental programs are underway to help aid better diagnosis, such as endoscopy, ultrasound, CT scans, and CEA. Doctors agree that ultrasound looks promising in diagnosing small pancreatic cancers earlier.

What is a laparotomy?

A laparotomy is a surgical operation to open the abdominal cavity either to make an inspection or to perform surgery.

What does the incision look like, and where is it?

The incision for a laparotomy is about 4 or 5 inches long and is located in the upper abdomen.

The doctor says I'll need more than one operation. Why?

Sometimes operations for cancer of the pancreas are done in several steps.

How long does the operation take?

The operation to remove a localized tumor or cyst of the pancreas takes one to three hours. If the entire pancreas is to be removed, the operation can take anywhere from three to six hours.

What happens when the entire gland is removed?

The operation to remove the entire gland and the adjacent duodenum, called a pancreaticoduodenectomy, is one of the most extensive in all surgery. The bile duct and the stomach are both connected into the small intestine. This is a high-risk operation, not often performed. It can be successful in those cases in which the tumor has not spread to other organs.

Can you live with only part of the pancreas or without the pancreas?

Yes, an active, comfortable existence is possible when medicines are prescribed to substitute for the function of the pancreas.

What happens if the cancer has spread beyond the pancreas?

If the cancer has spread and is in places where it cannot be removed, the prognosis is very serious.

Would the doctor advise against surgery?

Since this cancer is so difficult to diagnose, surgery is usually a necessity. If cancer is not the cause, the surgery will determine this happy diagnosis. If cancer is the cause, the doctor can at least relieve the jaundice and the exasperating itching through surgery, even when the cancer cannot be removed. Sometimes, when the patient is elderly or has other health problems which put him in a high-risk category, surgery will not be attempted.

What sort of operation is performed?

If possible, the tumor of the pancreas, the surrounding bile duct, and part of the stomach and intestine are removed, and everything is rejoined. If that is not possible, a new opening is made for the bile, to relieve the jaundice and help in the digestive process.

What are the chances for cure of cancer of the pancreas?

Of course it depends upon many factors. However, it is important for the patient with pancreatic cancer to understand the seriousness of the condition and the risks. Because it is usually found late and has many times spread to nearby organs, the five-year survival rate at the present time is only one percent; of 21,900 cases estimated in 1978, approximately 20,000 will die within the five-year period.

Will I need transfusions and other intravenous medication?

Yes. This is an extremely serious operation. Blood transfusions may be needed during and after the operation. Intravenous feedings, medications, and special drugs will be used to help speed recovery. You will usually not be allowed out of bed until several days after the operation.

What are the aftereffects when the pancreas is removed?

The recovery period will be a long one and a permanent low-sugar, low-fat diet will be essential. Vitamin K will probably be prescribed. Because of the restricted diet, it is very difficult to gain weight, which makes recovery slower than usual.

When will I be able to get back to work?

Convalescence will take from two to six months. Physical exercise should be postponed for four to six months. About two months after the wound is completely healed, you will be able to resume some of your normal activities.

Will radiation therapy or chemotherapy be prescribed?

Sometimes radiation therapy is used after surgery. In other cases chemotherapy is used, either alone or in combination with the radiation therapy. The drug 5-Fluorouracil has been used with some success; other drugs are being evaluated.

Are most doctors qualified to diagnose and operate for pancreatic cancer?

This is a difficult diagnosis and a very specialized area. Major medical centers, especially those specializing in cancer treatment, have had more experience than smaller local hospitals. You should ask your doctor to check with the clinical cooperative groups in your area for information on new treatments or to see if you can be admitted into one of the controlled studies being conducted on pancreatic cancer. (See Chapter 23.)

chapter 16

Cancer of the Female Reproductive Organs

Questions to Ask Your Doctor Before Any Operation on the Female Reproductive Organs

- What size is the tumor and where is it located?
- Is it a cancerous tumor or is it benign?
- Has there been any spread?
- Will the ovaries be removed?
- Will this operation impair my ability to have a baby?
- Is there any chance that the ovaries can be saved?
- Will this operation impair my urinary function or control?
- Is the operation really necessary or is it elective?
- Is there an alternative way of treating this condition? Radiotherapy? Implant? Chemotherapy?
- In what condition are my bladder and rectal walls?
- Where will the scar be — and will it be horizontal or vertical?
- Will you show me on the diagram exactly where the problem is and what you are planning to remove?
- Will I still be able to have sexual intercourse?

Is the National Cancer Institute supporting any studies on cancer of the female reproductive organs?

The National Cancer Institute's clinical cooperative groups presently have studies of new treatment methods for cancer of the cervix, ovary, uterus, and vulva as well as some general studies on gynecologic tumors. (See Chapter 23.)

What kind of doctor should I see if I have cancer of the female reproductive organs?

Either a gynecologist or a surgeon whose specialty is in the area of gynecological cancer should be responsible for the primary treatment of your case. If you will have a radium implant, a therapeutic radiologist will also be involved. If you are being treated with chemotherapy you will probably be referred to an oncologist or hematologist.

Which organs are involved in cancer of the female reproductive system?

Six main organs are involved in cancer of the female reproductive system:
- Vulva
- Vagina
- Cervix (neck of uterus)
- Womb or endometrium (body of uterus)
- Fallopian tubes
- Ovaries

What is the vulva?

The vulva is the external fatty tissue around the outside of the vagina. It is made up of several structures, including the clitoris, the labia, and the hymen.

What is the vagina?

The vagina is the barrel-shaped female organ through which a woman has babies. It is also known as the birth canal.

What are the cervix and the endometrium?

The cervix and the endometrium are both part of the uterus, which is a hollow, pear-shaped muscular organ in which the fertilized egg attaches itself and develops during pregnancy. It is also called the womb. The cervix is the lower part of the uterus, located at the top of the vagina. It is the mouth of the womb. The endometrium is the lining of the body of the uterus.

What are the ovaries?

The ovaries are two almond-shaped female organs that produce estrogen and that once a month release an egg during ovulation.

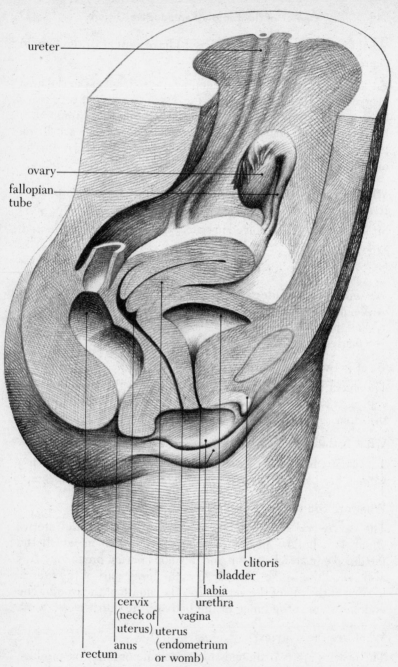

ureter

ovary

fallopian
tube

clitoris

bladder

labia

urethra

cervix
(neck of
uterus)

vagina

anus

uterus
(endometrium
or womb)

rectum

Female reproductive organs

428

Cancer of the Female Reproductive Organs

Type	High Risk	Symptoms	Diagnostic Tests	Treatments
Vulva	55–65 age group	Itching, burning, pain	Pap smear, simple biopsy, colposcopy, dermatologic punch	Vulvectomy and/or surgical removal of inguinal lymph nodes, radiation therapy, chemotherapy
Vagina	50–55 age group; young women whose mothers took DES	Painless bleeding following intercourse or exam, bladder pain, frequent urination	Pap smear, colposcopy, iodine or Schiller's test recommended for high-risk women	Radiation, radioisotopes, surgery
Cervix or neck of uterus (cervix, cervical canal, or entrance to womb)	40–49 age group; more than 5 pregnancies; early intercourse; young women whose mothers took DES	Unusual bleeding or discharge; pelvic pain	Pap smear, colposcopy, biopsy, conization. Note: Pap smear 97% accurate for this type of cancer	Radiotherapy, surgery, chemotherapy and hormones, cryotherapy, electrocoagulation
Body of uterus or womb (endometrium)	50–64 age group; women with diabetes or high blood pressure; overweight; those who have never been pregnant; family history of this type of cancer; late menopause	Unusual bleeding especially if past menopause; lower abdominal and back pain. Note: Fibroids and other nonmalignant conditions may cause same symptoms.	Vaginal pool smear, aspiration curettage, D&C. Note: Pap smear only 50% accurate for this type. Diagnostic results unreliable in menopausal women using estrogen.	Hysterectomy or preoperative radiation followed by hysterectomy and oophorectomy. Hormone therapy with surgery. Difficult to cure.

Cancer of the Female Reproductive Organs (continued)

Type	High Risk	Symptoms	Diagnostic Tests	Treatments
Fallopian tubes (uterine tubes)	Extremely rare	Profuse, intermittent watery discharge or bleeding	Diagnosis difficult. Positive Pap smear; usually requires operation to identify.	Hysterectomy and bilateral oophorectomy, radiation and chemotherapy
Ovary	50–64 age group; history of ovarian imbalance or malfunction	No symptoms except vague abdominal discomfort or indigestion. Advanced symptoms: abdominal pain and swelling.	Diagnosis difficult. Physical exam only method for detection. Positive diagnosis requires exploratory laparotomy.	Hysterectomy and oophorectomy. Radiation sometimes used. Chemotherapy used following surgery. Difficult to cure.

Operations for Cancer of the Female Reproductive Organs

OPERATION	PROCEDURE	YOU SHOULD KNOW
Surgical conization or cold-knife conization	Removal of localized preinvasive lesion	More extensive than simple biopsy, performed under general anesthesia. If successful can be done instead of hysterectomy. Pregnancy possible but should be discussed.
Subtotal or supracervical hysterectomy	Uterus is removed, but cervix remains	Will be unable to bear children. Normal sexual relations.
Vaginal hysterectomy	Uterus removed through vagina	Not advisable if uterus is enlarged or not fully movable. More difficult to perform than hysterectomy.
Total hysterectomy	Removal of cervix and uterus	Unable to bear children but will continue to menstruate, have normal menopause. Normal sexual relations.
Radical hysterectomy, also called Wertheim's operation	Removal of uterus, tubes and ovaries as well as much of tissue surrounding uterus, regional lymph nodes, part of vagina	Because of extent of operation, greater chance of postoperative complications. If done on premenopausal woman, causes abrupt menopause. Will be unable to bear children. Normal sexual relations.
Myomectomy	Fibroid tumors removed from wall of uterus but uterus left intact	Usually recommended for younger women with fibroid tumors who wish to retain ability to become pregnant.
Oophorectomy, also called ovariectomy	Removal of one or both ovaries	Abrupt menopause if both ovaries removed. If only one ovary removed, may still become pregnant; will continue to menstruate. Normal sexual relations.

Operations for Cancer of the Female Reproductive Organs (continued)

OPERATION	PROCEDURE	YOU SHOULD KNOW
Salpingectomy or bilateral salpingo oophorectomy	Removal of both fallopian tubes and ovaries	Menstruation ceases, unable to reproduce. Normal sexual relations.
Simple vulvectomy	Removal of skin of major and minor lips of vulva and clitoris	Normal sexual relations still possible.
Radical vulvectomy	Removal of vaginal lips, clitoris, skin surrounding vulva and lymph glands	Preoperative radiotherapy often prescribed prior to operation. Normal sexual relations still possible.
Pelvic exenteration	Radical hysterectomy plus removal of rectum and bladder	For very advanced cancer of cervix. Leaves patient with both bowel and urinary openings on abdomen. Very extreme operation.
Vaginectomy	Removal of vagina	Vagina may be smaller or shorter after surgery. Plastic surgery may be necessary.

What are the fallopian tubes?

The fallopian tubes, also called uterine tubes, run from the ovaries to the womb. The fallopian tubes transport the egg from the ovaries to the uterus.

What is the most common place for cancer cells to grow in the reproductive organs?

The most common place is in the cervix. If the cancer starting there is not found or is not treated, it can grow and spread to other reproductive organs and to other body organs.

Who is at risk for cancer of the vulva?

Usually women with cancer of the vulva fall into the 60–80-year-old age group, though it can occur in premenopausal women. It is a fairly uncommon disease. Eighty-five to 90 percent of the cases of vulvular cancer which are surgically treated and which have not metastasized to other parts of the body are considered curable.

What are some of the symptoms?

Common symptoms include itching, burning, pain, and bleeding. A Pap smear and a biopsy are necessary to help diagnose whether these symptoms indicate cancer or whether an infection is present which may be causing the same symptoms.

How is a biopsy taken in the vulvular area?

The doctor will give a simple injection of local anesthetic. A small dermatologic punch is usually used to obtain a biopsy. The procedure is simple and almost painless. The doctor may use a colposcope in his routine checking of a suspicious growth in this area. This allows him to have a photographic recording of the site for future reference.

What are the doctor's considerations in deciding how to treat cancer of the vulva?

The physican must tailor treatment to the individual patient. He considers the size of the growth, whether it has spread from the original site, whether radical surgery is practical for the patient on the basis of her age and health, or whether radiotherapy is feasible. If the disease has progressed to a stage that is not treatable by either surgery or radiotherapy, the doctor may consider the use of chemotherapy.

The General Stages of Cancer of the Vulva

STAGE	OTHER CLASSIFICATION	EXPLANATION
Stage I	T1	Tumor 2 centimeters or less, confined to vulva
Stage II	T2	Tumor larger than 2 centimeters, confined to vulva
Stage III	T3	Tumor of any size with spread to urethra, vagina, or anus and/or nodes obviously involved but mobile
Stage IV	T4	Tumor invading bladder or rectum, bone, or any fixed nodes or distant metastasis

What operations are performed for cancer of the vulva?

If a biopsy indicates leukoplakia (a condition which usually causes intense itching), a simple vulvectomy will usually be performed. If untreated, 50 percent of those with leukoplakia will later develop cancer of the vulva.

What is leukoplakia of the vulva?

Leukoplakia is *not* a cancerous condition, though in some cases it may be a precancerous condition. Leukoplakia can appear in various parts of the body with mucous-membrane lining—such as the inside of the mouth, the anal region, and the genital areas. It is characterized by moist white patches that are raised and may contain grooves or clefts and have sharply defined edges. In the vulva, leukoplakia can cause itching. Because it can progress through the formation of fissures to a cancerous condition, it should be watched carefully by the physician and removed surgically if it does not disappear.

What is a simple vulvectomy?

This operation includes the removal of the skin of the major and minor lips of the vulva and clitoris. New skin will grow in the area to replace the skin removed by the surgery. X-ray treatments may be given in conjunction with the surgery.

What is a radical vulvectomy?

This operation is performed when the biopsy shows that cancer has invaded the skin of the vulva. The operation includes the removal of the vaginal lips, clitoris, skin surrounding the vulva, and the lymph glands. Separate incisions are usually made in both groins to remove lymph glands.

Can cancer of the vulva be treated with radiation?

Yes. However, surgery is the preferred treatment, since tissues in the area are sensitive to radiation. The radiation is uncomfortable and the area is difficult to treat with radiation. Radiotherapy is sometimes used prior to the operation to reduce the size of large, infected lesions.

Are any other treatments used for cancer of the vulva?

Surgery is the preferred method of treatment, as indicated by the excellent survival rates when this method is followed—up to 85–95 percent, even in Stage II disease. However, if the cancer has metastasized beyond the regional lymph nodes, radiation therapy is usually used. In the very early stages, a chemothera-peutic cream (5-FU) has been used over a ten-week period in patients whose immune response is shown to be functioning well. In some cases this treatment appears to cause the lesion to disappear. Biopsies will usually be performed at intervals during and after this treatment. If the disease remains, the patient can be retreated with the 5-FU. However, if the cancer persists after two trials of 5-FU and it is small and in one area, local removal of the cancer is usually recommended. If the pathological workup indicates spread of the cancer, vulvectomy will be recommended.

Are radium needle implants used for cancer of the vulva?

Radium needle implants are sometimes used to treat cancer in this area. Usually it is when the cancer cannot be operated on or has metastasized from another location.

What type of anesthesia is used for a vulvectomy?

Usually a general anesthesia or a spinal.

How long must the patient remain in bed after a vulvectomy?

Usually the patient will remain in bed for two days, depending on the extent of the surgery.

How long is the hospital stay after a vulvectomy?

This, too, depends upon the extent of the surgery. In a simple vulvectomy, the patient will usually be allowed to return home after two weeks.

Are there any complications that one should be alerted to following vulvectomy?

In a radical vulvectomy, because of the removal of a large number of lymph nodes, fluid collects under the skin and may be a problem for quite some time following the operation until other lymph channels have become established. It is extremely important for the patient to start on deep-breathing, coughing, and leg exercises immediately after surgery to reduce the possibility of complications such as infections, pneumonia, leg edema, or lung complications. Usually, the doctor will leave orders for the patient to be turned frequently, and for pillows to be placed so as to lessen tension on the operation. Frequent irrigations with sterile saline solution, heat lamp, and sitz baths may be used to promote healing of the wound.

Can a woman become pregnant after having a vulvectomy?

Yes, a patient who has had a vulvectomy can become pregnant. Delivery might be a problem and a cesarean section would probably be done. However, since most of the people who require this operation are in the older age group, the problem does not arise often.

Is sexual intercourse possible after vulvectomy?

Yes, intercourse is still possible, because the vagina is still present. You may have to change position or technique. For example, the woman may have to keep her thighs close together to lengthen the distance from the vaginal cavity so that although the penetration is not as deep, it can still be satisfying. Most important is whether or not the two people care enough about each other to work at finding new ways to satisfy each other.

Are cancer of the vulva and cancer of the vagina common?

Neither cancer of the vulva nor cancer of the vagina are common cancers. Most frequently they appear in women over the age of 65. Some 500 new cases are diagnosed in the United States each year of these two cancers. In the past few years, it has been found that some teenage girls were developing cancer of the vagina. The drug DES (diethylstilbestrol) given to pregnant women between 1945 and 1970 has been suspected of causing abnormalities in this area.

How is cancer of the vagina diagnosed?

Pelvic exams, Pap smears, colposcopy, and iodine or Schiller's tests are used to diagnose cancer of the vagina. Women who have previously had either in situ or invasive carcinoma of the cervix are likely to develop premalignant conditions of the vagina. Leukoplakia of the vagina is usually regarded as a precancerous condition.

Are biopsies usually performed to diagnose cancer of the vagina?

Yes. Biopsy is always necessary to confirm a diagnosis of cancer. Careful diagnosis is important in vaginal cancer, since a biopsy sometimes shows the condition to be a metastasis from another kind of cancer. A biopsy is also important because treatment for each stage of vaginal cancer varies.

What are the treatments for vaginal cancer?

The treatments are surgery, either removing the cancerous areas or doing a total hysterectomy and/or a total vaginectomy and vulvectomy, depending on the stage of the cancer and its location. Sometimes radiation therapy—both external and radiation implants in the vaginal cavity—is used.

What is the treatment for cancer in situ of the vagina?

The cancer is either removed surgically or treated by radiation implant.

The General Stages of Cancer of the Vagina

Stage	Other Classification	Explanation
Stage I	T1	Tumor limited to the vaginal wall
Stage II	T2	Involves subvaginal tissue but not extended to pelvic wall
Stage III	T3	Extended to pelvic wall
Stage IV	T4	Extended beyond pelvis or invading bladder or rectum or other organs
Stage IVA	T4a	Spread to adjacent organs
Stage IVB	T4b	Spread to distant organs

Is there any special care which must be taken when having a radiation implant in the vagina?

Description of the procedure for radiation implants will be found in Chapter 7. However, there are a few points which must be remembered if you are having vaginal radiation-implant treatment. For two weeks following the implant, the patient should not use tampons, should not have intercourse, and should not douche or take tub baths. After the two-week period, it is necessary, in the interest of proper healing, for the patient to either use a dilator or to have intercourse in order to prevent the vaginal cavity from closing and/or forming adhesions.

Is sexual intercourse possible following a radiation implant in the vagina?

Yes. The first time you have intercourse following the implant, be sure to use a water-soluble lubricant. Do not allow penetration of more than 1 to 2 inches. Most women find that a lubricant must always be used for comfortable intercourse.

Is plastic surgery ever used after a vaginectomy or after other treatment for vaginal cancer?

This depends upon the extent of the treatment. One of the problems with treatment in the vagina is that some deformity occurs in many cases. The doctor's first priority is to try to cure the cancer. Once this is accomplished, he will try to reconstruct the organs. An artificial vagina can be constructed by making a cavity and lining it with a skin graft or an intestinal transplant. Sometimes the vagina is smaller or shorter after surgery, but the patient finds that she can still have reasonably adequate sexual relations without reconstruction.

Who is at greater risk of cervical cancer?

At a greater risk of cervical cancer are women who have unusual bleeding or vaginal discharge between periods, had frequent sex before the age of 20, have had sex with many partners, have had more than five pregnancies, and have poor genital hygiene.

Is cancer of the cervix easy to detect?

Yes. Cancer of the cervix is detected through a Pap smear, which is a very simple examination. Cancer of the cervix is virtually 100 percent curable in its earliest stages.

How is the Pap test done?

Living cells are collected from the vaginal fluid by gently scraping the surface of the cervix. These cells are preserved with fixative solution, stained, and put on a microscope slide to be read by a pathologist. The test is done by a gynecologist or another physician in his office or it can be done at a clinic.

Is it necessary to have a Pap test every year?

Since the early 1950s American women have been urged to have an annual Pap test. There are many doctors and health institutions who now question the necessity of a yearly Pap test. For people with limited funds, some physicians are now recommending Pap smears annually beginning at the start of sexual activity or at age 20. After two or three negative Pap tests within a year of each other, smears need be taken only at three-to-five-year intervals. However, until there are more definite guidelines (the National Cancer Institute is holding meetings to find a consensus on the subject), be guided by your own doctor.

Besides the Pap test, how else can cervical cancer be detected?

There are usually no visible symptoms or signs in the early stages of cancer of the cervix. As the cancer grows, there may be unusual bleeding or discharge. You may have a longer menstrual period than usual, a heavier flow, bleeding between periods or after intercourse, or bleeding after menopause. The bleeding is usually described as bright-red and unpredictable as to time, amount, or duration. Although these symptoms may not be cancer, they should be checked by a doctor.

At what age is a woman most apt to get cervical cancer?

The age varies, with the peak for cancer in situ being between 30 and 40 and for invasive cancer between 40 and 50. However, cervical cancer may occur at any age. About 15 percent is seen before the age of 30. Statistics indicate that there is an increasing number of patients diagnosed at the age of 20 years or below.

Isn't the cervix part of the uterus?

It is. The cervix is the lower part or neck of the uterus. It protrudes into the vagina and is the segment of the uterus which can be seen by the doctor during a pelvic examination. Cancer of the neck of the uterus or cervix and cancer of the body of the uterus (endometrium) present two very different sorts of problems, so it is important for you to ask the doctor exactly where the problem lies.

Can a Pap smear detect cancer of the uterus?

A Pap smear can accurately detect cancer of the cervix, but it is sustantially less accurate for detecting cancer of the body of the uterus (endometrium), the fallopian tubes, or the ovary. In cases where these types of cancer are discovered through a Pap smear it is because the cancer cells have passed down through the tube into the cavity of the uterus and continued out through the cervix and into the vaginal discharge.

In other words, the Pap test is really designed only to detect cervical cancer?

That is correct. And women who have regular Pap smears can view cervical cancer as a preventable disease. Since cells from the cervix are continually being sloughed off into the normal discharge from the cervix and vagina, the Pap smear makes it possible for cancer to be detected before it has had an opportunity to invade or spread.

Is it painful to have a Pap smear?

No. There is little or no discomfort—and most doctors include it as a part of the regular pelvic examination. It is a good idea for all women over the age of 20—and most especially for women of menopausal age—to have regular Pap smears. If you have a special, high-risk situation, your physician may require a smear to be taken more often than once a year.

How can I be sure I'm getting an accurate Pap smear?

The accuracy of your Pap smear depends on the quality of the laboratory interpreting the glass slide which is sent by the doctor—and so it is important to have a doctor who is fussy about the lab he uses. However, women themselves can ensure a more accurate reading if they follow these suggestions:

- Don't douche for at least three days before your Pap test. If you do, there won't be enough loose cells in your vaginal fluid for an accurate test.
- Use shower instead of tub bath for at least 48 hours before the test.
- Don't use tampons, birth-control foams, or jellies for five days before your appointment.
- Try to arrange your appointment for day 15–20 of your menstrual cycle.

Is it necessary to have a Pap smear after a woman has had a hysterectomy?

That depends upon why the hysterectomy was done and what was removed. If the cervix is still present, Pap tests are necessary. If the hysterectomy was done because of cancer, it is absolutely necessary to have a regular Pap test. You should discuss this with your doctor.

I usually douche before going to the doctor for a gynecological exam. Is this wise?

No, it is not. Since the Pap smear is based on an examination of the actual vaginal discharge, a smear would not be accurate if you have douched during the few days prior to the examination. You should not douche for at least three days prior to the day of your examination because a douche washes away the vaginal discharge which the doctor needs for his examination.

When should a woman have her first Pap smear?

A woman's first Pap smear should normally be done when she reaches the age of 18. If her mother took the hormone DES while pregnant, a Pap test should be performed at the start of her menstrual periods.

What do the different classes of Pap test mean?

Pap test results are usually assigned numbers from 1 to 5, although some laboratories use slightly different systems. The usual meaning of the tests is:

- *Class 1:* Smear completely normal. No abnormal cells.
- *Class 2:* Some atypical cells present but none suggest a malignancy. Inflammation and/or possible infection. Pap test should be repeated between three and six months.
- *Class 3:* Some abnormal cells present, suggestive of but not definitely malignant cells. The degree and kind of abnormality is greater than Class 2 test. Suggest followup smear and biopsy.
- *Class 4:* Smear contains some malignant cells. There are signs of early cancer. Followup smear and biopsy needed.
- *Class 5:* Smear contains malignant cells more disorganized than Class 4. Immediate treatment necessary.

What does the doctor do if I have a Class 2 Pap smear?

It depends on other conditions. A Class 2 Pap smear can be the result of a bacterial infection or inflammation, for example. If there is some evidence of inflammation, the doctor would probably treat you for that condition and then repeat the smear.

What does the doctor do about a Class 3 Pap test?

It depends upon what else the pathologist told the doctor about his findings. If no lesion is seen, usually a Class 3 would call for another Pap smear test. If the second test was also a Class 3, a biopsy would probably be performed. Sometimes the Class 3 level is referred to as dysplasia, which is still a noncancerous condition. The relationship between cancer and dysplasia is not entirely clear. Class 3 cells can return to normal cells for no obvious reason and without treatment.

What would the doctor do about a Class 4 or a Class 5 test?

In both cases, a biopsy would be done. Class 4 means the degree of abnormality has reached the level at which a biopsy should be taken to determine whether or not cancer is present. Class 5 means that the cells appear to be even more bizarre and are apt to be associated with a more aggressive and more widely spread tumor. Remember, as noted before, the classification of the Pap test varies from one laboratory to another. Normally, your physician would discuss the findings with you. Rarely would you be given a numerical classification without an explanation.

Why must a biopsy be done? Can't the Pap smear tell whether or not I have cancer?

The Pap smear is only a screening tool. Although it is very accurate as a screening device, a biopsy must be done to give a definite diagnosis of cancer. The biopsy also is essential for staging the disease. If the cell samples from the Pap smear show abnormality, additional diagnostic tests are performed. They may include colposcopy or conization.

I have read the terms "dysplasia" and "hyperplasia" used in reference to cancer of the uterus. What do they mean?

"Dysplasia" is a term used in describing a condition in the cervix. The cells covering the cervix usually go through mild to severe changes before becoming cancer. These changes are called dysplasia. Similar changes in the tissue lining the uterus are called hyperplasia.

Does dysplasia or hyperplasia always lead to cancer?

No. These precancerous conditions do not necessarily lead to cancer. It is important, however, that any woman with such a condition be treated and then examined by a physician at regular intervals.

What is carcinoma in situ?

Carcinoma in situ is the earliest stage of cancer. It means that the cancer is confined to its original site. If not detected and treated properly, the cancer cells go into deeper layers of the uterus, then spread to neighboring organs such as the vagina, bladder, or rectum and eventually metastasize to other parts of the body.

Is there any way the doctor can examine the cervix, the vulva, and the vagina without an operation?

Yes. The colposcope allows the doctor to look into parts of a woman's reproductive system—the cervix, vulva, and vagina—without operating. Previously, an operation was needed to see these organs. The colposcope is basically a microscope on a stand which gives a lighted, magnified view showing greater detail than can be seen by the naked eye. Since using the colposcope properly requires special training, many doctors refer their patients to physicians who are specialized in this technique. Doctors can also biopsy the organs with this technique. No anesthesia is needed. The procedure usually takes only 10 or 15 minutes.

How is the colposcopy done?

In doing a colposcopy, the doctor proceeds with the usual pelvic examination. With the speculum (the instrument used to separate the walls of the vagina to expose the cervix) inserted into the vagina, the doctor points the magnifying lens and a powerful light at the opening of the vagina and looks through an eyepiece. The cervix and/or vagina are swabbed with a special solution. The solution, along with a green lens placed on the colposcope, makes the abnormal area appear as whitish spots. Biopsies of these white spots or any abnormal areas are usually taken for examination. The sensation of a biopsy is similar to a mild menstrual cramp. A TV attachment on the side of the colposcope beams a picture to a nearby monitor. If he wishes, the doctor can make videotapes of the cells to study changes over a period of time. No part of the instrument is inserted into the vagina.

When is a colposcopy done?

Sometimes a colposcopy is done when you have had an abnormal Pap smear. With the colposcope the doctor can see if there is an abnormal pattern to the blood vessels in your cervix and whether there is a lesion there. Using the colposcope, the doctor can very often identify the abnormal tissue from which abnormal cells on the Pap smear have been scraped. In many instances such abnormal tissue may then be destroyed or removed painlessly in the office, often avoiding other surgical procedures.

Is a colposcopy painful? Will it affect my ability to have children?

No, the colposcopy is neither painful nor will it in any way affect your ability to bear children.

Will I have a discharge after I have a colposcopic examination?

Sometimes. The biopsied area is usually swabbed with a brown solution to prevent bleeding. This solution can cause a slight brownish vaginal discharge for one or two days. The solution may be irritating to your partner so the doctor will usually advise you to abstain from intercourse for a day or two.

Is the colposcope used for DES daughters?

Yes, the colposcope is also used as an examining tool for girls whose mothers took DES during pregnancy.

How much does colposcopy examination usually cost?

It ranges from about $50 to $100.

What is conization?

Conization is a surgical procedure to remove a cone-shaped specimen of tissue from the cervical canal. It provides a larger tissue sample than is removed for a biopsy. It is used sometimes when the area causing the abnormal Pap smear is a large one or if it extends into the cervical opening. Conization involves removing the central portion of the cervix and its other opening. The amount of tissue removed depends on the size and location of the abnormal area. It is a minor surgical procedure that must be done in the hospital, usually using general anesthesia.

Is conization used instead of colposcopy?

Before the colposcope, conization was used to do a biopsy of the cervix. Today, colposcopy is the preferred method because conization costs more and takes more time. Conization can also cause difficulty with future pregnancies. However, conization is used as a diagnostic tool if colposcopy fails to determine the source of the abnormal Pap smear.

The General Stages of Cancer of the Cervix

STAGE	OTHER CLASSIFICATION	EXPLANATION
Stage 0	TIS	Carcinoma in situ as demonstrated by biopsy
Stage I	T1, T1a, T1b	Tumor confined to the cervix
Stage II	T2, T2a, T2b	Extends beyond the cervix but not to the pelvic wall; involves vagina but not as far as lower third
Stage III	T3, T3b	Extends to one or both pelvic walls or lower vagina, or ureteral obstruction
Stage IV	T4, T4a, T4b	Extends beyond true pelvis or involves bladder or rectum, spread to adjacent or distant organs

If the biopsy shows that I have cancer of the cervix, what other tests will the doctor perform before he begins the treatment?

Before treatment is started, the doctor will usually perform a cystogram, an intravenous pyelogram, and barium enema examination. Depending upon the stage of the disease, he might also perform some body scans to check for involvement in the bone or liver or a lymphangiogram to look for lymph-node involvement. The stage of the tumor is the principal factor in determining the particular treatment which will be used, so the tests the physician performs are very important.

What kind of treatment is used for cervical cancer?

The treatments used for early-stage cervical cancer include minor surgery such as conization, cryosurgery (freezing), or sometimes removal of the uterus. The important point is that cancer of the cervix if discovered early is 100 percent curable. Sometimes in the precancerous stage cervical changes are treated by electrocoagulation—the destruction of tissue through intense heat delivered by electric current. In some early cases, childbearing function can be maintained.

What kind of treatment is used to treat advanced cervical cancer?

In the more advanced stages, extensive surgery or radiation is required to treat cancer of the cervix.

Is cryosurgery often used in place of conization?

It depends upon the extent of the abnormality. Cryosurgery is effective in eliminating abnormal cells in carefully selected patients. If the abnormal area is large or goes into the cervical opening, then conization is usually used. Sometimes, if cryosurgery does not eliminate all the abnormal cells, conization will be done.

Is the conization used for treating early cervical cancer the same procedure as used in diagnosing it?

Yes. A conization takes a cone-shaped piece of tissue and involves removing the central portion of the cervix and its outer opening. The amount of tissue removed depends on the size and location of the abnormal area.

Will a conization mean that I can no longer have a baby?

This will depend upon the amount of tissue removed and on the future progress of the disease. The conization alone usually does not rule out future pregnancy. This is a question you should definitely discuss with your doctor so he can discuss it with you in relation to your particular case.

When is cryosurgery used?

Cryosurgery is often recommended to treat abnormal Pap smears due to early changes in cell structure called dysplasia. The procedure is often done in the doctor's office. It takes about 15 minutes to perform the treatment, no medication is needed, and it can be done with an IUD in place.

How is cryosurgery done?

After you are positioned on the examining table, the doctor will use a speculum to expose the cervix. A probe is used to transmit the gas used for freezing from the tank to the cervix. The gas, usually nitrous oxide or carbon dioxide, is applied for three minutes or longer while an ice ball forms.

Will I feel anything during the procedure?

You might feel some cramping, like mild menstrual cramps. After the procedure is finished you might feel "weak in the knees."

Will I have any kind of discharge after the cryosurgery?

You will probably have a heavy, watery discharge for two to four weeks. It might be blood-tinged, be irritating to the skin, and have an odor. If you wish, you can wear a sanitary pad to absorb the fluid. Do not use tampons. You may take warm tub baths as often as you like to relieve the irritation. The mild cramps may also continue for a few hours or a few days. The doctor will probably prescribe medication to relieve the discomfort.

Will there be a change in my periods because of the cryosurgery?

You might experience a temporary change in the pattern of your periods—it might be early or late. Bleeding may be heavier or lighter than normal.

Are there any side effects of the cryosurgery I should report to the doctor?

There are some side effects you should call to the attention of the doctor immediately:
- Fever and chills
- Heavy vaginal bleeding with clots
- Extreme pain in the lower abdomen or back

Can I have intercourse after cryosurgery?

You cannot have intercourse for ten days after cryosurgery, since the treatment has temporarily injured the cervix. You must be careful in order to protect yourself against infection and bleeding. During those ten days you should not douche or use tampons.

Can the cryosurgery be done while I have my menstrual period?

No, it cannot. It is best done within one week after your menstrual period ends.

What followup is necessary after cryosurgery?

You should have a Pap smear done about three months after the cryosurgery and again in three more months. Then, if the smears are normal, you will probably have Pap smears every six months from then on.

What happens when cervical cancer is discovered in a pregnant woman?

The treatment depends upon the extent of the cancer and upon how pregnant the woman is when it is discovered. A punch biopsy can be taken at any time during pregnancy if there is a lesion on the cervix. If no lesion is present but the smear is suspicious, most doctors wait until the end of the third month to carry out a conization, thus reducing the risk of abortion. If a Class 3 smear is discovered late in pregnancy, a vaginal delivery may be possible with delay of conization until several weeks after the birth. If a Class 4 or Class 5 smear is discovered, conization is usually postponed, an early cesarean birth is planned, and conization or hysterectomy is performed several weeks later, followed by radiation therapy.

How is cancer of the endometrium detected?

The Pap test is only about 40 percent effective in detecting endometrial cancer—that is, cancer in the womb or lining of the body of the uterus. Two other techniques are used in diagnosing this cancer: dilation and curettage (D&C) and aspiration curettage.

How is dilation and curettage (D&C) performed?

After the patient is anesthetized, usually with light, general anesthesia, the doctor gently stretches the cervix and inserts an instrument called a curette, which he uses to scrape the wall of the uterus. Tissue samples are removed for study under the microscope. The procedure is usually done in the hospital, often on an outpatient basis.

What is aspiration curettage?

The doctor, in his office, takes a tissue specimen from the lining of the uterus. A device, called an endometrial aspirator, consists of a disposable tube connected to a syringe. The tube is inserted through the cervix into the uterus and scrapes a piece of tissue from the uterine lining. The tissue samples are then studied under the microscope for abnormal cell changes.

What do the results from the aspiration curettage show?

If analysis of the tissue shows endometrial hyperplasia (an overgrowth of lining cells), the doctor usually advises the patient to have a D&C to help prevent future problems. If there is a history of uterine cancer in your family, or if you are overweight, have high blood pressure, have been on estrogen replacement therapy, and/or are going through the menopause, ask your doctor about having this kind of analysis.

What is endometriosis?

Endometriosis is a condition in which the kind of tissue which normally lines the uterus is found in abnormal places, such as on the surface of the ovaries, the outside of the uterus, in operation scars in the lower abdomen, in tissue between the vagina and rectum, etc. It is not a cancerous condition, but it does cause painful menstrual periods, abnormal bleeding, and general discomfort. Surgery is usually required.

What is hyperplasia?

Endometrial hyperplasia is an overabundance of cells lining the uterus. It is not cancerous. However, among certain women who are predisposed toward cancer of the uterus, hyperplasia can develop into cancer. Though every case of hyperplasia does not develop into cancer, uterine cancer always goes through a hyperplastic stage before becoming cancerous. Therefore, hyperplasia is a warning that cancer may develop.

What are the symptoms of hyperplasia?

If the uterus is hyperplastic, bleeding will occur. In addition to heavy menstrual periods, there will be bleeding at irregular intervals.

What is the treatment for hyperplasia?

A good gynecologist will test for hyperplasia by aspirating cells from the uterus, by "jet" washing out of uterine cells for analysis, or by performing a D&C (dilation and curettage). A Pap smear is not a conclusive test for uterine cancer. The Pap smear is designed to detect cervical cancer. If the doctor finds that you do have hyperplasia, he may prescribe progesterone for one week of each month. The progesterone is designed to cause the lining to shed the built-up cells. Or the doctor may decide that the proliferation is due to menopausal causes and will withhold treatment until menopause has occurred. If the condition doesn't improve after menopause, then the doctor may recommend a hysterectomy.

What causes bleeding between periods?

Bleeding between periods can be caused by many different conditions: polyps in the cervix or uterus, fibroid tumors, overactivity of the endometrial lining, and vaginitis in which the skin of the vagina thins and bleeds easily, to name just a few. Bleeding between periods is *abnormal* and indicates that you should be examined to determine the cause. Any bleeding that occurs six months after your period has ceased should be investigated by your doctor.

Is it normal to have heavy clotting during premenopause?

Heavy bleeding and clotting are very common during pre-menopause. As the ovarian function decreases, the pituitary gland attempts to make the ovaries respond and a large amount of estrogen is produced by the body. The endometrium becomes filled with tissue, and when the buildup starts to shed, heavy clotting and bleeding result.

Why does the doctor prescribe progesterone when I have heavy bleeding and clotting?

He does this to test the reason for the heavy bleeding and clotting. After you have taken progesterone for one week, the uterus can usually be stimulated to return to a more normal menstrual rhythm. If normal periods return, the doctor knows that the heavy periods were caused by a lack of ovulation and progesterone. If the heavy bleeding and clotting continue, further investigation is necessary.

The General Stages of Cancer of the Endometrium or Uterus

STAGE	OTHER CLASSIFICATION	EXPLANATION
Stage 0	TIS	Carcinoma in situ
Stage I	T1, T1a, T1b	Confined to the uterus
Stage II	T2	Extends to the cervix
Stage III	T3	Has extended outside uterus but not outside true pelvis
Stage IV	T4	Extension beyond pelvis or invading bladder or rectum or other organs

Stage I may also have a G rating—G1, highly differentiated; G2, moderately differentiated; G3, undifferentiated.

What is the treatment for cancer of the endometrium?

Cancer of the endometrium or uterine cancer is generally treated by surgery or radiation or by a combination of the two. In the precancerous stages, endometrial changes may be treated with the hormone progesterone. It is important for the doctor to assess the extent of the disease before treatment begins, since treatment differs depending upon the stage of the cancer.

What is a hysterectomy?

Technically, hysterectomy means only the removal of the uterus. It does not refer to the removal of ovaries or fallopian tubes, which are sometimes removed at the same time. However, most women use the term vaguely, and many do not know exactly what was removed. You should be sure to ask your doctor to explain exactly what he is planning to remove and why.

Are most hysterectomies performed because cancer is present?

No. Most hysterectomies are performed because of fibroids and hyperplasia.

What is a fibroid tumor?

A fibroid tumor is a noncancerous growth composed mostly of

muscle and fibrous connective tissue. Fibrous tumors are most common among women who are over 35 years of age, and are not usually dangerous unless they grow very large. It is estimated that about 40 percent of women over 50 have fibroid tumors. Most fibroid tumors shrink after menopause. If a fibroid tumor grows large, it will usually cause bleeding and may cause pressure on the bladder, rectum, or ureter. Estrogen replacement may cause them to continue to grow. If you have fibroid tumors, they should be checked by your gynecologist. However, unless they are causing problems, they do not need to be removed.

What kind of tests are done before a hysterectomy is performed?

A complete blood count, urine analysis, electrocardiogram, and x-rays of the chest. Usually an intravenous pyelogram and a barium enema are used as part of the preoperation tests.

What kinds of problems do doctors run into in making a diagnosis about hysterectomy?

Because it is difficult to examine the entire area fully, diagnosis is often complicated. Fibroids, for instance, can completely fill the uterus. They can be quite solid, but if they begin to degenerate, they become soft. X-rays will detect a large mass, but cannot differentiate between a large fibroid and an ovarian cyst.

What is a vaginal hysterectomy?

That is when the doctor performs the operation through the vagina, so that no incision is necessary.

What organs other than the uterus are usually removed during a hysterectomy?

It depends on why the doctor is performing the operation. In the cancer field, for example, if your cancer involves just the cervix, the surgeon may take out only the uterus and the lymph nodes that drain that area. If the cancer is more widespread, much of the tissue surrounding the cervix, sometimes including the bladder and/or the lower part of the bowel, may have to be removed. If the cancer involves the body of the uterus, the uterus as well as the tubes and the ovaries might have to be taken out.

Will I have menstrual periods after the hysterectomy?

No. After a hysterectomy, you will not have any more menstrual periods, nor will you be able to become pregnant.

Will I still be able to have sexual intercourse after a hysterectomy?

Yes. Your hysterectomy should not change your ability to have intercourse, and because the fear of pregnancy is gone, many women say they enjoy intercourse more after their hysterectomy.

How long does it usually take to perform a hysterectomy?

It usually takes between 45 and 90 minutes to perform a hysterectomy.

What type of anesthesia is usually used?

General anesthesia is usually used, but spinal anesthesia may be recommended.

How long will I have to be in the hospital?

Usually from 10 to 14 days.

Will I have problems with urination or bowel movements following the operation?

As with most abdominal surgery, patients find it difficult to urinate at first following the operation. It will be several days before the bowels resume their normal functioning.

Can I expect to have vaginal discharge and bleeding following the operation?

Do not be alarmed if there is vaginal discharge or bleeding following your operation, but be sure to report it to your doctor. The discharge or bleeding is usually a part of the healing process.

How soon can I take a tub bath?

It is usually wise to wait for about a month after the operation before taking a tub bath, but it is safe to take a shower once the abdominal incision has healed.

What kind of incision is made for a hysterectomy?

Usually a 4-to-8-inch incision is made in the lower abdomen, below the navel. Some surgeons place the incision vertically, others do a horizontal incision. If you have a preference in this matter, you should mention it to your doctor so you can discuss it with him. Some hysterectomy procedures, especially when vaginal repair is necessary, are performed through the vagina so that no incision is required.

Is a catheter used following hysterectomy?

Yes. A catheter to empty the bladder is usually used for several days following either abdominal or vaginal removal of the uterus. If stretched muscles of the bladder and rectum are tightened at the time of the hysterectomy, a catheter may be left for as long as six to eight days.

Will removal of the uterus mean that I'll gain weight?

No. There is no evidence that there is any change in metabolism because of the removal of the uterus.

What happens to the body when both ovaries are removed?

When both ovaries are removed, menstrual periods cease and symptoms of the menopause develop.

What happens when one ovary is removed?

There are no noticeable effects when only one ovary is removed.

When cancer is found in one ovary, can the other ovary be saved?

Both ovaries are removed if there is cancer in one of them.

Is radiation ever used before a hysterectomy to treat cancer?

In some cases, radiation treatment is done before the operation to try to shrink the tumor or to contain it. Radiation is also sometimes used after surgery.

What is choriocarcinoma?

This is a rare type of cancer of the placenta, sometimes preceded by the appearance of a hydatidiform mole, which usually occurs during childbearing years. A microscopically similar cancer can occur as testicular cancer in men. It spreads very rapidly, metastasizes to other parts of the body—particularly to the lungs—and until ten years ago was considered fatal. It was, however, the first malignancy which proved to be curable by chemotherapy after it had metastasized. Today, thanks to the use of chemotherapy, these cancers are considered to be highly curable. However, since it is a rare disease, very few doctors outside treatment centers have had the opportunity to treat this type of cancer, and it is recommended that treatment be sought through a large medical center to ensure that the necessary expertise is available to handle the treatment. The cancer may start early in pregnancy, result in a miscarriage, and be followed by the development of a tumor. It may also occur after the delivery of a normal child. Physicians are able to cure between 95 and 100 percent of women in whom the disease is detected in an early stage and 75 percent of women with advanced choriocarcinoma.

Who gets cancer of the fallopian tube?

Primary cancer of the fallopian tube is the rarest cancer of the female genital tract. Usually the patient is between 50 and 60— but the range is 18 to 80 years. Symptoms can include excessive bleeding or yellowish or blood-tinged vaginal discharge. Some patients complain of a colicky pain prior to the discharge of fluid.

What is the treatment for cancer of the fallopian tube?

Where the cancer is localized, hysterectomy and removal of the ovaries and fallopian tubes are usually recommended. Radiotherapy usually follows the operation. Chemotherapy is also sometimes used.

What is an ovarian cyst?

An ovarian cyst is a hollow swelling containing fluid which grows in the region of the ovary.

Is an ovarian cyst often cancerous?

Most ovarian cysts—especially in younger women—are found to be benign. Cancer of the ovary is infrequent in patients under the age of 35; it is most frequent between ages 50 and 59. However, ovarian cancer develops silently, with no symptoms until it is often so far advanced that it is difficult to remove it successfully. The risk of having ovarian cancer is higher if close relatives have had it.

How can the doctor tell there is a cyst on the ovary?

Most ovarian cysts are first found by the doctor during a routine pelvic examination—and this is a very good reason for having a routine internal examination each year.

What symptoms make the doctor suspect an ovarian cyst?

Cysts of the ovary are quite common. The majority of them are benign, but some are cancerous. Cysts appear to grow quickly and often cause the abdomen to become distended. The patient may notice that she needs to urinate frequently or may complain of constipation or swelling in the legs. Interestingly enough, ovarian cysts often grow to the size of an orange or grapefruit before they are discovered. The ovaries are normally shaped like almonds; they are attached loosely to the undersurface of the fallopian tubes and have space around them, so a benign cyst of a fairly good size can be present for years without the woman being aware of its presence. When it starts to increase in size, it pushes the loose, flexible bowel away and fills in the space around it, causing a sensation of fullness or heaviness in the lower pelvic area.

Do ovarian cysts ever disappear?

Sometimes they do. Called physiological cysts because they are involved with the menstrual cycle, these cysts can sometimes cause the patient to miss a period. Normally, the sac that contains the egg ruptures about halfway between periods. If the sac fails to rupture, it begins to swell and fill with a clear liquid or jellylike material and increase to the size of an egg or even larger. That is why the doctor will sometimes wait for a few weeks before suggesting surgery. If the cyst fails to disappear, then surgery will be recommended.

What if the cyst does not disappear?

If the cyst does not disappear, or is very large and is causing other problems, surgery will be necessary. A benign cyst in a woman under 30 is often treated in a different way than one in a middle-aged woman or an older woman. If the cyst has not destroyed the ovary, the doctor can remove the cyst and leave the part of the ovary not affected by the cyst. There are decisions that need to be made and options that need to be discussed before going into surgery so that both the patient and doctor understand each other. Ask these questions of yourself:

- Should the doctor remove the uterus and other ovary if he finds nothing wrong with them?
- Since the operation is being done, do I prefer to have a hysterectomy at this stage in my life even if it is not necessary?
- Do I want the other ovary left if it is healthy so that I can have a normal menopause and avoid the need for taking hormones? (Hysterectomy does not cause you to have instant menopause unless both ovaries have been removed.)

The General Stages of Cancer of the Ovary

STAGE	OTHER CLASSIFICATION	EXPLANATION
Stage I	T1 T1a, IAi, IAii, T1b, IBi, IBii, T1c	Growth limited to ovaries
Stage II	T2, T2a, T2b, T2c	Growth involving one or both ovaries with pelvic extension or extension to uterus, tubes and/or pelvic tissues
Stage III	T3	Spread outside pelvis or to retroperitoneal nodes or both
Stage IV	T4	Spread to distant sites

What operation is performed if the cyst is cancerous?

If the ovarian cyst is cancerous, regardless of the patient's age, a hysterectomy and oophorectomy (removal of both ovaries) is usually performed. Sometimes radiation therapy or chemotherapy will follow the operation.

Why are ovaries removed?

Ovaries are removed surgically because they are diseased or not functioning properly. Ovaries are also often removed in patients with breast cancer if the cancer has been found to be estrogen-dependent. Sometimes the ovaries are destroyed by radiation as an alternative to surgery. Some physicians remove healthy ovaries as a preventive measure against ovarian cancer in doing hysterectomies if the woman is past menopause.

What happens when the ovaries are removed?

When the ovaries are destroyed—either surgically or by radiation—the body no longer produces estrogen. The result is that menopause occurs, bringing with it sudden and severe symptoms, usually more severe than would have happened if menopause occurred naturally. Most premenopausal women who have an oophorectomy (removal of both ovaries) are given estrogen replacement therapy to help avoid severe menopausal symptoms.

Would the doctor prescribe estrogen if my ovaries were removed because of cancer?

No. If there is any sign of a cancerous condition, estrogen would probably not be prescribed.

What is the estrogen controversy?

Estrogen is a female hormone produced by the ovaries. Scientists have also developed chemical estrogen. Both regulate the development of female sexual characteristics. For a number of years, estrogens have been prescribed for women during and after menopause to make up for the decline in this hormone normally produced by the ovaries. Estrogen has been found to be helpful in controlling hot flashes or in regulating the thinning of the vaginal lining, which can be painful during menopausal years. However, because cancers of some women with breast disease have been known to recede when the women are given additional estrogens, while other breast cancers have been found to grow more rapidly with the same treatment, the role of estrogen in the cancer picture is the subject of disagreement among many doctors. Within the last few years, much discussion has surrounded the use of estrogens—particularly as it was widely prescribed for postmenopausal women during the last ten years. Most doctors are usually reluctant to prescribe estrogen for postmenopausal women in whose families there is a high incidence of breast cancer.

If the doctor prescribes estrogen therapy for my postmenopausal symptoms, should I expect to continue taking estrogen forever?

No. Patients who are using estrogen therapy should have a thorough physical checkup, including breast and pelvic examination, before starting estrogen therapy and every six months thereafter. You should also examine your breasts monthly for lumps or changes in appearance that may be warning signs of cancer. You should be sure to ask the doctor to reevaluate the situation at each examination.

Have estrogens been proved to cause cancer?

Studies are still underway, and as yet there is no "proof." However, the use of estrogen during or after menopause has been linked with cancer of the uterus. Some studies have shown that women taking estrogen for menopausal symptoms have roughly five to ten times as great a chance of developing uterine cancer as women who take no estrogen. The risk of uterine cancer increases with duration of estrogen use and seems to get greater when larger doses are taken. If a woman has had her uterus completely removed (total hysterectomy), there is no danger of developing cancer of the uterus.

Is there any link between estrogens and breast cancer?

There has been one study, according to the National Cancer Institute, that has suggested that the use of menopausal estrogen may increase the risk of breast cancer 10 to 15 years after it is first taken. Particularly high breast-cancer risk was noted in estrogen users who had benign breast disease—that is, cysts or nodules that are not cancerous.

Are there problems with using vaginal estrogen cream? I am using it to relieve vaginal dryness that has accompanied my menopause.

The warning about the increased risk of uterine cancer related to the use of postmenopausal estrogens for prolonged periods does include the vaginal creams as well as the estrogens taken by mouth or injection. Estrogens are manufactured in several forms, including tablets for oral application, liquids for intravenous and intramuscular injection, and vaginal creams for external application. They can be manufactured synthetically in the laboratory or derived from animal sources. Estrogens, whether naturally occurring, animal-derived, or man-made, presumably have similar benefits, side effects, and risks associated with their use. You should discuss the questions of estrogen replacement with your doctor. The two of you can decide whether continued use of the cream is advisable in your particular situation. Your doctor will probably advise you to take the lowest dose that will control the symptoms and attempt to discontinue the medication or decrease it at designated intervals.

Does a face cream that contains estrogen cause cancer?

Hormone creams have to be carefully used, and your own individual situation should be discussed with your doctor. Estrogen in the cream can be absorbed into your body. The action once in the body is the same as if you had swallowed a pill by mouth. Use of this kind of cream is not advised for anyone with a history of cancer.

Aren't estrogens good for preventing bone loss?

There is some evidence that estrogens prevent bone loss—and perhaps fractures—in postmenopausal women. Some doctors feel that women who are at high risk for bone loss should be given estrogens as preventive medicine. The individual doctor and patient must weigh the risks against the benefits.

Is it true that the FDA has put warnings on estrogen products?

It is important for all women to be aware that estrogen replacement therapy should be questioned and sound and satisfactory answers given before taking estrogen in any form. The FDA has recently ruled that all prescriptions for estrogens include a brochure with the following warnings:

- There is probably an increased risk of cancer of the uterus if a woman uses estrogens for more than a year in treating symptoms of menopause.

- Patients should have their estrogen treatment reevaluated every six months.
- Estrogens should not be taken by women who have cancer of the breast or of the uterus, who have undiagnosed abnormal vaginal bleeding, or who have clotting in the legs or lungs.
- Estrogens should not be used in treating simple nervousness or depression during menopause, because it has not been proved effective for those purposes nor has it been proved that estrogens keep the skin soft or help a woman feel young.

The brochure also recommends that users of menopausal estrogen be monitored closely by their doctors, that they use estrogen only as long as necessary, and that they take the lowest dose that will control symptoms.

Is the FDA brochure also required to accompany oral contraceptive pills?

Yes. The Food and Drug Administration requires that a special brochure accompany each prescription of oral contraceptives. In addition to explaining other risks, the brochure warns that oral contraceptives should not be used by women with known or suspected cancer of the breast or sex organs, pregnant women, or those who suspect they are pregnant. The brochure also advises women with benign breast disease or a family history of breast cancer to see their doctors frequently for an examination if they elect to use oral contraceptives instead of another method of birth control. All women taking oral contraceptives should examine their breasts monthly for lumps or changes of appearance that may be warning signs of cancer.

Is there any conclusive proof that cancer is being caused by oral contraceptives?

No. There is no conclusive evidence that cancer is being caused by oral contraceptives on the market today. However, one study has suggested that these pills have increased the risk of breast cancer in women with benign breast disease—that is, women with cysts or nodules which are not cancerous—and other studies have found an increased rate of early cervical cancer in groups of women using oral contraceptives. A few cases of cancer of the liver have been reported in women using oral contraceptives, but it is not yet known whether the drug caused them. Oral contraceptives do cause—although rarely— a benign tumor of the liver. These tumors do not spread, but they may rupture and cause internal bleeding, which can be fatal. Oral contraceptives on the market today contain either a combination of estrogen and progestogen or progestogen alone. The former are more commonly used. Laboratory studies have shown that when certain animals are given estrogen for long periods, cancer may develop in the breast, cervix, vagina, and liver.

When did we discover that the estrogen drug DES might cause problems?

It was in 1971 that doctors discovered a link between DES (diethylstilbestrol) and cancer of the female reproductive system. Clear-cell adenocarcinoma of the vagina or cervix was found in a very small number of young women whose mothers had taken DES-type drugs during pregnancy.

What was the purpose of giving the drug to pregnant women?

During the 1940s and on into the 1960s the drug was given to women to prevent miscarriage. It was one of the first synthetic estrogen-type hormones developed that was inexpensive and could be given by mouth. Many of the women who took it had lost babies, were spotting or bleeding, or had other complications such as diabetes.

Is the drug DES still being used today?

It is no longer being used for pregnant women. It is available, by prescription, and is used in treating certain kinds of cancer, for unusual menopausal problems, and in the "morning after" pill. When patients with cancers of the breast and prostate are treated with DES, the tumors in some cases have been known to shrink, and there is often dramatic relief of pain. It is thought to be 100 percent effective as a "morning after" pill, and there is no evidence that it causes cancer when used in this manner. Usually the prescription is for 50 milligrams a day for five days. However, the FDA emphasizes that the use of the pill as a contraceptive is to be considered an emergency measure and explicitly warns against routine or frequent use.

What are the DES-type drugs that may have been prescribed for pregnant women?

There are a good many:

Nonsteroidal Estrogens

Benzestrol	Estrosyn	Palestrol
Chlorotrianisene	Fonatol	Restrol
Comestrol	Gynben	Stil-Rol
Cyren A.	Gyneben	Stilbal
Cyren B.	Hexestrol	Stilbestrol
Delvinal	Hexoestrol	Stilbestronate
DES	Hi-Bestrol	Stilbetin
DesPlex	Menocrin	Stilbinol
Diestryl	Meprane	Stilboestroform
Dibestil	Mestilbol	Stilboestrol
Dienestrol	Methallenestril	Stilboestrol DP.
Dienoestrol	Microest	Stilestrate
Diethylstilbestrol	Mikarol	Stilpalmitate
Dipalmitate	Mikarol forti	Stilphostrol
Diethylstilbestrol	Milestrol	Stilronate
Diphosphate	Monomestrol	Stilrone
Diethylstilbestrol	Neo-Oestranol I	Stils
Dipropionate	Neo-Oestranol II	Synestrin
Diethylstilbenediol	Nulabort	Synestrol
Digestil	Oestrogenine	Synthoestrin
Domestrol	Oestromenin	Tace
Estilben	Oestromon	Vallestril
Estrobene	Orestol	Willestrol
Estrobene DP.	Pabestrol D.	

Nonsteroidal Estrogen—Androgen Combinations

Amperone	Metystil	Tylandril
Di-Erone	Teserene	Tylosterone
Estan		

Nonsteroidal Estrogen—Progesterone Combination

Progravidium

Vaginal Cream—Suppositories with Nonsteroidal Estrogens

AVC cream with Dienestrol
Dienestrol cream

Does the risk of cancer depend upon the amount of the DES-type drug taken during pregnancy?

The amount does not seem to be the important factor. The exposure during the first five months of pregnancy seems to be more of a determining factor than the amount.

What does research show was the most dangerous time for taking DES?

If DES or other hormones were taken before the 8th week, some effects may show up, but most probably will not be of a serious nature. The most critical time is when hormones were given between the 8th and 18th week. These are the cases where vaginal abnormalities are more likely. If taken after the 18th week, defects are extremely rare.

What are the doctors finding in DES daughters?

They are finding unusual tissue formations in the vagina or cervix of the daughters. Normally, the uterus is lined with a red (vascular) and moist (glandular) tissue that meets the pink, drier tissue of the vagina at the outer opening of the cervix. In DES daughters, this red tissue frequently extends into the cervix and is called eversion. Some DES daughters have spots of the red moist tissue on the walls of the vagina as well. This is called adenosis. This misplaced tissue is not harmful but may cause an unusually heavy vaginal discharge. Many DES daughters have an extra rim of tissue around the cervix. Depending on whether this rim is partial or complete, it might be referred to as a rooster's comb, cock's comb, hood, collar, or pseudo-polyp. At this time, these tissue abnormalities have not been found to be harmful.

Will any of these conditions affect sexual activity or future pregnancies?

These conditions do not affect sexual activity. To date, there have been no known problems with pregnancies. Women who have been exposed to DES-type drugs during their mothers' pregnancies have given birth to normal children. Information is still being accumulated, however, since the total number of women of child-bearing age is still relatively small.

Do DES daughters have to worry about infertility?

Though a number of these women have already had normal children, there does seem to be a higher rate of infertility and menstrual irregularities among these young women.

Are there any symptoms that DES-exposed daughters should be aware of?

The only symptom which is occasionally seen is an increase in vaginal discharge due to adenosis. Although this symptom is also found in women not exposed before birth to DES-type drugs, in DES-exposed daughters there seems to be more than the usual amount of tissue and more than the usual amount of vaginal discharge.

If I took a DES drug during pregnancy, should my children be examined?

Yes. But not until puberty has begun. Unless vaginal bleeding or discharge occurs before that time, the examination need not be done for girls under 14 years of age who have not yet begun to menstruate. Some doctors prefer an earlier examination—and this can be done with tact and understanding; many young girls whose mothers took DES have been examined without trauma. You must balance within your own mind the risk of cancer versus the risk of emotional upset.

What kind of examination will the doctor do?

The doctor will take a medical history, including information about any illnesses, hospitalization, or pregnancies. (Be sure to give the doctor a complete rundown on your DES background. It is helpful to get a copy of records from the doctor who administered the DES so you know exactly what was prescribed, when, and for how long.) The doctor will ask what medications are being taken, including birth-control pills, the pattern of the menstrual periods, and information about sexual activity. These questions are not meant to embarrass, but are an essential part of the record. The doctor will then perform a complete physical, including breast examination, pelvic exam, Pap smear, and a painless staining of the vagina with a dye. He may use a colposcope to examine the cervix and vagina. The examination is not painful.

This seems very frightening to me. How should I handle it with my daughter?

Though the idea of this sort of an examination on a young girl may sound frightening, you should explain to your daughter in a matter-of-fact way what your concerns are and what she can expect when the doctor does his examination. You should know, first of all, that the incidence of cancer is very slight—out of over a million women who took DES, fewer than 150 cases of vaginal or cervical clear-cell cancers have been found among their daughters. The risk is truly very small and you should not allow yourself to become upset and frightened. You should, however, be certain that you discuss the matter with your doctor and make arrangements for your daughter to be examined when she reaches puberty.

How long should DES-exposed daughters be examined for cancer?

Since the oldest women exposed to DES drugs before birth are in their middle 30s, it isn't possible to predict whether there will be other problems as these women grow older. Regular semi-yearly or yearly examinations are definitely in order.

What if the doctor finds abnormal tissue in the vaginal lining?

If the doctor should find abnormal tissue, he will probably want to take a biopsy and have it examined by the pathologist. The biopsy will usually be performed in the doctor's office and will cause little or no discomfort.

What kind of treatment will usually be necessary?

If the pathologist finds no clear-cut cancer (and, as explained before, chances of his finding it are slight) but only finds tissue abnormalities as noted earlier (eversion, adenosis, or rooster's comb), no treatment will be necessary. The doctor will recommend followup examinations at regular intervals. Follow-up is very important—and examinations should be scheduled at 6-to-12-month intervals.

What if the doctor recommends preventive surgery for adenosis due to DES exposure?

If the physician's examination shows that your daughter is free from cancer, but he suggests surgery for preventive reasons, without question you should get another opinion. Preventive surgery in these cases has been practiced in some areas, but doctors who have treated many DES patients feel that this surgery is unnecessary unless it is proved that cancer is present. This is particularly true since it now seems that adenosis and other benign abnormalities are diminishing with maturity.

Can a DES daughter safely take other hormones?

We would suggest that this question be investigated completely with your doctor. Remember that oral contraceptives and the morning-after pill would introduce "more of the same" into your daughter's already complicated hormonal situation.

Are sons of mothers who took DES-type drugs affected?

Although studies have been underway, there are no findings as of this date which indicate that any boy or man has developed cancer as a result of his exposure before birth to DES. There has been some evidence of abnormalities in the genital tract. However, the abnormalities are common ones and the evidence that they were caused by DES is still inconclusive.

What kind of cancer has developed in the daughters of mothers who took DES?

An unusual cancer of the vagina or the cervix has developed in a very small number of young women whose mothers took DES-type drugs during pregnancy. When this was first reported, it was expected that many more such incidents would be found. However, very few DES-exposed daughters have actually developed this cancer, called clear-cell adenocarcinoma.

What is the treatment if cancer is found in a DES daughter?

Removal by surgery or radiation therapy is the usual treatment — naturally, it would depend upon where the cancer was situated. Cancer of the vagina or cervix is not a happy prospect for anyone, and especially not for a young woman when it may mean that she will not be able to bear children. However, the cancer may be cured, especially if detected early. All efforts should be made in such cases to find the most experienced doctor for this surgery. Remember, however, that unnecessary *preventive* surgery has been done in some cases on DES daughters. If surgery is recommended be sure to get a second opinion.

Should the mothers who took DES take any special precautions?

Yes. Studies are now underway to determine whether women who took DES during pregnancy may be at either a higher or earlier than average risk of breast or gynecologic cancers. DES-exposed mothers should have an annual pelvic examination including a Pap smear. The examination should also include breast palpation. In addition, monthly breast self-examination should be practiced by the DES-exposed mothers and any abnormal findings reported promptly to the doctor.

Should a DES-exposed mother have routine mammograms?

If there are no symptoms of breast cancer, mammography is not recommended under the age of 35 even for DES-exposed mothers. (It is suggested only for women between 35 and 39 who have a personal history of breast cancer or immediate relatives with a history of breast cancer.) For women over 50, mammography may be considered for the annual examination.

Should a DES-exposed mother take estrogens?

As with the daughter, the DES-exposed mother should avoid further exposure to DES or other estrogens, particularly in the form of the "morning after" pill for birth control. In addition, DES-exposed mothers should not use DES after childbirth to dry up breast milk. In addition, the use of any oral contraceptives or estrogens prescribed for postmenopausal conditions should be discussed thoroughly with the doctor in light of prior exposure to DES.

Are any special studies being done of DES daughters?

Yes. The National Cancer Institute is sponsoring a five-year study with a sample group of exposed offspring. Institutions and principal investigators participating in this study are:

Massachusetts General Hospital
Harvard Medical School
Boston, Mass.
Drs. Ann Barnes and Stanley Robboy

University of Southern California
Los Angeles, Calif.
Dr. Duane E. Townsend

Baylor College of Medicine
Houston, Tex.
Dr. Raymond H. Kaufman

Mayo Clinic
Rochester, Minn.
Dr. Kenneth Noller

Mayo Clinic
National Coordinating Center
Dr. Leonard T. Kurland

Is there anywhere where I can get information on DES?

There is a group called DES Action which is a self-help support organization of volunteers. The group is active in public education and legislation related to the DES problem, serves as a resource for mothers and daughters confronted with the DES problem, and maintains a telephone hotline. For further information contact: DES Action, P.O. Box 1977, Plainview, N.Y. 11803; tel. 516-775-3450. For information regarding the availability of colposcopy in your area: The American Society for Colposcopy, Medical College of Wisconsin, 8700 W. Wisconsin Avenue, Milwaukee, Wis. 53226.

chapter 17

Cancer of the Male Reproductive Organs

Tests for Prostate Cancer

- Rectal examination
- Urine studies
- Blood studies (especially acid phosphatase)
- Needle biopsy
- Kidney-function tests
- Chest x-ray
- EKG
- Skeleton survey
- Bone scan
- Intravenous pyelogram (IVP)

Tests for Cancer of the Testicle

Note: Investigative biopsy prior to removal of affected testicle *should never* be done. The tests that are done are:
- Physical examination—with careful attention to testes with patient in standing position, neck, breasts, abdomen, and groin
- Blood studies
- Urinary studies
- Chest x-ray
- Intravenous pyelogram (IVP)
- Excretory urogram
- Lymphangiogram
- Venacavography

Cancer of the Male Reproductive Organs

TYPE	HIGH RISK	SYMPTOMS	TREATMENT	REMARKS
Prostate	Over 55, black males, married	Urination problems, blood in urine, pain in lower back, pelvis, upper thighs	Surgery, chemotherapy, radiation, radioisotopes, cryosurgery; removal of testicles, or pituitary gland; injection of female hormones sometimes used to suppress male hormones.	Most tumors found in prostate are *not* cancerous.
Testicle	Age 20-35, white males, those with undescended testicles	Enlargement or change in consistency of testicles; dull ache in abdomen, dragging or heaviness; enlargement of breast, tender nipples	Surgical removal of entire affected testicle. Follow-up treatment can include radiation, node removal, chemotherapy.	Very fast-growing tumor; often metastasizes while original growth is still small. Immediate attention imperative. *Do not allow investigative biopsy.* Extremely important before treatment to be certain doctor has latest information from studies being supported by National Cancer Institute.
Penis	Uncircumcised males, ages 50-70	Pimple, sore, nodule, wart, ulcer, etc. on penis, usually tip. Bleeding associated with erection. Erection without sexual desire.	Surgical removal of tumor; radiation not usually effective except for very small tumors.	Very rare. Curable in early stages.

Questions to Ask Your Doctor Before Treatment for Prostate Cancer

- What type of treatment do you suggest?
- Is there treatment other than surgery that would be possible for me?
- Could I be treated with radium implants or radiation?
- Are you planning hormone therapy?
- Can I be treated with chemotherapy?
- If surgery ask:
  - Do you ever use treatment other than surgery?
  - How often do you do this type of surgery?
  - How extensive do you expect the surgery to be?
  - Where will the scar be?
  - Will the surgery leave me impotent? Can the surgery be done so it will not leave me impotent?
- If the scar is to be behind the scrotum, ask:
  - Why are you planning to make the incision in that area?
  - Can you cut through the abdominal wall instead?

Questions to Ask Your Doctor Before Treatment for Cancer of the Testicle

- Are you planning to do a needle or simple biopsy? (*If answer is yes, see another doctor.*)
- Will only one testicle be removed?
- Is the tumor confined to one testicle?
- If the tumor is confined to the testicle and the cell type is seminoma, will you remove the lymph nodes or will you use radiation therapy?
- Will this operation leave me sterile?
- Will you make arrangements for sperm to be collected for a sperm bank for me just in case I become sterile?
- Can an artificial testicle be implanted during surgery?
- Are you planning to follow the operation with chemotherapy or radiation therapy?

Is the National Cancer Institute supporting any studies on cancer of the male organs?

Yes, there are studies being conducted on cancer of the male organs. Most are involved with the use of chemotherapy for prostate and testicular cancers (see Chapter 23).

Treatments for Cancer of the Prostate and Testicle

TREATMENT	PROCEDURE	RESULTS	REMARKS
Transurethral resection (TUR)	Does not require external incision. Used only for very small tumors. Requires very skilled surgeon.	Does not reduce sexual potency.	No incision.
Suprapubic prostatectomy	Bladder neck is cut to reach prostate. Catheter and drain left in place about ten days. Vasectomy usually performed at same time.	Most uncomplicated from surgeon's viewpoint, allows correction of any bladder problems. Produces infertility but no loss of potency.	Incision is made above pubic bone.
Retropubic prostatectomy	Bladder neck and nerve and muscle attachments left intact. Catheter to bladder for about ten days.	Less cutting, less surgical shock, more difficult to perform, takes longer than suprapubic. Usually no loss of potency.	Incision is below pubic bone over penis.
Perineal prostatectomy	Between legs, through surface separating the scrotum and anus, operation similar to retropubic.	Difficult for surgeon to perform. Patient lies with legs in stirrups, knees above waist, placing weight upon chest, creating breathing difficulties. Nerves involving erection often severed.	Little postoperative discomfort; incision is usually half-circle around inner side of anus.

Treatments for Cancer of the Prostate and Testicle (continued)

TREATMENT	PROCEDURE	RESULTS	REMARKS
Total prostatectomy	Removal of prostate	Suprapubic, retropubic, or perineal method is used.	Nerve and muscle connections between gland, bladder neck, and urethra removed. Impotency results.
Radiation	Linear accelerator or cobalt 60 directed directly at prostate.	Often used in early stages; useful in shrinking tumors in later stages.	If carefully given should not affect fertility.
Radium implants	Pellets inserted into prostate.	Used for early small cancers or to reduce size of tumor and relieve pain.	
Chemotherapy	Usually hospitalized during early stages of treatment.	Experiments still being conducted to determine most effective dosages. Several drugs including 5-FU, Cytoxan, effective in relieving painful symptoms of advanced prostate cancer.	Usual side effects.
Cryosurgery	Catheterlike probe destroys cells through freezing.	Destroys malignant tissue, may develop antibodies against cancer. May be repeated.	Still experimental.

Treatments for Cancer of the Prostate and Testicle (continued)

TREATMENT	PROCEDURE	RESULTS	REMARKS
Hormone and drug treatment	Variety of by-mouth treatments including estrogen, DES, Cortisone, stilbestrol, and L-Dopa, being used.	Discrepancies in effect on different patients.	Not ordinarily used as primary treatment.
Hypophysectomy	Removal of pituitary gland	Reduces production of male hormone.	Used on patients who have shown previous response to estrogen therapy.
Adrenalectomy	Removal of adrenal glands	Reduces production of male hormone.	Used on patients who have shown previous response to estrogen therapy.
Orchiectomy	Removal of one or both testicles	If both removed, patient will be sterile, but not impotent.	Used in testicle cancer; plastic replacement of testicle is possible.
Bilateral orchiectomy	Removal of both testicles	If both removed, patient will be sterile, but not impotent.	Done to control hormone production in prostate cancer.

What are the most common cancers of the male reproductive organs?

Cancer of the prostate is the most common cancer of the male reproductive organs. Next to lung cancer, cancer of the prostate has the highest incidence of any form of male cancer. After age 75, it is the main cause of cancer deaths among men. Cancer of the testicles is one of the commonest cancers in males between 20 and 40. Cancer of the penis occurs infrequently, and usually in uncircumcised males in the 50–70-year-old group.

Who usually gets cancer of the prostate?

The risk of developing cancer of the prostate increases with age. Cancer of the prostate is primarily a disease of older men and occurs most often in those over 55 years of age. After age 75, prostate cancer is the main cause of cancer death among men. Black men have two times more cancer of the prostate than white men.

How can I protect myself against cancer of the prostate?

There is no real protection, except through early detection and treatment. Every man over 40 should have a rectal exam as part of his regular physical checkup, since this is the only way this cancer can be spotted. Cancer specialists are working to improve diagnostic techniques and new methods of treatment are being tested. More than half of all prostatic cancers are discovered while still localized within the general region of the prostate. The cures for early prostate cancer are encouraging.

What is the prostate and what does it do?

The prostate, a gland a bit smaller than a golf ball, weighs about ¾ ounce and surrounds the outlet of the urinary bladder. Physicians in referring to the prostate separate it into five lobes. The posterior lobe, the one which is felt when the doctor does a rectal exam, is the one which seems to be most susceptible to cancer. Its main purpose is to secrete the fluid in which the sperm cells are ejaculated. Not all the gland's functions are fully understood, but it is sometimes possible to slow growth of the cancer through some variety of hormone therapy.

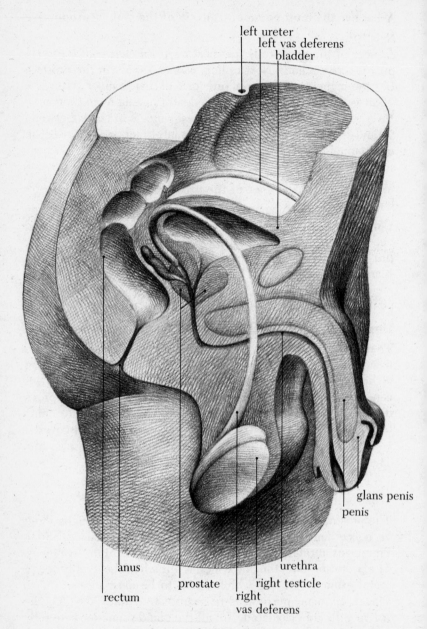

left ureter
left vas deferens
bladder

glans penis
penis

anus

prostate

urethra
right testicle

rectum

right
vas deferens

Male reproductive organs

Are most prostate tumors cancerous?

No. The most common tumors found in the prostate are *not* cancerous. The most common prostate problem is called benign prostatic hypertrophy (BPH). More than half the men in the United States over 50 suffer from this enlargement.

What are the symptoms of cancer of the prostate?

Symptoms which should not be ignored include a weak or interrupted flow of urine, inability to urinate or difficulty in starting urination, need to urinate frequently (especially at night), blood in the urine, urine flow that is not easily stopped, painful or burning urination, and continuing pain in the lower back, pelvis, or upper thighs. These symptoms are often the same symptoms that indicate other prostatic problems such as BPH, but they are symptoms which should be checked by the doctor, because only a doctor can tell the difference between a cancerous and noncancerous enlargement of the prostate.

How does the doctor check the prostate?

The initial step is through a digital examination of the gland through the rectum. The doctor inserts a gloved finger into the rectum and feels the gland. It often can enlarge to the size of an orange. The doctor suspects a cancerous growth if the gland is stony and hard to the touch, rather than rubbery. If there is an enlargement of the prostate gland, the doctor will usually order urine and blood analyses and x-ray.

Do most prostate glands enlarge as a man gets older?

This happens to the majority of men, beginning in the 40s and increasing in each subsequent decade of life. The enlargement itself becomes a problem only if it produces serious side effects, obstructing the flow of urine, but it should be checked yearly by the doctor. Surgery is necessary only in those whose symptoms become acute or where cancer is present.

How is cancer of the prostate diagnosed?

The presence of cancer can be confirmed by the removal of a small piece of prostate tissue for microscopic examination. Often a needle biopsy is used. In other cases, biopsy can be obtained during surgical procedures required for dealing with complications caused by the enlargement of the prostate. Blood tests are also important in diagnosing since prostatic cancer cells secrete a chemical substance known as acid phosphatase, which finds its way into the bloodstream. This chemical may help to identify the disease and may help to determine whether or not the cancer has spread beyond the prostate. However, about half the cancers of the prostate do not show acid-phosphatase changes so the doctor cannot rule out cancer when the level is normal. Irritation of the prostate or a rectal exam can raise levels even when cancer is not present. Therefore, the acid-phosphatase test alone is not a definitive test and must be used with other indicators to determine diagnosis.

Are new tests being developed to routinely discover prostate cancer?

Two new tests for prostate cancer are presently being tested by the National Prostate Cancer Project of the National Cancer Institute. One, which employs counterimmunoelectrophoreses (CIEP), is said to be capable of signaling prostate cancer before metastasis. The other, using radioimmunoassay, which is a more expensive and more complicated method, is claimed to be even more sensitive than CIEP. The hope of the researchers is that a simple test, like the Pap test, will someday be available for detection of prostate cancer. Your doctor can get further information about the latest developments by checking with the Prostatic Cancer Project chairman listed in Chapter 23.

Is it common for prostate cancer to spread to other parts of the body?

Yes. About 90 percent of prostate cancers are found only after they have spread to other parts of the body.

How is cancer of the prostate staged?

Prostate tumors are classified as follows:
- *T1:* Tumor encapsulated within gland, surrounded by normal gland.
- *T2:* Tumor confined to gland, deforming contour, and invading capsule.
- *T3:* Tumor extends beyond capsule.
- *T4:* Tumor fixed or involving neighboring structures. If a

number plus the letter "m" follows, this indicates multiple tumors and how many there are. "N" plus a number indicates involvement of nodes.

What treatments are available for prostate cancer?

Treatment varies depending on such factors as whether cancer has spread to other areas, its rate of growth, and the patient's age and general health. New treatments with radiation, radioisotopes, and cryosurgery are being experimented with in many of the larger cancer centers. Though all urologists do not agree about the success of these treatments, many advances are being made. In most cases at present, if the cancer is confined to the prostatic gland, surgical removal is usually recommended. If the cancer has spread, it can often be checked for long periods of time by surgical removal of the testicles, by removal of the pituitary gland, or by injections of female hormones to suppress the production of male hormones. Chemotherapy is also being used alone or in combination with surgery or radiation.

What is a prostatectomy?

A prostatectomy is the surgical removal of all or part of the prostate. A total prostactectomy is the removal of the entire prostate.

What is suprapubic prostatectomy?

This is removal of all or part of the prostate in which the incision is made in the area above the pubic bone. The operation makes it possible for the surgeon to explore the urinary bladder and gives easy access to the prostate. It is probably the most common operation for prostate surgery.

What is a retropubic prostatectomy?

Retropubic prostatectomy is the removal of all or part of the prostate when the incision is made just below the pelvic bone and over the penis. The surgeon performs the operation without opening the bladder.

What is a transurethral resection or TUR?

This operation permits removal of a tumor without an incision. It is recommended only for very small tumors. This new approach to prostate surgery is accomplished by inserting an extremely sophisticated instrument through the penis and up into the bladder area. Because it requires tremendous skill and expertise, this procedure should be done only by a surgeon who uses the technique regularly.

What are the aftereffects of total prostatectomy?

Although the cancer may be controlled, there are three consequences you should be aware of:

- Since the prostate gland produces most of the fluid released at the time of sexual intercourse and climax, most patients are sterile following this operation, just as they would be following a vasectomy.
- Many of the nerves that are involved with sexual function may be damaged, so that following surgery, many patients will no longer be able to have an erection.
- A few patients find that the operation causes them to lose their ability to control urine. Strengthening of muscles through simple exercise during recovery can usually help to return control.

Is it true that after prostatectomy I will no longer ejaculate?

Yes. After prostatectomy, the ability to ejaculate through the penis is lost. What happens is that ejaculation continues but it is directed backward into the bladder, rather than forward through the urethra. The semen remains in the bladder until urination, and is carried out via that route. The man who ejaculates in this manner has the very same sensations during sex that he had before except that there is no discharge through the penis.

Is radiation ever used alone to treat prostate cancer?

Yes. A recent study of 405 patients treated exclusively with external radiation therapy for cancer confined to the prostate which had advanced beyond the stage where surgery was indicated, showed a five-year survival rate of 72 percent and a ten-year survival rate of 44 percent. Many of these patients appear to be completely cured.

What types of radiation treatments are used?

The basic principle of radiation therapy is to bombard the cancer with rays at doses which damage or destroy the cancer yet produce only a minimum of damage to the surrounding normal tissues. This can be done either with external radiation or with internal radiation.

What type of external radiation is used?

External radiation employs either a linear accelerator or a cobalt-60 source to pinpoint the delivery of the radiation dosage. Some doctors use radiation as the primary treatment for prostate cancers in early stages. Others use it as additional therapy for some patients with later-stage disease. Radiation is usually given four or five times a week over a period of six or seven weeks. It is important that the patient be in good enough general physical condition to tolerate this heavy concentration of high-energy radiation.

How are radium implants used in prostatic cancer?

Though still a controversial investigational method, radium implants are being used in treating prostatic cancer. Radioactive gold and iodine (I-125) isotopes have been used in treatment of prostate cancers. With the patient anesthetized, a physician inserts thin metal tubes through the pubic region into the prostate. Then, through these tubes, he inserts the radioactive pellets, which remain in the patient's prostate. In some cases, radioactive implants have proved effective in decreasing the size of the tumor and in relieving pain. After the initial hospitalization, this type of radium implant is not considered dangerous in any way. Even in the hospital, forceps, linens, bandages, etc. are handled in the normal way. The patient does not endanger others and is advised that he may resume his normal living habits, having normal sexual relations, and can be near children and pregnant women without any fear for their health or safety due to potential contamination.

Is chemotherapy used in treating prostate cancer?

Chemotherapy may be used alone or in combination with surgery or radiation for treatment of prostate cancer. New treatments and refinements of treatments which have been under study are changing the guidelines of treatment in many cases.

What are the advantages of radiation therapy over prostatectomy?

Radiation therapy is being used to treat some prostate cancers in investigational studies, and the success rates indicate that this treatment is as effective or more effective than radical surgery, depending upon the spread of the disease. Since potency is maintained in 75 percent of patients following radiation, this is a consideration, particularly in men who are still sexually active. It is important that you discuss this question with the doctor before undergoing treatment.

How is cryosurgery used in prostatic cancer?

This method of treatment, though controversial and experimental, has been used in treating both small benign and malignant prostatic growths. Though not commonly used, some experiences seem to suggest that cryosurgery not only destroys malignant tissue but may help develop antibodies against cancer. A catheter-like probe containing a liquid-nitrogen system and a heating coil is inserted into the bladder. The probe is positioned with the liquid-nitrogen element against the area of the urethra upon which the prostatic cancer is pressing. The temperature is dropped and the surrounding tissue frozen. The heating coil then thaws the area surrounding the probe just enough to permit the probe to be extracted. The tissue that was frozen soon deteriorates and is carried out of the body in the urine.

What is an orchiectomy?

An orchiectomy is the removal of the testicle. Removal of both testicles is a bilateral orchiectomy. This procedure is sometimes used in the treatment of prostate cancer which has spread. Doctors have found that the spread of cancer can often be controlled for years by removing the testicles—man's natural source of the male sex hormone.

Isn't an orchiectomy the same as castration?

Some men have the mistaken belief that removal of the testicles will leave them with feminine voices and enlarged breasts. This is simply not so if the man has passed puberty. If both testicles are removed, orchiectomy does leave the patient sterile—but usually he does not lose his ability to have an erection.

Aren't sterility, impotency, and the lack of ability to ejaculate the same thing?

Sterility is the opposite of fertility and means that you are no longer able to father a child. Men who have had a vasectomy are sterile but are still potent and can ejaculate. Impotency refers to the inability to achieve erection. Prostatectomy may or may not leave a man impotent, depending upon whether the nerves governing erection are severed. Prostatectomy will often leave a man incapable of ejaculating, as the seminal fluids are forced backward into the bladder, from which they subsequently are excreted in the urine. If both vas are also severed, he will also be sterile.

What types of hormone treatments are used in dealing with prostate cancer?

Hormone treatments fall into several categories, including the use of estrogen and cortisone, the surgical removal of the testicles, and the surgical removal of the pituitary or adrenal gland.

Can hormone treatment cure cancer of the prostate?

No. Hormone treatment cannot cure cancer of the prostate but is often used to control the activity of the disease and lessen pain. Many patients also recover appetite, gain weight, and return to normal activities. The tumor often shrinks, as well. However, in some patients, for reasons as yet not understood, the hormones may lose their effectiveness and the original symptoms may return.

Is the pituitary gland sometimes removed in treatment of prostate cancer?

Yes. Some research has indicated that the removal of the pituitary gland, called a transphenoidal hypophysectomy, can arrest the spread of prostate cancer in 50 percent of patients. Thanks to a relatively new operation, developed because of the high risk of previous pituitary surgery, which required opening the skull to reach the pituitary gland, removal has been simplified. The pituitary gland is removed by an operation performed through the upper gum and into the nasal passage to the pituitary below the brain. An unexpected result of the surgery is the disappearance of pain in about 75 percent of patients. The pain disappearance usually occurs within 48 hours and is usually permanent.

If a man has undergone surgery for a tumor of the prostate, does this mean he can no longer have prostate cancer?

No. Most operations performed for prostate problems other than cancer do not remove the whole prostate. Unless a man has undergone a total prostatectomy, he should remember that it is still possible for him to develop prostate cancer. Remaining prostatic tissue should be examined as part of every annual physical examination.

Are blood transfusions needed during prostate operations?

Yes. There is considerable blood loss, which is replaced by blood transfusion.

Where is the incision made for a prostatectomy?

This depends on the type of operation. Lengthwise or horizontal incisions are made either in the lower abdomen or behind the scrotal sac and in front of the rectum. Be sure to ask your doctor where the incision will be made and what his reasons are for the decision.

Is pain very great after prostatectomy?

Usually, moderate pain is felt.

How is the urine drained after the operation?

Usually by a catheter placed in the urethra or bladder.

What are the testes and how do they function?

The testes, egg-shaped glands, are situated in the scrotum and produce spermatozoa. The sperm is collected at the back of the testicles in a maze of coiled tubes called the epididymis and then travels up toward the seminal vesicles and prostate through a long tube known as the vas deferens.

What is a retroperitoneal lymphadenectomy?

This is the operation which removes the lymph nodes that affect the testicle.

Is testicular cancer a common type of cancer?

No, it is not—but because of the young age group which usually has this type of cancer, this disease attracts attention. It is most commonly seen in patients ranging in age from 20 to 35. Testicular cancer actually accounts for only 1 percent of all cancer in males and about 3 percent of cancer of the male urogenital organs. Young men whose brothers or fathers had testicular cancer are more likely to have it.

What are the symptoms of testicular cancer?

The first sign is usually a slight enlargement or change in the consistency of the testes. There may be a dull ache in the lower abdomen and groin, accompanied by a sensation of dragging or heaviness. If the tumor is growing rapidly and hemorrhage is present, there may be sharp testicular pain. Enlargement of the breast or tenderness of the nipples may also be noticed.

Does removal of one testicle affect potency or fertility?

No, providing the remaining testicle is normal.

After removal of a testicle (orchiectomy) and x-ray therapy, is it still possible for a man to father a child?

If the radiation can be calculated to pinpoint the specific site without damaging surrounding tissues or organs, it is possible to avoid sterility. Sperm can also be frozen and stored in a sperm bank for later use in case the patient does become sterile. Be sure to discuss the entire question of fertility, radiation, and sperm storage in depth with your doctor before treatment.

How is testicular cancer staged?

Tumors are staged as follows:
- *T1:* Tumor limited to the body of the testis
- *T2:* Extends beyond the tunica albugines
- *T3:* Involvement of the rete testis or epididymis
- *T4:* Invasion of spermatic cord
- *T5:* Invasion of scrotal wall

Are there different kinds of testicular cancer?

Yes. Actually, there are many different kinds, but they are generally placed in four categories:

- Seminoma (typical anaplastic, spermatocytic)
- Embryonal carcinoma
- Teratoma (with malignant areas termed teratocarcinoma). Spread and treatment similar to embryonal carcinoma.
- Choriocarcinoma (rare)

Are different treatments recommended for the different types of testicular cancer?

Yes. Surgery—the removal of the suspected testicle—is usually the first step in all cases. Treatment of the affected lymph nodes varies according to the type of cells found in the tumor. For seminoma, which represents 40 percent of all testicular cancers, the preferred treatment following surgery is radiation therapy. Surgical removal of the nodes, sometimes with radiation and sometimes with the addition of chemotherapy, is often recommended for most of the other types.

Is testicular cancer more common in those who have undescended testicles?

Yes. In the male fetus, the testes are formed farther up in the body, near the kidneys, and, in normal development, descend to the scrotum shortly after birth. If they never make this descent or descend after the age of six, the chances of testicular cancer developing in later years is forty times more likely than if they properly enter the scrotum.

Can an artificial testicle be implanted to replace the testicle which has been removed?

An artificial testicle made of medical plastic can often be inserted at the time of surgery, or the procedure can be done at a later date. Great improvements have been made in the type of implant used. Originally, a hard plastic was used. Today, gel-filled implants with the weight and feel of a normal testicle have been developed which are more satisfactory.

Can I go to my local doctor for treatment of testicular cancer?

Since this is a rare form of cancer, the patient with suspected testicular cancer would be well advised to seek out a urologist specializing in cancer in one of the large medical centers to be certain that he receives the optimal treatment for this disease. Close cooperation and exchange of information among surgeon, radiotherapist, and medical oncologist is a must to ensure the successful outcome of this type of cancer.

Is a biopsy usually done before a testicle is removed?

No. This is one of the cases where the usual simple biopsy is not used for diagnosis. Doctors are warned against using needle aspiration or cutting into the tumor. In most cases, the doctor will schedule you for an operation to remove the testicle. Further therapy is based on results of a permanent section biopsy—not on a frozen-section examination.

What is the role of chemotherapy in testicular cancer which has metastasized?

Chemotherapy was first found potentially curative for testicular cancer in the late 1950s. Many trials and protocols have been tested in the past ten years—and it is important that your doctor be aware of the latest treatments being used. Several drugs have been found to be effective and some patients with metastatic testicular cancer can now be cured with combination chemotherapy. The treatment is difficult; however, and requires experienced medical oncologists to administer it.

Is testicular cancer usually curable?

The outlook for patients with cancer of the testes varies considerably, depending upon the extent of the disease when diagnosed, the tumor cell type, and the growth rate. For example, in men with seminomas (the most common type of testicular cancer) confined to the testes, a ten-year survival rate of 93 percent has been reported.

Does cancer of the penis ever occur?

Cancer of the penis is quite rare. It usually occurs on the tip of the penis and is almost exclusively found in uncircumcised males between the ages of 50 and 70. In others, cancer of the penis is found to be a metastasis from the bladder, prostate, lung, pancreas, kidney, testicle, or ureter.

What symptoms should alert a man to the possibility of cancer of the penis?

A pimple or sore, small nodule, white thickened patches, raised, velvety patch, wart or ulcer—especially a painless ulcer—are all suspicious symptoms. Bleeding associated with erection or intercourse, persistent abnormal erection without sexual desire, foul-smelling discharge, or a lump in the groin should all be carefully investigated.

What is the usual treatment?

The usual treatment is surgical removal of the tumor. Most cancers of the penis have been found to be resistant to radiation. Radiotherapy also can cause shrinking of the penis and collapse of the urethra, leading to urinary difficulties. Approximately 90 percent of patients with cancer of the penis, when found in the early stages, will be cured through the surgical removal of the tumor. If the cancer has spread to the groin, nodes in the groin will usually be removed.

What is the treatment for a metastasis that appears on the penis?

The treatment in this case would usually involve surgical removal of the tumor followed by radiation to relieve the pain which this type of metastasis usually causes.

chapter 18

Cancers of the Head and Neck

Questions to Ask Your Doctor Before Agreeing to Any Treatment

- Who will be performing surgery?
- Where will the incision be and what will the scar look like?
- How disfiguring will the surgery be?
- What will I look like?
- Will I still be able to eat, talk, and swallow after the surgery?
- Can radiation or radium implant be used instead of the surgery? Chemotherapy?
- Will radiation or chemotherapy be used in addition to the surgery?
- What kind of reconstructive surgery can be done?
- How many operations will that entail?
- What are the effects?
- How long will it all take?
- Will it cure me?
- How expensive will it be?
- Who else will be on the treatment team?
- Can I talk with them before I have any operation?

What kind of doctor should I see if I have symptoms of head and neck cancer?

The doctors who usually specialize in the treatment of head and neck cancer include otolaryngologists (ENT—doctors who treat ear, nose, and throat, air tubes to the lung, and neck regions), plastic surgeons (who do operations involving skin grafts, facial injuries, and tendon and nerve repair), and some general surgeons. Depending upon the type of cancer, the oral surgeon, maxillofacial prosthodontist (who specializes in replacing lost facial features), speech therapist, radiotherapist, and chemotherapist might also be part of the team.

Is the National Cancer Institute supporting any studies on head and neck cancer?

Yes. There are many clinical cooperative group studies being conducted by the National Cancer Institute on head and neck tumors. A variety of different trials, most of them involving radiation therapy or chemotherapy, either alone or in combination and either with or without surgery, as well as immunotherapy and neutron radiotherapy are being used (see Chapter 23).

Are cancers of the head and neck common?

Head and neck cancers constitute only about 5 percent of all cancers. They are not common cancers, especially in comparison with cancers of the breast, lung, or colon-rectal areas. However, since they are difficult to manage and the team approach is most important in treating them, we discuss the major types of head and neck cancer in some detail in this book.

What is head and neck cancer?

Cancer of the head and neck is a catchall phrase for an assortment of cancers which occur above the collarbone. Usually the term does not include the brain and the esophagus. It usually includes cancer in the ears, salivary glands, upper airway and food passages, nose, paranasal sinuses, nasopharynx, lips, oral cavity, tongue, tonsils, pharynx, hypopharynx, larynx, and cervical esophagus, neck, thyroid and parathyroid glands.

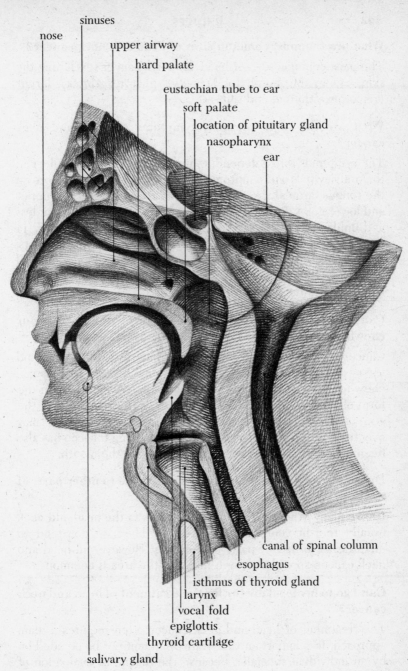

nose

sinuses

upper airway

hard palate

eustachian tube to ear

soft palate

location of pituitary gland

nasopharynx

ear

canal of spinal column

esophagus

isthmus of thyroid gland

larynx

vocal fold

epiglottis

thyroid cartilage

salivary gland

Head and neck

493

What are the most common sites of head and neck cancer?

The most common sites of head and neck cancer (excluding the skin) are in the mouth (oral cavity), pharynx (throat), larynx (voice box), thyroid and sinuses.

What are the most common symptoms of head and neck cancer?

The symptoms differ depending upon the site. A small ulcer in the oral cavity is one symptom. It may first appear somewhere on the tongue, around the tonsils, or along the edges of the upper and lower gums. It may look like a cold sore. It is usually painless and unlike a cold sore it does not heal by itself. Difficulty in swallowing, continued hoarseness, a sore throat that persists, neck swelling, and a lump on the side of the neck are all symptoms which, if they last for more than two weeks, should be checked by a doctor.

Can a person develop head and neck cancer from smoking or chewing tobacco?

Cancer of the lip, tongue, mouth, and pharynx (the space behind the nose and mouth) do occur more often in people who smoke, chew tobacco, or use snuff. Snuff, particularly when used in the form of a pellet and held for long periods of time between the gum and the cheek, frequently causes irritation and may eventually produce cancer at the spot. Chewing tobacco has also been linked to the development of cancer of the mouth.

Do cancers of the head and neck metastasize to other parts of the body?

Unlike many other types of tumor, tumors in the head and neck usually remain confined to that area. They do not tend to metastasize to distant parts of the body. However, in head and neck cancer, spread to lymph nodes in the area is common.

Can I go to my local doctor for the treatment of head and neck cancer?

The treatment of head and neck cancer often requires a team approach. It is important that your treatment not be decided on by an individual specialist because the diagnosis, evaluation of the extent of the disease, choice of primary treatment, and effective rehabilitation require special talents that cross over conventional lines. There are several doctors who have special interest and training in the management of head and neck cancer problems—the general surgeon, otorhinolaryngologist, plastic surgeon, oral surgeon, radiotherapist, and oncologist. The total care requires collaboration among these specialists as well as with the neurosurgeon, prosthodontist, speech therapist, and other allied health personnel.

What kind of treatment is used in head and neck cancer?

As is true with most other types of cancer, treatment includes all three disciplines: surgery, radiotherapy, and chemotherapy. Surgery is the treatment most often used. Usually early tumors are treated by surgery with adjoining tissue taken out. If the neck nodes are involved, a radical neck dissection may be done. Radiation therapy is used either before or after surgery. Sometimes chemotherapy is combined with immunotherapy in treating head and neck cancer patients.

Is reconstructive surgery usually necessary for head and neck cancer?

It depends upon the kind of cancer, the extent of the tumor, and the kind of surgery which is performed. In many cases of cancer of the head and neck, reconstructive surgery is not necessary. However, where needed, skillful skin and bone grafting allows persons who have had radical surgery to return to as normal an appearance and function as possible.

Are there any new treatments being tried for head and neck cancer?

There are several new treatments being tested, especially for large tumors of the head and neck region or tumors that have spread beyond the area. Chemotherapy, immunotherapy, a combination of the two treatments, chemotherapy used before surgery to shrink the tumor, chemotherapy and/or radiotherapy after surgery, chemotherapy followed by radiation therapy are all being tried with some success. Radium implants are being used in the treatment of tongue cancer.

Head and Neck Cancer

Type	Symptoms	Diagnostic Tests	Treatment
Nose (including sinus, nasopharynx)	Reddish, easily bleeding mass in nasal passage or cheek. If in paranasal sinuses, pain or swelling of cheek, inability to wear dentures	Head and neck examination, x-rays, biopsy	Surgery, preceded or followed by radiation. Nasopharyngeal radiation and/or surgery followed by radium implant. Reconstructive surgery.
Salivary glands (including parotid gland)	Lump below ear and jaw; occasionally pain or tenderness, hard consistency, facial palsy	Manual examination, x-rays, biopsy	Surgery to remove tumor. Radical neck dissection if lymph nodes involved. Radiation, chemotherapy sometimes used. Estrogen with or without radiation treatment. Treatment may involve facial nerve. Reconstructive surgery.
Mouth (including tongue, gums, floor of mouth, lip, cheek)	White patches, sore that does not heal, lump or thickening, bleeding, difficulty in chewing or swallowing food, restricted movement of tongue or jaw, discomfort in wearing dentures	Manual examination by doctor and dentist, smear tests, x-rays, biopsy	Surgery, radiation, radium implants, alone or in combination. Chemotherapy may be used. Reconstructive surgery.
Oropharynx (including soft palate, tonsil, walls back of tongue)	Velvety red patches, open sores in mouth, difficulty in breathing, earaches	Manual examination, x-rays, laryngoscopy, biopsy	Radiation, surgery, alone or in combination. Chemotherapy may be used. Reconstructive surgery.

Head and Neck Cancer

TYPE	SYMPTOMS	DIAGNOSTIC TESTS	TREATMENT
Hypopharynx (lower pharynx)	Difficulty in swallowing, lumps in neck, difficulty in breathing, earaches, cough, bad breath	Manual examination, laryngoscopy, biopsy	Radiation, surgery, alone or in combination. Chemotherapy may be used. Reconstructive surgery.
Thyroid	Lump in neck, persistent hoarseness, difficulty in swallowing	Thyroid scan	Thyroid hormone, surgery, postoperative hormone treatment, radiation, chemotherapy
Larynx	Hoarseness, lump in throat, difficult or painful swallowing, pain in ear, shortness of breath, harsh and noisy breathing	Indirect laryngoscopy, laryngogram, direct laryngoscopy, biopsy, diagnostic x-rays	Surgery, radiation, chemotherapy
Esophagus	Difficulty in swallowing, pressure, burning or pain in middle chest	Barium swallow, x-rays, esophagoscopy	Surgery, radiation

What is a radical neck dissection?

This means that along with the primary cancer (of the lips, tongue, larynx, etc.) the lymph nodes in the neck are removed. A radical neck dissection (sometimes called a radical neck node dissection) is done under general anesthesia. The operation may require up to five or six hours when it is done along with the removal of the primary cancer.

What kind of incision is made with a radical neck dissection?

The incision depends upon what the surgery is for. It can run from below the ear to the collarbone. Everything in the front of the neck on one side or on both sides may be removed. This includes the lymph nodes, blood vessels, nerves, and the salivary gland under the jawbone.

How long must I remain in the hospital for a radical neck dissection?

Your doctor usually lets you get out of bed within a day or two. You can go home from the hospital in about ten days.

When is a radical neck dissection performed?

A radical neck dissection is performed to remove the lymph nodes in the neck. Cancers such as those of the lips, tongue, and larynx sometimes spread to the lymph nodes, requiring them to be removed.

Is a tracheostomy done as part of the operation for radical neck dissection?

A tracheostomy (opening made in the windpipe) is usually necessary if the doctor is going to perform a radical neck dissection. After a few days the tube will be taken out and the opening will close.

Is a radical neck dissection a major operation?

Yes, it is. It may require up to five or six hours to perform when it is done along with the removal of the primary cancer.

Why is it important to exercise after I have had radical neck dissection?

In a radical neck dissection, the nerve mainly responsible for arm motion, which connects with one of the most important muscles in your neck and upper back, is cut. It makes it harder for you to raise your arm over your head or out to your side. If the surgery is on both sides of your neck, you will probably have some trouble raising both arms. However, there are special exercises which will help you get some of the strength back again.

How will I know what exercises to do?

Don't do any exercises until your doctor or your physical therapist tell you to. You may need to be seen by a physical therapist, who will determine your condition and give you exercises which will help your particular case. He or she will show you how to do them and tell you how often they should be done. It is important to make sure you do these exercises regularly. If they are not done, you may find the shoulder on the operated side will fall forward and look lower than the other side. And if the surgery was on both sides of the neck, you might find that both shoulders are falling forward and you will be standing and sitting in an uncomfortable, slumped-over position which may cause shoulder pain.

What kinds of facial defects might a head and neck cancer patient have?

Patients with head and neck cancer may be left with defects of various facial structures, including eyes, ears, nose, mouth, lips, cheek, and neck.

What kind of work is done to correct these facial defects?

The defects are corrected either by reconstructive surgery or with the use of maxillofacial prosthetics.

How will the decision be made as to what will be done?

The choice of methods depends upon the kind of defect which needs to be corrected, and discussion between the patient and the doctors involved.

What is reconstructive surgery?

Reconstructive surgery is the reconstruction of features from the patient's own tissue. A plastic surgeon does reconstructive surgery.

What does the reconstructive surgeon do?

The reconstructive surgeon usually has two roles: he attempts to minimize the deformity which results from the treatment of the tumor and he initiates and coordinates an overall rehabilitation program.

What techniques can the reconstructive surgeon use?

The reconstructive surgeon must be familiar with the use of skin, cartilage, and bone grafts. He must be able to transfer tissue from a distant site to the tumor area. He helps people who have limited ability to speak, hear, see, eat, or even move, live more normal lives.

What are maxillofacial prosthetics?

The field of maxillofacial prosthetics grew out of prosthetic dentistry. It means using an artificial part to correct a defect in the body. The new plastics, vinyl and silicone rubber, are used to make parts to replace what is taken out in the surgical operation. There are some specialized centers in the United States which have the facilities to construct these prosthetics for the rehabilitation of patients with facial defects. A listing of the rehabilitation research projects being funded by the National Cancer Institute is listed in Chapter 23.

What kind of doctors create maxillofacial prosthodontics?

Doctors who specialize in this field belong to the American Academy of Maxillofacial Prosthetics. Training programs are presently being funded by the National Cancer Institute to train fully qualified maxillofacial prosthodontists and prosthetic technicians.

What does a maxillofacial prosthodontist do?

The job of the maxillofacial prosthodontist is to restore the patient's appearance and function. He uses the remaining tissues that the patient has to support the prosthesis. He manages the dental and paradental structures to prevent loss of the supporting tissues. You may need a maxillofacial prosthesis to speak or eat or swallow. Or it may be necessary because you have lost an eye, your nose, or some part of your face.

When does the maxillofacial prosthodontist see me?

Many times the prosthodontist will be part of the team you see before surgery or radiation therapy. Sometimes, after surgery the prosthodontist will not see you until the sixth or seventh day. He may give you a temporary prosthesis for use until the permanent prosthesis is fitted and made.

What is an obturator?

An obturator is a "cork" which plugs a hole or seals off an opening. It is the basis of most prostheses. It fits into the defect which was made by the surgery. It may help make a part function naturally or may help build out the face cosmetically when some parts have been removed.

When is an obturator put in?

Sometimes the obturator is inserted at the time of surgery, sometimes about a week after.

If I am missing part of the face, how is the prosthesis made?

If you need to replace a missing part of the face such as the nose, eye, ear, or a combination of these, the missing or defect areas are sculpted in clay or wax on casts of the defect. Molds are then made and the prosthesis is created of a flexible plastic from the mold. The prostheses are tinted to match your skin. If you wish, you can have more than one prosthesis made—tinted to match the skin color at different seasons.

Must I wear the obturator all the time?

It depends upon where the surgery is performed. If you have had oral surgery, the doctor will tell you to try to wear the obturator most of the time, even at night, and remove it only for cleaning the mouth. The obturator allows you to eat, speak, and swallow, and will keep the wound from contracting.

Do most head and neck patients need dental prostheses?

It is estimated that more than half the head and neck patients will need some kind of dental care—some form of prosthesis to restore function or appearance or both.

What kinds of areas can be fitted with prostheses?

There are several areas in the head and neck region where prostheses are used.

For instance:
- An ear can be replaced by plastic material.
- An eye and even portions of the cheek can be replaced.
- Parts of the nose or the complete nose can be made either with a graft or with a prosthesis.
- Parts of the mouth and lip can be reconstructed.
- Teeth and parts of the palate are filled by prostheses which allow the patient to eat and to talk.

The doctors can simulate skin tones, ruddy complexions, freckles, and veins. They can fit parts which remain permanently in place. They use lightweight materials which are easily cleaned, are durable and compatible with the nearby tissue.

Is it true that many patients with head and neck cancer get very depressed and discouraged?

Again, it depends upon the site of the cancer and the attitude of the patient. Many patients whose operation has caused facial disfigurement or a great change such as a laryngectomy naturally go through some depressed periods. However, when they find out that they can live their lives in much the same fashion as they did before—with reconstructive surgery and help in learning to speak—most head and neck patients find that life is still worth living. However, most people need support and help from family and friends to get through the difficult period of adjustment.

What are the cancers of the mouth?

The cancers of the mouth (oral cavity) include the lip, tongue, floor of the mouth, cheeks (buccal mucosa), and gums (gingivae).

Who is at high risk to get cancer of the mouth?

This cancer is predominantly found in men between the ages of 60 and 70. People who are heavy smokers, have a heavy alcoholic intake, are over 40, and have a family history of this kind of cancer are at a higher risk to develop cancers of the oral cavity, the mouth, and the throat.

Is cancer of the mouth easily found?

Yes, it is usually discovered early, since it can be seen easily. White patches (leukoplakia), velvety red spots (erythroplasia), or dark patches are symptoms which should be seen by a doctor, who should do a biopsy of them. Many cancers of the mouth are first discovered by dentists.

What are the symptoms of oral cancer?

The warning signs of oral cancer are:
- Sore spot or ulceration of lips, tongue, or other area inside the mouth that does not heal in two weeks
- White scaly area inside the mouth
- Swelling of the lips, gums, or other area inside the mouth, with or without pain
- Repeated bleeding in the mouth with no apparent cause
- Numbness or loss of feeling in any part of mouth.

What is leukoplakia?

Leukoplakia is a fairly common condition among people who smoke. It is not cancerous, but it can become cancerous if it is continually irritated, as by smoking. It occurs as a white thickening or patches on the lip, on the tongue, or in the mouth. Sometimes it is called smoker's tongue or smoker's patches. Poorly fitted dentures can also be irritating to leukoplakia. If you have this problem, it is important to have the dental defect taken care of.

Are the white patches usually removed?

It depends upon the extent of the patches. The patches may be removed with an electric needle, using local anesthesia. If there are many of them, you will need several treatments to take them all out. You can also have them removed surgically or with cryosurgery. They usually require either local or general anesthesia and an overnight stay in the hospital.

What is Plummer-Vinson syndrome?

Plummer-Vinson syndrome is a wasting away of mucous membranes of the mouth, pharynx, and esophagus caused by deficiencies in the diet. It is a noncancerous condition that tends to become malignant. It frequently precedes mouth cancer.

What is torus palatinus?

Torus palatinus is a bony growth in the middle of the hard palate in the roof of the mouth. It is a benign tumor which can grow to an inch or more in diameter. It grows slowly and you may not notice it. Unless you are having some problem with it, such as in fitting dentures, it is usually left alone. If necessary, it can be surgically removed. The operation can be done under local anesthesia. The membrane of the palate will be opened, the excess bone chiseled away, and the membrane stitched together.

Is bleeding in the mouth a sign of cancer?

Repeated bleeding of the mouth without cause is a sign of some kind of problem. If it has been going on for two weeks, you should have it checked by a doctor or a dentist. Most cases of bleeding in the mouth are not cancerous.

Can I examine myself for oral cancer?

Yes, it is possible for you to examine yourself for oral cancer.

There are six areas of the mouth—lips, cheeks, gums, tongue, roof, and floor—which should be examined. A well-lit mirror, a gauze pad or handkerchief, and clean hands are all that are needed.

- Check your lips, cheeks, and gums, looking for changes in the normal color. Look for areas of red, white, or blue. See if there are any scabs, cracks, ulcers, or areas of swelling or bleeding. You should feel for sore spots, numbness, bumps, or thickening within the tissues of your lips and cheeks. Feel your gums to see if there is any swelling, numbness, soreness, or a loose tooth.
- Look at your tongue. Stick it out as far as you can. Examine the tip, the top, the bottom, and edges. You are looking for white patches, velvety-red spots, ulcers, or swellings. Feel the tongue to see if there are any lumps, sore spots, or lack of movement. Extend the tongue in all directions by grasping it with the gauze pad or handkerchief.
- Check both the floor and the roof of your mouth. Look for lumps, swellings, or soreness. Feel along the sides and as far back as you can go. Tilt your head back and look at the front and back of the roof of your mouth in the mirror. If you have any problems that last for more than two weeks, you should

see your doctor or your dentist. Although these signs don't
always mean cancer is present, they are warning signals.

Will habitual biting of the inside of my cheek cause cancer?

No one really knows. Regular irritation has been suspected as a
possible cause of cancer. Maybe the dentist can help with
suggestions for stopping this habit. Sometimes chewing gum can
help. If there are white, red, or darkened patches inside the
cheek, see the doctor.

How does the doctor diagnose cancer of the mouth?

Mouth cancer, like any other cancer, is diagnosed by biopsy. As a
preliminary step, some doctors and dentists will scrape cells from
a suspicious area, as they do in taking a Pap smear, for
examination under a microscope. If the smear shows signs of
cancer, a biopsy is done to confirm the diagnosis.

How is cancer of the mouth treated?

Surgery and radiation are the principal methods for treating
cancer of the mouth, depending on the site and stage of the
disease. Sometimes radiation is used to shrink tumors of the
cheek or floor of the mouth before surgery. Radium needles are
also used in treating some mouth cancers—they may be
implanted for cancer of the upper lip, tongue, cheek, or floor of
the mouth. Sometimes external radiation is used before the
radium implant. The use of chemotherapy together with
radiation therapy is also being tested.

Is radical neck dissection used for treating mouth cancer?

If involvement of lymph nodes in the neck is suspected, a radical
neck dissection is sometimes performed.

Does plastic reconstructive surgery usually accompany an operation for mouth cancer?

It depends upon the extent of the surgery. Sometimes, to make
sure all the malignant tissue is taken out, extensive surgery may
be necessary. Although such procedures are sometimes disfiguring, highly developed techniques of reconstructive surgery can
be used to rebuild or repair facial features or other affected
areas. If a complete reconstructive procedure is not advisable at

the time of cancer surgery, temporary artificial devices of a cosmetic nature can be used.

Are most tumors of the lip cancerous?

No, most tumors on the lips are benign. They are usually warty growths or tumors of the blood vessels. Most of these can be cured by one of several methods: cutting them out and stitching the cut edges together, burning them with an electric needle, freezing them, or treating them with x-ray.

Where does cancer of the lip occur most commonly?

Lip cancer usually occurs in the lower lip, in men between the ages of 60 and 70. Chapping, overexposure to sunburn, and smoking (especially pipe smoking) are thought to be factors in developing this cancer. Cancer of the lip is fairly common and usually highly curable, especially if there are no neck-node metastases.

How is lip cancer treated?

Sometimes surgery is used, usually a procedure called a V-lip excision. Sometimes radiation therapy is used, but surgery seems to be simpler and more convenient, especially for smaller cancers. Very large lip cancers are usually treated with radiation therapy because major reconstructive work would be necessary after surgery.

Lip cancer, because it is slow-growing and visible, is usually discovered in the early stages. It often takes lip cancer months to spread to the lymph nodes in the neck.

Will I have disfiguring scars after a partial removal of the lip?

The lip regains almost normal appearance, even after large sections of it have been taken out.

How is the reconstruction done if surgery is performed on a large lip cancer?

Usually the reconstruction is done with the use of a skin graft taken from the forehead.

What is a lip shave?

A lip shave removes the mucous membrane on the lip. It is usually performed as a preventive measure for persons who have extensive leukoplakia (white patches) on the lower lip—even if the patches are not cancerous.

Is neck dissection done with lip cancer?

If the biopsy shows that the lymph nodes are involved, a neck dissection may be performed on the involved side.

Does lip cancer metastasize?

Lip cancer rarely metastasizes. When it does, it goes to the lymph nodes in the region. However, swollen lymph nodes can be an inflammatory reaction to lip surgery.

Do benign lip tumors ever turn into cancer?

Sometimes. Warty growths have a tendency to become cancerous and should be removed.

Who is at high risk to get cancer of the tongue?

Cancer of the tongue appears mostly in men who are over 40.

Where does most tongue cancer occur?

Most cancer of the tongue is situated at the tip or along the side of the tongue. It can usually be discovered early.

What are the symptoms of tongue cancer?

You might see deep-red patches. Sometimes there are white patches. Sometimes the deep-red patches turn bluish white. This is called leukoplakia, which represents an overgrowth of cells. There may be only a few spots or they may be on the whole tongue. Sometimes they will not hurt. They may be irritating and uncomfortable. The greatest danger of these patches is that if they are not treated, some of the area might turn into cancer. Some people complain of pain, which they usually think is a sore throat. It gets worse when they talk and swallow. Sometimes the pain goes to the side of the head or the ear.

Can the red or white patches on the tongue be removed?

They can be removed with an electric needle or by surgery. They are thought to be caused by tobacco smoking, alcohol, sharp-edged or diseased teeth, and faulty-fitting or sharp-edged dentures.

Can these patches recur? Do they turn into tongue cancer?

Leukoplakia has a tendency to recur and the recurrent areas can be retreated. The appearance of an ulcer or hard growth in one of these patches often indicates a cancerous change. An ulcer or cracking or peeling develops in the leukoplakic area and the surrounding region becomes firm and hard. The doctor will take a biopsy of these tissues.

What does cancer of the tongue look like?

Cancer of the tongue usually appears as a painless, thickened, ulcerated area along the margin of the tongue. As it gets bigger, it may be swollen and tender and may bleed occasionally.

Does tongue cancer tend to spread?

Tongue cancer does not tend to spread rapidly. Although most tongue cancer remains confined for months to the original site before spreading to the lymph nodes of the neck, symptoms should not be ignored. If the cancer is toward the back of the tongue, it tends to spread to lymph nodes on both sides of the neck.

How is cancer of the tongue treated?

Cancer of the tongue can be treated by surgery, by radiation, or by radium implant.

What operations are performed for cancer of the tongue?

Cancers located on the side of the tongue are usually treated by either removing a wedge or half the tongue (hemiglossectomy). If the cancer is on the top of the tongue or in the middle forward portion of it, the doctor will usually remove the front two-thirds of it. Cancers of the base of the tongue are almost always treated with radium and x-ray treatments. If the tongue cancer has spread to the lymph nodes, neck dissection will be needed to take out the nodes in the neck. If it has spread to the floor of the mouth, the areas under the tongue which have been affected will be removed. Sometimes the jawbone will be involved. If so, it may be replaced with a bone graft or a metal splint.

Is one treatment preferred above the others?

It depends upon the size of the tumor, the extent of the cancer, and the patient's and doctor's preference. Some cancers can be removed by taking out a wedge of the tongue. Another treatment involves inserting radium needles into the tongue. You should discuss with your doctor the advantages and disadvantages of all treatments before any decision is made.

Will I be able to swallow, speak, and eat normally if I have parts of my tongue removed?

It depends upon the extent of the operation. If a large portion of your tongue is taken out, swallowing can become awkward, but you can still do it. Speech may also be slightly impaired. If 75 percent of the tongue is removed, chewing may become very difficult, making it necessary for you to live on a soft diet. Again, speech may be impaired.

What kind of anesthesia is used for a tongue operation?

General anesthesia is usually used. A tube is placed in the trachea. Often there is a need for blood transfusions for this operation. Special nurses may be needed.

When will I be able to eat after the operation?

You will be on fluids, given through the tube placed in the nose and extending to the stomach, for the first few days. Then you will be able to eat soft foods.

Will I be able to speak if I have a part of my tongue taken out?

Yes, you will still be able to speak. If you have a small wedge taken out, the deformity is not great. If you have a larger cancer which might remove as much as a third of the tongue from the tip back, your speech will be changed but will remain understandable. With training, many patients, even when more than half the tongue has been removed, learn to talk again. Radium implants or x-ray treatments, if they can be done for your type and stage of cancer, do not ordinarily involve any speech deformity.

Will I have a large scar after tongue surgery?

If you have had neck dissection along with the tongue operation, part of the jawbone and the glands in the neck are removed, leaving a visible scar.

How is cancer of the floor of the mouth diagnosed?

The doctor will look at and feel the tumor. He will take x-rays and do a biopsy to confirm the diagnosis.

Does cancer of the floor of the mouth metastasize?

Yes. This is one of the oral cancers which metastasizes to the lymph nodes in the neck in a good number of patients.

What treatment is used for cancer of the floor of the mouth?

In early-stage cancers, the treatment is usually radiation or surgery. Cancers that are more advanced are usually treated with surgery followed by radiation and sometimes chemotherapy.

Who is at high risk for cancer of the cheek?

Cancer of the inside of the cheek (sometimes referred to by doctors as buccal mucosa) occurs more often in males over the age of 55. It is believed that persons who chew tobacco and betel nuts or who bite their cheeks are at a higher risk of getting cancer of the cheek.

What are the symptoms?

The symptoms include a sore inside the cheek which does not heal, bloody saliva, and white patches inside the cheek. There is usually no pain.

Does cancer of the cheek metastasize?

Cancer of the cheek is usually slow-growing. It also has a relatively low rate of metastasis.

How is cancer of the cheek diagnosed?

It is diagnosed by direct inspection and feeling by the doctor. Final diagnosis is by biopsy.

How is cancer of the cheek treated?

Early stages of cancer of the cheek are treated with radiation or by surgery. Advanced cancer of the cheek is treated by surgery, followed by radiation and sometimes chemotherapy.

Who is at high risk for cancer of the gums (gingivae) and hard palate?

Women are at a higher risk for cancer of the gums and hard palate. The average age for this cancer is 60 years old. Most occur in the lower gums.

What are the symptoms?

The symptoms are painful ulceration and difficulty in wearing dentures.

What is the treatment method?

Early stages are treated by radiation or by surgery. Late stages are treated by surgery, followed by radiation and sometimes chemotherapy.

What are the parts of the nose?

The nose is made up of connective tissue (cartilage) and bone. It contains two cavities, which are separated in the middle by a septum. The nose serves as the organ of smell and is the airway for breathing. It filters, warms, and moistens the air which is breathed in.

What are the sinuses?

The sinuses are air spaces within the bones of the face and the skull. They connect through small openings (ostia) into the air passages in the nose. The soft, moist mucous lining which coats the inside of the nose goes into the sinuses. There are four types of sinus: frontal (within the bone just above and behind the eyebrows), maxillary (in the bones of the cheeks beneath the eyes), ethmoid (near the side of the nose and inner part of the eyes and going back into the skull), and sphenoid (in the skull above the level of the nose).

Is cancer of the sinuses common?

No. Cancer of the sinuses is very rare. Most often it is the maxillary sinus that is involved in the disease.

What are the cancers of this area called?

The cancers in the nose area are called cancer of the nasal fossa (nasal cavity), paranasal sinuses (sinus), and nasopharynx (tube which connects the mouth and nose with the esophagus).

What are the symptoms of cancer of the nasal area?

One symptom is a reddish, easily bleeding mass in the nasal passage. Sometimes paranasal sinuses will produce pain and pressure in the cheek, a toothache, or persistent draining of the sinus after tooth extraction, a nasal quality to the voice, a lump in the cheek, or bloodstained discharge from the nose.

How is this tumor diagnosed?

The doctor uses a head light and a small mirror or a nasopharyngoscope (a flexible optical instrument) to look in the passages. He may also order x-rays of the facial bone. He can take a biopsy or a brush scraping with the nasopharyngoscope.

What is nasopharyngeal fibroma?

This is a tumor of the nasopharynx which is found mainly in youngsters. It is a benign tumor but may destroy bone and soft tissue about it as it enlarges. It should be diagnosed early. It is curable but sometimes several operations are needed. Sometimes radium implant, radiation, or cryosurgery is used to remove these tumors.

Are the tumors in the area of the nose and sinuses always malignant?

No. There are many noncancerous tumors in the area of the nose and the sinuses. Warts, polyps, and small blood-vessel tumors are often found and are usually nonmalignant.

How is cancer of the nose and sinuses treated?

The growth is usually removed by surgery. Surrounding tissue may also be removed. Sometimes sections of the nose, the roof of the mouth, the floor of the eye socket, or the face and the cheek must be excised. Radiation can be used before or after surgery. Cancer of the nasopharynx is usually treated by radiation alone or by a combination of radiation, surgery, and radium implant.

Why is such drastic surgery performed?

The main goal is to get beyond the cancer. Many lives have been saved with this kind of surgery, and the advances in plastic surgery mean that people can be restored to normal appearance.

How is cancer of the nasopharynx treated?

Cancer of the nasopharynx is usually treated with radiation therapy or with surgery or both, depending upon the extent of the disease.

What is cancer of the oropharynx?

Cancer of the region of the oropharynx includes the soft palate, tonsil, walls of the pharynx, and back third of the tongue. The most common site for this cancer is on the tonsil.

How is cancer of the oropharynx diagnosed?

The doctor will diagnose it by looking at it and feeling it if it is in an area that can be reached. In other areas he will use laryngoscopy. As with other cancers, biopsy is essential for a definite diagnosis.

What are the symptoms of cancer of the oropharynx?

The symptoms are similar to those of oral cancer—velvety red patches appear. Some are open sores. There is usually little or no pain associated with them. Some people complain of difficulty in swallowing, lumps in the neck, difficulty in breathing, and earaches.

What is the treatment for cancer of the oropharynx?

Primary treatment for this cancer is radiation therapy in most early cases. In more advanced stages treatment may be surgery, radiation, and sometimes chemotherapy. If there is involvement with the bone or neck nodes, radiation will usually be followed by surgery.

What is cancer of the hypopharynx?

Cancers of the hypopharynx are tumors of the lower pharynx. They are found mostly in males from the ages of 49 to 60.

What are the symptoms of cancer of the hypopharynx?

The symptoms include difficulty in swallowing, lumps in the neck, difficulty in breathing, earaches, cough, and bad breath.

How does the doctor detect cancer of the hypopharynx?

He looks at it and feels it if it is in an area that can be reached. He will probably use a nasopharyngeal mirror or a laryngoscope (flexible optical instruments which allow him to look into the lower pharynx). He will do a biopsy to get a final diagnosis.

How is cancer of the hypopharynx treated?

Radiation therapy is used sometimes alone, sometimes followed by surgery. Part of the pharynx and/or part of the larynx may be removed.

Where are the salivary glands?

The major salivary glands are in the sides of the face, in front of and slightly below the ears. These salivary glands are also known as parotid glands. The saliva gets from these glands to the mouth through parotid ducts, which open on the inner surfaces of the cheeks. There is also a pair of glands in the lower jaws (submandibular glands) and under the tongue (sublingual glands). The ducts from these glands open into the floor of the mouth underneath the tongue.

Where are tumors of the salivary glands found?

Tumors of the salivary glands are most often found in the parotid glands. Most often these tumors are not malignant. They are either on the outer surface of the parotid gland, which is near the ear, or in the inner surface, which is in the mouth. Benign parotid-gland tumors are usually painless and slow-growing. Malignant tumors of the parotid tend to grow rapidly. Sometimes a tumor seems to be benign for many years and then suddenly becomes malignant. Tumors of the parotid gland are relatively rare. Of those tumors that are found, 80 percent are benign. If a person has a lump in the neck which does not quickly disappear, or which grows, he should go to a doctor. A second opinion by a doctor specializing in head and neck surgery should also be sought.

What are the symptoms of cancer in the parotid gland?

Usually the most common complaint is the presence of a slowly growing lump in the cheek next to the ear. Sometimes there is a rather dull and indefinite but progressive pain and facial-nerve paralysis.

How does the doctor operate on the salivary-gland tumors?

He makes an incision running from in front of the ear to the neck. The doctor must be sure the incision is long enough to let him carefully separate the gland from the facial nerve so that the nerve is not cut. If the nerve is cut, distortion and paralysis of that side of the face may occur. Sometimes, such as when the tumor is malignant, the nerve must be cut. In many cases the treatment for cancer of the salivary glands is removal of the complete gland, the affected area around it, and sometimes the facial nerve.

Is it difficult to recover from an operation on the salivary glands?

No. The doctor will leave the drain in for a few days after the operation. You will probably be out of bed the day after that and home in a week or less. You may have to remain on a fluid diet for several days because it may be painful to chew solid foods, but after that you will have an unrestricted diet. Usually the scar heals in about ten days.

Where are the incisions made in operations on the salivary glands?

The incision placement depends upon which glands the doctor is operating on. If it is a parotid-gland operation the incision is made in front of the ear and along the angle of the jaw. If it is the submaxillary gland it is made parallel to and along the undersurface of the lower jaw. The incision for the sublingual gland is in the mouth or in the skin just below the chin.

Does the doctor take out the whole gland?

Again it depends upon the gland and on the problem. Usually if cancer is present, the whole gland is taken out. If the parotid tumor is benign, and can be completely taken out, the rest of the gland will be left.

Is radiotherapy used in treating cancer of the salivary glands?

Sometimes radiation is used in this type of cancer. It may be given to persons who cannot be operated on or to reduce the size of the tumor. Sometimes it is used after the operation on a portion of the facial nerve.

Can the facial nerve be replaced?

Yes it can. However, some return of facial-nerve function has been seen in patients without a nerve graft. If the paralysis is due to the shock of the operation, the function usually returns within 6 to 8 weeks.

Will my hair be shaved for an operation on the parotid tumor?

Yes. Because of the location of the parotid gland, the hair around the ear must be shaved. Sometimes the hair is brushed up and back, if possible, or cut so that the top hair may be arranged to cover the ear when you are ready to go home.

Will I have to have special care after the operation?

You will probably be on a fluid diet for the first few days because it may be painful to chew solid foods. You may be given antibiotics in large doses to control infection. Special attention will be paid to your mouth and to your teeth.

Does this kind of cancer usually recur?

Parotid tumors can recur. Sometimes they are treated with surgery again. The whole area may be treated with radiation.

If the doctor removes one of the salivary glands, will I still have normal saliva production?

Yes. The remaining glands will take over for the gland that the doctor has removed.

Questions to Ask Your Doctor About Thyroid Cancer

- How many thyroid operations have you performed in the last year? What are the usual results?
- Is there any indication that there is spread beyond the thyroid area?
- Is the nodule soft or hard?
- What tests are you planning for me?
- What type of cancer do you suspect?
- Will it be necessary to operate?
- Will it be possible for you to remove only the one nodule?
- If not, how extensive do you expect the operation to be?

Questions to Ask Your Doctor About Thyroid Cancer (continued)

- Do you think it will be necessary for you to remove both lobes?
- Will the diagnosis be made from the frozen section, or can we wait for a permanent section before proceeding with the removal of the thyroid?
- Are you planning to remove the regional lymph nodes?
- Will there be permanent hoarseness?
- Will I have trouble swallowing? For how long?

What is the thyroid?

This ductless gland, located in the front of the throat, below the Adam's apple and just above the breastbone, is roughly U-shaped and has two lobes—one on each side of the windpipe. The thyroid serves as the body's thermostat. It regulates the rate at which the body uses oxygen, the rate at which the body uses food, and the rate at which various organs function.

How is cancer of the thyroid usually discovered?

The patient may become aware of a growth in the neck, or the doctor may discover it during a regular examination. The lump usually is not painful or tender. A hard, irregular lump that does not seem to move is the most suspicious to the doctor's touch. Softness, mobility, the indication of more than one lump, and slow growth usually indicate a benign condition. There may also be enlargement of the nearby lymph nodes either above or below the level of the thyroid nodule. Any noticeable lump should be checked by a doctor, especially if it begins to increase in size. Sometimes there may be a history of persistent hoarseness or difficulty in swallowing.

Are all lumps in this area cancerous?

No. Only about 10–20 percent of patients with suspicious nodules actually prove to have cancer of the thyroid. Most of the tumors are cysts. However, removal is usually recommended because of the location.

Who is at a higher risk to get cancer of the thyroid?

Cancer of the thyroid is found twice as often in women as in men, more often in whites than in blacks, and more often in the older age group. People who had radiation to the head and neck area when they were children are also at a higher risk for thyroid cancer. Cancer of the thyroid is not a common cancer—it accounts for less than 1 percent of all cancers. It is also one of the least frequent causes of death from cancer.

Why do people who had radiation treatment to the head and neck in childhood or adolescence get thyroid cancer?

X-ray treatment was used beginning in the 1920s and continued over 25 years to treat noncancerous conditions. Among the conditions which were treated with x-rays were ringworm of the scalp, enlargement of the thymus glands in infants, various types of ear inflammations, deafness due to overgrowth of the lymphoid tissue around the eustachian tubes, enlargement or inflammation of the tonsils and adenoids, inflammation of the sinuses, head and neck lumps, and acne. At the time the treatment was used, no one anticipated the aftereffects of the radiation.

Are x-rays to the head and neck still being used in treatment of children?

No. This kind of treatment is no longer prescribed for these childhood conditions.

Am I more likely to get thyroid cancer than the general population if I had x-ray treatment as a child?

You are at a higher risk, but only a small percentage of the people irradiated at an early age develop thyroid tumors. Most of the tumors are slow-growing. Most of the tumors are benign. Even those which are cancerous usually remain limited to the neck for many years and can be successfully removed by surgery.

What should I do if I was exposed to x-ray treatment when I was a child?

You should tell your doctor as much as you can about the kind of treatment which you had. It is important to find out, if you can, the kind of treatment you were given, what form it took, how many doses you were given, and any other details. This information should become a permanent part of your medical record. People with a history of radiation should be reexamined every one or two years. The most important part of the examination is careful inspection of the neck to detect the possible presence of nodules in the thyroid. Remember, the risk is for people who had x-ray *treatments* during childhood, not for people who had x-rays for diagnosing an illness.

Is a goiter cancerous?

Goiter is a term which means overgrowth of the thyroid. There are two kinds of goiters: colloid goiter, which comes from insufficient iodine in the drinking water and food, which is now rarely seen, and nodular goiter, which in some 10 percent of the cases may develop into cancer.

Is it unusual for a child to have cancer of the thyroid?

Cancer of the thyroid does occur in children and young adults. In contrast to cancers of some other organs, however, the statistics show that 90 percent continue to live normal lives with fairly normal life expectancies. Even when the disease is locally advanced with extensive involvement of the lymph nodes in the neck, this still holds true.

What kinds of tests are used to detect thyroid cancer?

The doctor will probably do several things. First he will look at the thyroid area for abnormalities. He will feel the thyroid gland and nearby areas for any lumps or swellings. If he suspects a tumor he will examine the inside of the throat with a small instrument called a laryngoscope—it lets him look with a mirror into the vocal cords. He might give you a thyroid scan or do a needle biopsy. Depending on the size and extent of the growth the doctor might do a barium swallow to examine the neck or chest films and a skeletal survey to determine if there are distant metastases. However, as in most kinds of cancer, the only true test is through biopsy, which is usually performed as part of an operation to remove the tumor.

How is a thyroid scan performed?

You will swallow a tiny dose of radioactive material. An instrument is moved back and forth over your neck to determine how actively your thyroid tissue is absorbing this substance. If it is quite active, the lump is called "hot." If it is not absorbing the substance, the lump is called "cold." Cold lumps may be cancerous, slow-growing, and slow to spread. Hot spots usually indicate a benign growth. Even if your scan shows you have a cold spot, you should not worry, because about 80 percent of the time, cold spots, upon biopsy, prove *not* to be cancer. Sometimes two thyroid scan readings are taken—usually at 2 and 24 hours after administration of the radioactive material.

How long will the radioactive substance from the scan remain in my body?

The radioactive substance is quickly absorbed by the bloodstream and taken directly to the thyroid gland. It stays in the gland about one to three days—and then is excreted in the urine.

Are needle biopsies usually performed in the thyroid area?

Sometimes doctors take needle biopsies to get a small specimen of thyroid tissue to study under the microscope. However, needle biopsy should be done only where special expertise in this technique has been developed.

If a tumor is found in the thyroid gland does the doctor usually operate?

It depends. An operation is usually necessary if there is an indication that the tumor is causing pressure, if there is a single nodule which shows rapid growth, if there are any signs of new growth, or if the patient is a child or young male. Sometimes the doctor will give you a thyroid hormone which cancels the need for the thyroid to produce its own hormones and causes the gland to shrink. The doctor may also use this technique in unclear cases, to let him feel for nodules which may lie hidden deep in the gland. He will probably watch the results for several months. If the tumor gets bigger or additional nodules appear, he will then operate. If there is a past history of x-ray treatment during childhood or adolescence, many doctors feel it is wiser to operate.

Is surgery the main treatment for thyroid cancer?

Once diagnosed, surgery is usually the treatment of choice for thyroid cancer. In some cases the doctor will remove the entire thyroid gland. This procedure is called a thyroidectomy—either partial or total. Sometimes suspicious nearby lymph glands are also removed.

What is the difference between a lobectomy and a thyroidectomy?

Lobectomy (or hemithyroidectomy) indicates that one lobe of the thyroid (and sometimes the isthmus, or tissue connecting the two lobes) has been removed. Sometimes this is called a partial thyroidectomy. The total thyroidectomy includes removal of both lobes.

What is involved in a thyroidectomy?

There are several kinds. Subtotal thyroidectomy means the removal of parts of both lobes and of the isthmus of thyroid tissue over the windpipe or removal of a whole lobe and part of another. Total thyroidectomy means removal of all thyroid tissue.

How long will the thyroid surgery take?

Though not a dangerous procedure, this is a fairly complicated operation. If the entire thyroid is removed, it will take from two to four hours. The thyroid operation is complex as it can involve nerves, veins, windpipe, and esophagus as well as parathyroid glands which lie directly under the thyroid. Most times the parathyroid glands are allowed to remain.

What kind of anesthesia is given?

A general anesthetic is usually used.

When can I expect to return to work after thyroid surgery?

Usually recovery is swift, and the patient can return to work within a few weeks. Hospital stay is usually one week. Because of the location of the operation, it is less painful than abdominal or chest surgery. The throat will probably be extremely sore and hoarseness can be expected. A drain is usually left in place for two to four days and is removed with little or no discomfort.

What does the incision look like?

Generally a 3½-to-4-inch incision is made in the neck above the collarbone, usually in one of the creases of the neck. When the scar is healed it is barely noticeable, though the thin-line scar will never fully disappear.

Is thyroid cancer ever treated with radiation or chemotherapy?

Sometimes, if all the abnormal tissue cannot be removed by surgery or if the cancer has metastasized to other parts of the body, radiation therapy or chemotherapy may be used.

Can I continue to smoke after I have had a thyroid operation?

It certainly would be better if you stopped smoking. However, your doctor will probably tell you to stop for at least two weeks after the operation. This is because coughing can cause pain and stress on the muscles and skin close to the incision.

Will removal of the thyroid gland affect my sex life?

No. Removal of the thyroid gland should have no effect upon your sex life.

Will I have to take thyroid hormone if I have my thyroid gland removed?

If it is entirely removed (there are three portions of your thyroid gland) you will need to take thyroid hormones daily for the rest of your life. If, however, only a portion of the gland is taken out, the remaining tissue may be able to produce enough for your body. Tests will be performed after surgery to see if you need to replace the hormone. The replacement hormone is usually given in pill form.

What are the parathyroid glands?

The parathyroids are four small glands which are attached to the thyroid gland. They secrete a hormone, parathormone, which is involved with the balance of the body and the excretion of calcium and phosphorus necessary for bone growth and maintenance. They are part of the endocrine system.

What are other parts of the endocrine system?

Other parts of the endocrine system include the adrenal glands and the pituitary glands.

Can one get cancer of any of the parts of the endocrine system?

Yes, it is possible to have cancer of the parathyroid glands, the adrenal glands, or the pituitary glands. Cancer of the endocrine system is relatively rare and is complex to diagnose.

Is cancer of the endocrine system difficult to treat?

Cancer of the endocrine system is difficult to treat because of hormonally produced changes in the patient. It is important, since a general practitioner rarely sees these cancers, to have endocrine cancer treated by a specialist.

Is surgery performed on the parathyroids?

Yes, surgery can be performed. If a tumor is located in only one gland, it can be removed. The incision is similar to that for the thyroid operation—a 3½-to-4-inch incision is made in the neck above the collarbone. The doctor will take out as much tissue as necessary to remove the tumor. Recovery is quick from this operation. If the tumor reappears, surgery is usually performed again.

What is the larynx?

The larynx is the voice box. It is the upper part of the windpipe above the trachea. The larynx forms the Adam's apple in the neck. Air coming in passes through the larynx to the lungs. In front of the larynx are the vocal cords. Muscles move the vocal cords, which are made to vibrate by air exhaled from the lungs.

Who is at high risk to get cancer of the larynx?

Men are almost nine times more likely to get it than women, although the incidence in females is now rising. Most people who get it are in their 50s, although there are some cases in people in their 20s and 30s. People at high risk are those who smoke, drink to excess, and have frequent irritation to the larynx such as coughing frequently.

What are the symptoms of cancer of the larynx?

The symptoms of cancer of the larynx occur early. They are noticeable hoarseness, a lump in the throat, difficult or painful swallowing, pain in the ear, shortness of breath, and harsh, noisy breathing. Some of the symptoms of more advanced cases are badly swollen neck glands, weight loss, and sometimes bleeding. If you have constant hoarseness that lasts more than three weeks, it should be checked by a doctor.

Can cancer of the larynx be cured if treated early?

Yes. Hoarseness is an early symptom, and many of the cases of cancer of the larynx can be cured if seen at an early stage. It is estimated that 85 percent of larynx tumors could be cured, and the patient left with a fairly good speaking voice and a natural air passage, if diagnosed early and treated before there is spread to surrounding tissue.

Are all growths on the larynx cancerous?

No. Most tumors of the larynx are benign. Cancer of the larynx can be removed by surgery when found early and the voice may be saved. Nonmalignant growths can also be removed and the voice restored to normal.

What causes nonmalignant growth?

Noncancerous growths may be caused by allergy, irritation, infection, or overuse of the voice. Singers, teachers, and politicians often have nonmalignant growths or papillomas.

How is the nonmalignant growth treated?

Usually, a hospital stay is required. Using a general anesthesia or local anesthetic, the doctor puts a tubular instrument (laryngoscope) through your mouth to the throat. He uses special instruments to cut away the tumor. You will feel some discomfort—similar to a very sore throat. You will be on a liquid diet and will go home in two or three days. The doctor will not let you use your throat for a week or more. It is important to heed the doctor's advice in not using the voice in order to have this area heal properly. You can do permanent injury to your vocal cords if they do not heal properly.

Do nonmalignant growths ever recur?

Yes, certain nonmalignant growths—those that are wartlike— have a tendency to recur and are operated on again.

Where does cancer of the larynx occur?

Most cancer of the larynx occurs on the vocal cords. It can also occur in the cartilage, muscles, passage from the throat, or passage to the windpipe.

How does the doctor diagnose cancer of the larynx?

The doctor may do an indirect laryngoscopy—he looks down your throat with a long-handled mirror to see whether or not the voice box shows signs of cancer of the larynx. This can be done in the doctor's office and is painless. If he needs to examine your throat more carefully, he may do a direct laryngoscopy. For this examination your throat is numbed and the doctor inserts a rigid tube through which he can inspect the area and take samples of the tissue if he wishes. This examination takes only about fifteen minutes but must usually be done either in an outpatient clinic or in a hospital. Diagnostic x-rays are also sometimes used, including a laryngeal tomograph (laryngogram) and chest x-rays. As with other types of cancer, a biopsy is needed for a final diagnosis. The biopsy is essential before any treatment is planned.

How is cancer of the larynx treated?

It depends upon the exact location and site of the cancer. Surgery, radiation, and chemotherapy can all be used, either separately or in combination. Usually if the tumor is small, radiotherapy is used to shrink it enough so that your normal voice returns. Since it is less disfiguring and equally effective, radiation is more commonly used for small tumors. If the tumor is large, all or part of the voice box may be removed by surgery.

Will I have a change in my voice if I am treated with radiation?

No, you will in all probability be able to continue talking in much the same way as before the treatment. If you are going to be treated with radiation, be sure to read the information in Chapter 7 on radiation.

What is a laryngectomy?

A laryngectomy is the complete removal of the voice box. In a partial laryngectomy, only part of the voice box is removed and the voice is preserved; just one vocal cord, half of both vocal cords, or the epiglottis (the lidlike structure that covers the entrance to the larynx) is removed.

How is a partial laryngectomy done?

This operation is performed either under general anesthesia or local anesthesia. An incision is made in the neck, starting at the top of the Adam's apple and extending about 2½ inches. The doctor will split the cartilage of the larynx and then cut away the growth on the vocal cord.

Will I have an opening in my throat from a partial laryngectomy?

An opening in the windpipe (tracheostomy) may be performed as part of the partial laryngectomy if a considerable amount of tissue is removed. This is to make sure that there is an adequate airway. A metal tube will be inserted and taken out a few days later. The opening will then close normally without any stitches being taken.

Will I be in pain after having a partial laryngectomy?

You will probably have a very sore throat. You will probably be told to sit halfway up in bed for the first few days to help you swallow. Your stitches will be taken out within a week and you usually can go home in ten days to two weeks.

Does a partial laryngectomy ever involve radical neck dissection?

It depends upon the extent of the cancer. The partial laryngectomy can involve different things. If the tumor is widespread, a radical neck dissection may be involved. If the cancer is in the leaflike flap of cartilage between the back of the tongue and the entrance to the larynx and windpipe (epiglottis), all of the larynx above the vocal cords may be taken out. In that case, the voice is preserved but you might have trouble swallowing. The doctor may put in a temporary feeding tube through the nose to the stomach for a week or longer until the swallowing becomes easier.

Will my voice change as a result of a partial laryngectomy?

Sometimes some change in voice occurs. However, you will

probably be able to continue talking in much the same way as before the operation.

How is a total laryngectomy performed?

The total laryngectomy is done under general anesthesia. It is a much more extensive operation. The incision is along the center of the neck, but is longer than for the partial laryngectomy. The windpipe is cut above the collarbone and a tube is inserted so that the anesthetic gas goes to the windpipe. The whole larynx is taken out.

Will I be in much pain after the total laryngectomy?

You will have a very sore throat. Sometimes the doctor will put in a plastic feeding tube through the nose to the stomach so that the area can heal more easily. This is not always necessary and you may be able to swallow soft food within a few days. Your neck may feel weak, and it may be uncomfortable for you to move. You may need help to raise your head. You may have to have a special nurse or be in intensive care for a day or two. You should be able to go home from the hospital after two weeks.

Will I have a hole in my throat after a total laryngectomy?

Yes, you will. After a total laryngectomy you must breathe through a permanent opening in the neck. This opening is called a stoma.

I am afraid to have my voice box taken out. Is there any alternative?

If you have a large tumor there is probably no alternative, although you should talk to your doctor about it. It is only natural to be afraid, for you will be losing a part of your body which you use constantly. You should know, however, that many people who have had this operation have been able to resume their normal living. Most people have learned how to talk again. Many are people for whom talking is a livelihood, and they are able to talk fluently and understandably with their new voices.

What will I do while I am in the hospital and can't talk?

Some hospitals use simple charts with pictures of what you need and in the early stage you can point to what you want. Some people find it easier to write a note for what they want. The nurses usually place a marker over your signal at their desks so that they can tell your calls from calls of patients who can speak. If you wish, you can ask the nurse for a spoon and a water glass to signal with or you can bring a bell to the hospital with you. One patient and his wife worked out a code which he could tap on the speaker of the telephone so she could call him in the morning and find out how he was. A magic slate or small blackboard is useful.

Will my lips and tongue be the same as before the laryngectomy?

Ordinarily, your lips, teeth, tongue, and nasal passages remain the same as before surgery.

What is a person who has lost his voice box called?

A person who has had his voice box removed is called a laryngectomee. Most of these people are men and they have lost their ability to speak normally because they have had cancer of the larynx.

How soon will I be able to talk again?

That depends upon many factors—mainly it depends on you. You need to have determination and the willingness to practice the new way of speaking. Some people say some words within three or four weeks after the operation. Others take several months. It will take time to be able to talk fluently so that everyone can understand you.

How can I breathe and speak if I am going to have my voice box removed?

Because your operation to remove the voice box removes the connection between the lungs and the nose and mouth, air from the lungs is no longer used to speak. The person breathes through an opening, called a stoma, in the front part of the neck. You will have to learn how to speak again.

Who will teach me to speak again?

If you are going to have this operation performed, it is important to talk with the doctor and the speech pathologist before the operation. That will be a big help in understanding what changes can be expected after surgery. Laryngectomees usually learn to talk again with the help of a speech pathologist. Occasionally some laryngectomees teach themselves. Talk to your doctor and to the local unit of the American Cancer Society to find out the names of speech clinicians or trained laryngectomees available. After you have learned basic speech you may wish to take advantage of group therapy available through such organizations as the International Association of Laryngectomees (see Chapter 23).

Is there more than one way to speak if you have had a voice box removed?

Basically there are three new ways to talk. One is by using esophageal speech—the tongue is used to force air into the very top part of the food pipe and that same air is forced back out through the mouth. By doing this, a sound is made deep in the throat that is used to form words in much the same way as in normal speech. The second method is pharyngeal speech, which uses the limited amount of air that goes into the nose and mouth when you breathe through the tracheostomy tube. You block this air with your tongue, making it vibrate against the roof of the pharynx at the back of the mouth. You can practice and make this speech sound almost normal—your voice will sound ordinary, but slightly hoarse. The other way uses a battery-operated device called an electro-larynx for speaking. The electro-larynx is held in the hand against the neck. When a button is pushed, the sound travels from the vibrating surface of this device through the neck and into the mouth, where the sound is formed into words. (This device is available from the telephone company's special-equipment service.)

All the ways seem very difficult. How will I be able to do it?

You will need a lot of practice and it will be quite a challenge for you. But most people want to learn to talk again so they can go back to the things they did before surgery as soon as they can. And many people have learned to talk in these ways.

When can I begin speech therapy?

You can start learning the new method of speaking as soon as your operation has healed. Your doctor will tell you when you can do this, but it is usually shortly after you can safely swallow liquids and solid foods.

Why is the opening in the neck necessary for a laryngectomy?

Before the operation, breathing and food passages had a common passage in the throat. Farther down, they divided into the windpipe for breathing and the esophagus for carrying food to the stomach. The voice box controlled the entry of air and guarded against food particles. The voice box has been taken out. It is necessary to relocate the end of the air passage as an opening at the front of the neck. This is called the stoma.

Will I always have to breathe through this opening?

Yes, you will always have to breathe through this opening, and once you learn how, you will do it without thinking about it. At first, you may have much mucus and coughing, but later you will cough no more frequently than someone who has not had the operation.

Will I always have to wear a tube in my stoma?

Probably for some time. A tube shaped to fit the tracheal opening (laryngectomy tube) is necessary to keep the breathing passage wide open until the tissues are healed. The doctor will tell you when it can be removed safely and how long you should wear it. Some people wear it all the time. You will get instructions on how to take it out and put it back in.

What is a stoma button?

A stoma button is a short, soft plastic tube put into the opening in your neck. Some people use a button instead of the laryngectomy tube. Some people do not need either the stoma button or the tube.

Do I keep the opening in my neck covered?

Yes. The opening in the neck needs to be covered all the time so you get warm, clean, moistened air. Air that is dusty, dry, or cold can dry your windpipe and cause coughing and make it harder for you to breathe.

Will material collect around my stoma?

Mucus, which is the liquid which is secreted normally by the lining of the respiratory tract, will be present in your stoma and sometimes will dry on the rim of it. If the mucus thickens, dries out, or collects at the edge of the stoma it is called crustation.

How often do I have to clean my stoma?

It depends upon you. Some patients tell us they clean the stoma twice a day, once when they get up and again in the evening.

How do I clean my stoma?

You use plain water and soap and a soft cloth. It's usually easier if you are sitting down facing the mirror and leaning slightly forward. Do not use synthetic detergents or oil-based soaps.

Why is it important to have extra moisture in the air I breathe?

Before your operation, your nose helped to warm the air you were breathing and your respiratory tract helped to moisten it. Now there is no way to warm or moisten the air that comes into your lungs. It is a good idea to have a small vaporizer or a humidifier in your home so that the air you breathe is warm and moist. Some people keep a pot of water on the stove to moisten the air.

What do I do about blowing my nose?

You must remove the mucus manually. You can use a damp cloth to clean your nostrils but you cannot blow your nose. You also cannot suck on a straw, sip soup, gargle, or whistle because you cannot force air from your lungs out through your nose or mouth or force air through your mouth to your lungs.

How can I get rid of my secretions when I am wearing a shirt and tie?

Some patients tell us that they take off the second button on the shirt and sew it onto the buttonhole. That leaves an opening in which a handkerchief can be put to remove mucus. The shirt still looks as if it were buttoned.

Does my shirt have to be a bigger size than before?

Shirts usually need to be one to one and a half sizes larger than those worn before the surgery.

As a laryngectomee, can I take a shower?

You will have to be careful not to suck water into your lungs when you are bathing or showering. But baths and showers can provide moisture which you need. If you are taking a tub bath, pull the curtain around so that you keep the moisture in the air. Keep the drain partly open to keep the water from coming in high enough to get into the stoma. Keep a towel around your neck, and when you wash your face use a mirror so that you are sure water will not get into the stoma. If you are showering, adjust the stream so that it is chest-high. A special shower cover can be used to cover the stoma when you are in the shower.

Will I be able to swim?

No, you will no longer be able to swim when you are a laryngectomee. You should be careful when you are around water and you should not go boating.

Can I shave?

You must be careful if you are using a regular nonelectric razor. The area will be numb until the nerve endings return to normal and that might take six months. You could cut yourself without knowing it. Don't let the shaving lather or toilet water get into the stoma. You could have severe coughing if they get into the trachea.

Is a laryngectomee a physically handicapped person?

Absolutely not. A laryngectomee can do most jobs that most others can do. You can farm, do plumbing, do officework, work in a factory, and so on. You can also participate in most sports, such as golfing, hunting, and gardening.

Can I go back to my regular job after I have my voice box removed?

Most people find they can return to their regular jobs. Talk to your doctor about when you can go back to work. It is essential that you get back to normal routines as soon as you can and take every opportunity to try out your new speech patterns.

Where can I get help for all this adjustment?

The American Cancer Society sponsors Lost Cord Clubs (sometimes called New Voice Clubs), which are groups of laryngectomees and their families dedicated to helping new members get used to the same physical and emotional changes they have been through. Many of the clubs offer group speech therapy as part of scheduled meetings. Members also visit new patients on the request of doctors, to show them how they speak and to answer questions. Some clubs also teach laryngectomees and their families special first aid. Don't hesitate to call on them if you need a helping hand. Since all these changes are sometimes difficult to deal with by yourself, it is important that you let family and friends help you through this period. The more you go out with friends and practice the new way of speaking, the more confident you will feel. Let your family and friends help, but try to get back to doing everything for yourself just as you did before.

Where can I find out about these clubs and other information about laryngectomies?

You can call the nearest office of the American Cancer Society, or the Cancer Information Service in your area. You can also write to the International Association of Laryngectomees (521 West 57th Street, New York, N.Y. 10019).

Does a laryngectomee need a special kind of first aid if he becomes ill or is hurt in an accident?

A laryngectomee does need special first aid. First expose the neck. Give mouth-to-neck breathing only. Keep the person's head straight with the chin up. Keep the neck opening clear with cloth—don't use tissue. A laryngectomee should wear a special medic-alert identification bracelet or carry an emergency instruction card.

What is the esophagus?

The esophagus is the foodpipe. It is a long hollow muscular tube which goes from the back of the throat down to the stomach. It carries food and liquid to the stomach.

Are most tumors of the esophagus cancerous?

Yes. Most tumors of the esophagus are malignant. More men than women have esophageal cancer, and it occurs most often between the ages of 50 and 70.

Is difficulty in swallowing one of the symptoms of cancer of the esophagus?

Difficulty in swallowing could be due to a number of conditions. If the problem lasts more than two weeks, you should see a doctor, because cancer of the esophagus is one possibility. Because the tumors start in the lining of the membrane, the sensation may be that food, especially soft bread and meat, sticks behind the breastbone. Other warning signs of cancer of the esophagus include sensations of pressure and burning or pain in the upper middle part of the chest. However, the main symptom is difficulty in swallowing (dysphagia). The food doesn't feel as if it is going down properly—but the feeling is different from the one you get from a sore throat. Because of the difficulty in swallowing, weight loss is sometimes a symptom.

Does the difficulty in swallowing stay as a symptom?

Sometimes. Sometimes the sensation seems to get worse and then to get better. Sometimes it comes and goes.

What tests are used to detect cancer of the esophagus?

Usually the first test will be a barium swallow. This is an x-ray procedure. You swallow a liquid containing barium, which outlines the esophagus. X-rays are taken. If a tumor is present, the lining of the esophagus will appear abnormal or narrowed. The doctor will be able to tell whether or not a tumor is there, the size of the tumor, and the extent of its growth.

What is an esophagoscopy?

It is another way of detecting esophageal cancer. A long, thin tube with a light and lens at the end of it (esophagoscope) is slid down the throat and into the esophagus. The doctor can see the inside of the esophagus and can tell whether or not a tumor is present. Sometimes he can also tell the size of the tumor with this instrument. The doctor might also use a biopsy forceps with the esophagoscope to take a tiny bit of tissue from the areas which look suspicious during the esophagoscopy. Or he might gather loose cells from the esophagus with a brush. Either the tissue or the cells would then be studied under the microscope to determine the diagnosis.

The General Stages of Cancer of the Esophagus

STAGE	OTHER CLASSIFICATION	EXPLANATION
Stage I	TIS, N0, M0 T1, N0, M0 T1, NX, M0	Carcinoma in situ or tumor in any region of the esophagus that involves 5 centimeters of esophageal length, produces no obstruction, has no extraesophageal spread, does not involve the entire circumference, and shows no regional lymph node metastases or remote metastases
Stage II	Cervical esophagus: T1, N1, M0 T1, N2, M0 T2, N1, M0 T2, N2, M0 T2, N0, M0 Thoracic esophagus: T2, NX, M0 T2, N0, M0	A tumor of any size with no extraesophageal spread and with no distant metastases
Stage III	Any T3 Any N3 (cervical) Any N1 (thoracic) Any M1	Any esophageal cancer at any level with distant metastases, extraesophageal spread, fixed lymph node metastases.

How is cancer of the esophagus treated?

Cancer of the esophagus is treated either by radiation or by surgery. The surgical operation is called an esophagectomy. It is performed under general anesthesia. The doctor makes a 10-inch incision between the ribs on the side of the chest and removes the whole cancerous area, if possible. The passage must again be connected to the stomach, either by replacement with a plastic tube, by using the remaining healthy tissue, or by using a portion of the intestine. The earlier the disease is detected, of course, the more successful the operation.

How long must I stay in the hospital with cancer of the esophagus?

After the operation, you will usually stay in for two to four weeks. You will be in bed for from one to three days.

Will I be able to eat?

After the operation you will be fed with intravenous fluids and/or by a rubber tube passed through the esophagus into the stomach. A rubber tube is also placed in the chest for a few days after surgery to drain the chest. Within three to five days you will probably be able to take fluids and soft food by mouth.

Is this major surgery?

Yes, surgery for cancer of the esophagus is major surgery. You will probably be uncomfortable for many days afterward.

chapter 19

Cancer of the Brain and Spinal Cord

Persons Most Likely to Get Cancer of the Brain and Spinal Cord

- Young children and young adults to age 20
- People over 40; peak ages 50-60
- More men than women

Symptoms of Cancer of the Brain and Spinal Cord

The symptoms of cancer of the brain and spinal cord vary depending on where the tumor is located in the brain. Symptoms include:

- An unusual kind of headache, more painful than usual. A constant ache or soreness, located in the back, front or side of the head or behind the eyes, often present upon waking in the morning.
- Vomiting, usually in the morning
- Impaired speech
- Hearing loss or ringing and buzzing in ears
- Loss of smell
- Muscle weakness of the face
- Abnormality in functioning of the eye
- Balance problems, or lack of coordination in walking or movement
- Changes in personality

Symptoms of Cancer of the Brain and Spinal Cord (continued)
- Convulsion or epileptic seizure
- Inability to sleep for long periods
- Drowsiness

Tests for Cancer of the Brain and Spinal Cord

- Complete medical history and physical
- X-rays of skull
- Electroencephalogram
- Brain scan
- Ventriculogram
- Pneumoencephalogram
- Angiogram
- Spinal puncture
- Myelography

Questions You Should Ask Your Doctor Before Agreeing To Treatment for Cancer of the Brain and Spinal Cord

- Where is the tumor located?
- What kind of tumor do you suspect?
- Where will the operation be?
- Will you shave my hair off?
- Will it be painful?
- What kind of diagnostic tests will I still need? How painful or dangerous are they?
- Will you have to drill a hole in my skull? Will it be painful?
- How long will I have to stay in the hospital?
- Will I have any side effects?
- Will there be any additional treatments?
- When will I be able to go back to work?

What kind of doctor should I see if I have symptoms of brain or spinal-cord cancer?

This is a specialized field, and you should be sure you have a skilled, competent diagnostician and surgeon. The physician who specializes in diseases of the nervous system—brain, spinal cord, and nerves—is called a neurosurgeon.

Cancer of the Brain and Spinal Cord

TYPE	CHARACTERISTICS
Glioma	Family of tumors which starts within brain substance itself
Astrocytoma	Slow-growing, usually in shell-like capsule. May be malignant or benign. Found in both adults and children.
Glioblastoma multiforme	Most malignant type. Grows quickly. Term commonly used to describe a highly malignant astrocytoma.
Ependymoma	Begins in lining cells. Often benign. Usually occurs in children.
Medulloblastoma	Usually found in children. Usually malignant.
Congenital tumors	Include dermoids, teratomas, cholesteatomas, and craniopharyngiomas. More common in children.
Meningioma	Starts in membranous tissue. Can grow to large size and destroy bone. Mostly benign, occurs mostly in adults.
Neuroma (neurofibroma)	Arises in nerves. Usually occurs in adults over 40. Most common is acoustic neuroma, occurring in ear nerve. Benign, slow-growing.
Pituitary adenoma	Occurs in young or middle-aged adults. Almost always benign.
Metastatic	Starts somewhere else and spreads to brain. Usually comes from breast, lung, or melanoma.

Is the National Cancer Institute supporting any studies on cancer of the brain and spinal cord?

Yes, there are many clinical cooperative group studies being conducted by the National Cancer Institute on brain and other spinal-cord tumors. Numerous different drugs and radiation therapies are being used. For information on this subject, see Chapter 23.

What is meant by tumors of the central nervous system?

The central nervous system is made up of the brain and the spinal cord. Tumors can be found either in the brain or in the spinal cord. Sometimes brain tumors extend downward into the spinal cord. Usually, however, tumors of the central nervous system do not spread to any other part of the body. Cancer which starts in other parts of the body can, on the other hand, metastasize to the brain. About 80 percent of the central-nervous-system tumors involve the brain and about 20 percent the spinal cord.

What is the brain?

The brain is a soft grayish-white structure enclosed by the skull. It weighs about 3 pounds and has some 15 million nerve units which permit it to store memory images and learning. Its connections control more than 600 muscles in the body. The brain is the seat of consciousness, sensation, and emotion. It directs all voluntary acts and controls all higher mental processes.

What are the parts of the brain?

The brain has four main structures: cerebrum (the largest area, which is divided into four lobes and controls movement, speech, and visual functions), cerebellum (second-largest area, involving muscular coordination), pons (which receives and sends impulses from the cerebrum and cerebellum to the spinal cord), and medulla oblongata (which regulates breathing, heartbeat, and vomiting). The brain also has many nerve structures, including twelve cranial nerves.

Who gets tumors in the brain?

About 85 percent of brain tumors occur in adults, with a peak age of 50 to 60. The remaining affect infants or children, with a peak age of 10 years. More men have brain cancer than women.

Are brain tumors common?

No. Brain tumors are relatively uncommon. They account for only 2 percent of all cancer deaths.

What are the symptoms of brain tumors?

The symptoms vary depending on where the tumor is located in the brain. They are caused by increasing pressure inside the skull as the tumor grows. Most common is a headache, more painful than usual, which results in a constant ache or soreness. It may be in the back, front, or side of the head or behind the eyes. Patients

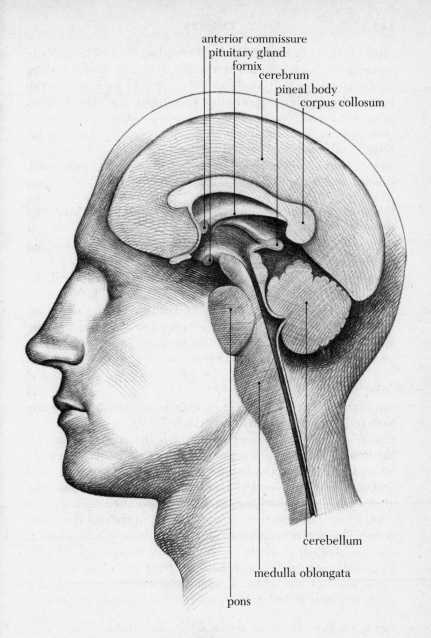

anterior commissure
pituitary gland
fornix
cerebrum
pineal body
corpus collosum

cerebellum

medulla oblongata

pons

Brain

report that the headache will be there when they wake up in the morning, or that it begins to ache right after they arise. Vomiting may accompany the headache. Some people note changes in personality or are more irritable than usual. Epilepsy is also a symptom, with convulsions, seizures, or short periods of unconsciousness. Sometimes patients say they hear strange sounds and smells that are not there or may fall into a dreamlike state. There may be a loss of hearing, sight, speech, taste, smell, and balance.

Do some symptoms relate directly to the part of the brain the tumor is in?

Sometimes the symptoms are produced by the tumor pushing into a particular area of the brain. Tumors which are located in the area controlling motion can produce weakness in the arm, the leg, or both. A tumor located in the cerebellum, for instance, might produce loss of coordination, balance, or the ability to walk. However, brain tumors are very hard to diagnose, since the symptoms are usually difficult to pinpoint, may appear only occasionally, and are similar to those of other diseases.

Are all brain tumors cancerous?

No. However, tumors in the brain must be thought of differently than tumors in other parts of the body. Tumors which would be considered benign in other parts of the body are more serious in the brain—not because they are cancerous but because they are located in a part of the brain where they cannot be taken out without doing irreversible damage. They expand inside the closed bony skull until they strangle essential centers. Even a small amount of growth occupying space can damage the nerve tissue. The doctor will often talk about a brain tumor which is encapsulated—that is, in a shell-like capsule—and can be completely removed. That is different from one which has roots like a plant or one which invades much brain tissue or is in a location where it cannot be removed completely by surgery.

Are those tumors which are in a capsule curable?

It depends upon the tumor. If it is discovered and removed when it is still in its capsule, the chances of cure are very good. If it goes untreated, it will eventually break through the capsule and spread cells into surrounding areas of the brain. When this happens, it is more difficult to treat. As with other cancers, the earlier it is discovered, the greater the possibility of successful treatment.

What causes the swelling in the brain?

Most tumors result in swelling (edema) of normal brain tissues. The swelling puts additional pressure on the brain and may cause a great deal of significant damage before the tumor grows to a large size. Sometimes steroid drugs are used to reduce the swelling in the brain. Steroid drugs are also sometimes used for pain of brain tumors, either alone or in addition to surgery or radiation.

How are brain tumors diagnosed?

There are several procedures which can help diagnose brain tumors. A complete medical history and physical, with the doctor looking for changes, watching movements, and looking at ear and eye nerves, and plain x-rays of the skull may sometimes give enough information. More specialized tests include:

- *Ventriculogram:* A burr hole is made in the skull and a needle is placed in one of the brain's ventricles (small cavities). A small amount of fluid is taken out and replaced by air, and x-rays are taken. A high-risk procedure.
- *Pneumoencephalogram:* A needle is placed into the spinal canal, fluid is taken out, and air is injected. X-rays are taken. A high-risk procedure. Following this procedure, many patients have headaches, nausea, vomiting, and fever which may last for several hours or days.
- *Angiogram:* A small amount of contrast material is injected into arteries of the neck leading to the brain. X-rays are taken. Some patients have a painful, burning sensation as the contrast material is injected. A high-risk procedure.
- *Electroencephalogram:* Wires are taped to the skull to record brain waves from that area. Can show abnormal brain functioning but does not show the tumor itself. Causes patient no discomfort.
- *CT scan:* Also called a CAT scan (computerized axial tomography). The patient takes a small amount of a radioactive isotope. A machine prints out a pattern showing

the concentration in the brain tumor of the radioactive substance. Causes patient no discomfort. Where equipment is available, this test has largely replaced the ventriculogram and pneumoencephalogram.

What are the different kinds of brain tumors called?

There are several kinds of brain tumors, which are usually broken down into the following types: gliomas, meningiomas, neuromas, pituitary adenomas, congenital tumors, and metastatic tumors. Gliomas and meningiomas can also occur in the spinal cord.

How do doctors classify tumors of the brain and spinal cord?

Classifying brain and spinal-cord tumors is extremely difficult because of the nature of the tumors and the location. Numerous methods are used, and most physicians and hospitals feel that the most critical features are the type of tumor, the extent of growth, and the location of the tumor. A "G" designation is sometimes used to indicate the biological activity of the tumor: G1, well differentiated; G2, moderately well differentiated with no mitoses; G3, poorly differentiated with occasional mitoses; G4, very poorly differentiated with frequent mitoses. "T" classifications are as follows:

- *T1:* Tumor less than 3 or 5 centimeters (size dependent on location), confined to one side
- *T2:* Tumor more than 3 or 5 centimeters (size dependent on location), confined to one side
- *T3:* Tumor invades or encroaches upon ventricular system. Greatest diameter may be less than 3 or 5 centimeters (depending on location in brain).
- *T4:* Tumor crosses the midline, invades opposite hemisphere, or extends into other sections of brain.

What are the gliomas?

About half of the tumors inside the cranium originate within the brain substance itself and are called gliomas. There are five types of gliomas:

- *Astrocytomas:* May be malignant or benign and are found in both adults and children. They grow slowly but penetrate into large areas. Sometimes astrocytomas are in a shell-like capsule and can be completely removed by surgery. Radiation and chemotherapy are sometimes used.

- *Glioblastoma multiforme:* The most malignant type of brain tumor. Accounts for more than half of all gliomas. It grows very quickly. It is treated by surgery but many times cannot be completely removed. Radiation and/or chemotherapy are used as secondary treatments.
- *Ependymomas:* Begin in the lining cells. Many of these are benign, but many cannot be removed because of location. Radiation and chemotherapy are sometimes used.
- *Medulloblastomas:* Most often found in children. Radiation and chemotherapy are often used.

What are congenital tumors?

The congenital tumors include dermoids (sometimes called dermoid cysts or cystic teratoma), cholesteatomas, and craniopharyngiomas. Craniopharyngiomas occur more commonly in children; they are benign but are sometimes difficult to remove because of their location.

What are meningiomas?

The meningiomas start in the meninges—the membranous tissue which surrounds, covers, and protects the brain. Some of these grow to a very large size and cause destruction of the bone. Most of them are benign. They vary in size from that of a small pea to that of a large grapefruit. They are usually distinct lumps. The meningiomas account for 10–15 percent of all tumors inside the brain and occur mostly in adults of middle age. They grow slowly. They are usually treated by surgery.

What are neuromas?

Neuromas, or neurofibromas as they are sometimes called, arise in the nerves of the brain. They rarely occur in persons under 40. They may develop at any nerve site, but the most common type is in the nerve of the ear, called acoustic neuroma. If left untreated it can cause deafness. Neuromas are benign, grow slowly, and produce limited symptoms for a long period of time. Many of the acoustic neuromas are discovered early because an early sign is difficulty in hearing, often accompanied by noises in the head. When discovered early, neuromas can be completely removed through the ear or through an opening in the back part of the skull. If they can be completely removed, they usually do not recur. Sometimes the patient's hearing can be saved.

What are metastatic brain tumors?

Metastatic brain tumors are different from other brain tumors because they are cancerous tumors which start somewhere else in the body and spread to the brain. Metastatic tumors make up about 10 to 15 percent of all brain tumors. They usually come from primary tumors of the breast, lung or from a melanoma. Radiation or hormone therapy are most often used.

Do tumors occur in the spinal cord?

Sometimes. Much that is true of brain tumors is also true of spinal-cord tumors because the spinal cord and the brain together form the central nervous system. Sometimes tumors of the brain may extend down into the spinal cord. There are also separate spinal-cord tumors but they are less often seen than brain tumors. Spinal-cord tumors may stop the flow of messages between the body and the brain in either one or both directions, similar to spinal cord injuries which occur from accidents.

Are most spinal-cord tumors cancerous?

Most of the spinal-cord tumors which start outside the cord itself (in the membrane around the cord or in a spinal nerve) are not cancerous. They cause pressure on the cord and the nerves. They can usually be completely removed by surgery.

Do tumors which are growing within the cord tend to be malignant?

Yes, tumors which are growing within the spinal cord are more often cancerous than those which start outside the cord itself. But they usually grow slowly. They are hard to remove without destroying a section of the spinal cord. However, they can be treated by radiation therapy, which stops the growth. Cancer in other parts of the body sometimes spreads and involves the spinal cord. Radiation treatment is usually used in these cases.

How are spinal-cord tumors diagnosed?

Several tests can be done to diagnose spinal tumors:
- *Spinal puncture:* This will usually show an obstruction to the free flow of the spinal fluid. Chemical analysis of the fluid often provides additional useful information.
- *Myelogram:* The doctor injects a radioactive substance into the spinal fluid and then takes x-rays.

How are brain tumors treated?

Surgery is almost always the first step in treating brain tumors. However, some brain tumors are not easily reached by surgery. In some cases, to get to them the doctor goes through vital brain tissues responsible for seeing, speaking, moving, or coordination. Therefore, the type, location, and extent of the tumor are very important in deciding the kind of treatment which will be used.

What is a craniotomy?

A craniotomy is the operation for exposing the brain. It is usually performed under general anesthesia, although sometimes local anesthesia is used.

What preparations will be necessary before the operation?

Your head will be shaved and your scalp will be cleaned with water and soap. An antiseptic will be put on the area and all but that portion to be operated on will be covered with sterile drapes.

How will the operation be done?

The doctor will make an incision in the shape of a semicircle facing downward in the skin on the affected part of the scalp. He will flap the skin down and drill holes in the skull. He will then connect the hole by sawing with a wire, air, or electric saw so that a block of bone (called a bone flap) can be taken out from the skull. In simple terms he has made a window into the skull through which to work. Directly underneath are the membranes which cover the brain. These will be cut so that the doctor can see the brain.

Will the block of bone be put back after the operation?

After the operation, the doctor will put the block of bone or flap back or he will use a metal or fabric mesh to cover the opening. The doctor will fix it securely and then sew the skin back in place.

Can the exact location of the tumor usually be determined before the operation?

Yes, with the many tests available the exact location can usually be pinpointed.

Can the doctor always tell before the operation whether a brain tumor is malignant or benign?

No, that is not always possible.

Do brain operations take a long time to perform?

It depends upon the location of the tumor, the procedure which will be used, and the surgeon himself. Some operations are done within an hour or two. Others may take three or four hours. Because of improvements in giving anesthesia, even the lengthy operations are safe.

Will I have intravenous feedings after my brain surgery?

Sometimes feedings are done with a tube in the stomach or into the vein. Often you can be fed by mouth.

Will I need special nurses after brain surgery?

Yes, you will usually either be in intensive care or need special nurses for several days.

How long must I stay in the hospital after brain surgery?

You will probably be in the hospital for about two weeks after a major brain operation.

Will there be any aftereffects of the brain surgery?

It depends upon your condition before your surgery and what the outcome of the surgery is. Many people who have had brain surgery live normal lives. Usually the doctor will be able to tell you before the operation if you will have any defects after the operation—such as poor vision, hearing loss, difficulty in speaking, or problems with arms or legs. The operation itself usually does not cause the problems—usually the problems are there before the operation. Many times, physical therapy will be recommended by the doctor especially to strengthen your arms and legs if they have been affected by your tumor. Many patients have learned to speak again if their speaking had been affected by the tumor.

Is radiation used in treating brain tumors?

Usually the surgeon will take out only as much of the tumor as is possible without damaging normal nerve tissue. The remaining tumor cells are often treated by radiation therapy. In many cases, radiation can stop the tumor from growing any further.

Will my head hurt as a result of the radiation treatments?

Your head itself probably won't hurt, but the skin may become sensitive, and it might be a good idea for you to plan on clothes and pajamas which button down the front or back so you won't have to worry about pulling things over your head.

Is chemotherapy ever used in treating brain tumors?

Chemotherapy in treating brain tumors is still in the experimental stages. However, since brain cells do not multiply, they are less susceptible to some of the chemotherapeutic drugs than are the fast-growing tumor cells. Among the drugs which have been used on an experimental basis are methotrexate carmustine, lomustine, and vincristrine. Relatively little information is available currently on the penetration of drugs into the central nervous system or into tumors of the brain.

What is meant by the blood-brain barrier?

The brain has a special mechanism, called the blood-brain barrier, which keeps substances which might be harmful to it from getting from the blood into the central-nervous-system tissue. Consequently, some chemotherapeutic drugs are not effective in treating brain tumors because they cannot penetrate the blood-brain barrier.

What is the Association for Brain Tumor Research?

The Association for Brain Tumor Research, also known as AFBTR, is a not-for-profit, tax-exempt, charitable organization which is working to raise funds to be used exclusively for brain-tumor research. It also publishes informational material. You can contact it by writing to Association for Brain Tumor Research, 6232 North Pulaski Road, Chicago, Ill. 60646; tel. 312-286-5571.

What is pituitary adenoma?

Pituitary adenoma is a tumor of the pituitary gland. It occurs in young or middle-aged adults.

What is the pituitary gland?

The pituitary gland is a small gland about the size of a pea which is at the base of the brain just above the back of the nose. It secretes several hormones and influences many distant parts of the body. This gland is sometimes called the master gland because it influences body growth, metabolism, and other functions.

Is the pituitary gland ever removed?

The pituitary gland can be removed, and treatment for a tumor of this site is usually surgery and radiation. The pituitary gland is normally related to brain cancer and its removal in that instance involves a craniotomy, which means the opening of the skull and pushing the brain aside to reach the gland.

Is the pituitary gland connected with breast and prostate cancer?

Some doctors are taking out the pituitary gland in breast-cancer patients and patients with prostate cancer because they believe that this eliminates various hormones that tend to support the growth of breast and prostate cancer. There is a new process in doing the operation for this purpose. Instead of a craniotomy the surgeon goes through the upper gum and the nasal passage into the pituitary chamber below the brain. This operation is called a transsphenoidal hypophysectomy.

chapter 20

Childhood Cancer

Acute lymphocytic leukemia (ALL)
- Complete blood count
- Bone-marrow aspiration
- Biopsy

Osteogenic sarcoma (bone tumor or Ewing sarcoma)
- X-rays
- Urinalysis
- Intravenous pyelogram
- Biopsy

Retinoblastoma
- Eye examinations
- X-rays
- CT scans

Wilms tumor
- Chest x-ray
- Complete blood count
- Urinalysis
- Intravenous pyelogram (IVP)
- Bone-marrow tests
- Liver and bone scans

Rhabdomyosarcoma

- X-ray
- Angiogram
- Intravenous pyelogram (IVP)
- Cystoscopy
- Brain scan
- Biopsy

What kind of doctor should be treating my child?

Ideally, an oncological pediatrician should be responsible for the primary treatment of your child. Your own pediatrician or surgeon will usually refer you to an oncologist, who may suggest that you take your child to one of the major medical centers for treatment. If you decide to use one of these, you could find total patient care; all the disciplines, including medical and other subspecialties, nursing, and social service, are orchestrated and individualized for the patient. However, the nineteen comprehensive cancer centers now supply extensive information services to the local medical community, and specialists from many of the centers work with local physicians in planning treatment. New treatment methods require teamwork among radiologists, surgeons, medical oncologists, pediatric oncologists, physiotherapists, nurses, and social workers.

Questions to Ask the Doctor

- What kind of cancer does my child have?
- Has the diagnosis been checked with another pathologist?
- What kind of treatment are you advising?
- Will I be able to get these treatments locally?
- Will my child be receiving treatment following one of the new protocols?
- Will my child be part of a clinical study?
- Is it advisable to go to an out-of-town hospital for treatment?
- If no, why not?
- Does the hospital have provisions for living facilities for the parents while the child is undergoing his hospital treatment?
- How long do you think the child will be hospitalized?
- Have you treated other children with this type of cancer?
- How many?

Childhood Cancer

TYPE	AGE	SYMPTOMS	TREATMENT
Acute lymphocytic leukemia (ALL)	Highest incidence under 6; boys more often than girls	Tired, pale, listless, swollen glands, easily bruised, infections that persist despite antibiotics	Chemotherapy, chemotherapy with radiotherapy. New drugs and combined treatments have extended lives and the picture becomes more hopeful each year.
Osteogenic sarcoma (bone tumors or Ewing sarcoma)	Teenage	Swelling or pain in lower leg or forearm	Surgery combined with radiation and chemotherapy are bringing good results in 60 percent of all cases.
Neuroblastoma		Swelling—abdomen, chest, or eye	Surgery and drugs used. Chances of recovery excellent in early stages.
Brain tumors		Blurred or double vision, dizziness, difficulty in walking, unexplained nausea	Surgery, or radiation, or chemotherapy. Many are curable if diagnosed early.
Lymphomas (Hodgkin and non-Hodgkin)	11 up	Swelling of lymph nodes in neck, armpit, groin; weakness, fever	Surgery, radiation, chemotherapy. Picture improving every year. See Chapter 14.
Retinoblastoma (eye tumors)	Under 4	Squint, widening of pupil of eye, cat's-eye reflex	Surgery or radiation, sometimes with chemotherapy, can cure 85 percent of cases.

Childhood Cancer (continued)

Type	Age	Symptoms	Treatment
Wilms tumor (cancer of kidney or nephroblastoma)	Under 7	Swelling or lump in abdomen	Surgery combined with radiation and chemotherapy; 80 percent of all patients are being cured.
Rhabdomyosarcoma	2-6	Swelling, bleeding, unusual mass — found in head, neck, eyes, genitourinary system, extremities, chest, and abdomen	Surgery, followed by chemotherapy and radiotherapy. High cure rate in early stages.

Is the National Cancer Institute supporting studies on childhood cancer?

A great many studies are under way by the National Cancer Institute's clinical cooperative groups, with oncologists, surgeons, pathologists, and radiologists participating. Included are leukemia, Wilms tumor, neuroblastoma, rhabdomyosarcoma, Ewing sarcoma, and other pediatric solid tumors. In Chapter 23 you will find the name of the chairman of each clinical cooperative group and the phone number for contact. The address listed is not an indication of where these groups are located. It is simply the information center for the specific type of study group. Your doctor or you may contact that person for information on what clinical trials are available in your area. You can get further information by calling the Cancer Information Service 800 number for your area listed in Chapter 23.

How common is childhood cancer?

Cancer is actually quite rare in children. Only 1 percent of all cancers appear in children. However, it is second only to accidents as a cause of death in children aged 3 to 14. Nearly half of the children with cancer are under the age of 5.

Are most tumors found in children cancerous?

No. Most tumors found in children are benign.

Is leukemia the most common childhood cancer?

Yes. Leukemia is the most frequent type of cancer found in children. Among the leukemias, acute lymphocytic leukemia, known by the abbreviation ALL, is the most common. Once fatal in 99 percent of cases, the outlook is now bright, thanks to research in the last decade.

Is cancer fatal to most children?

No. Many adults—and many physicians in practice today—were taught that most cancers in children were incurable. In the last ten years medical researchers have completely reversed this formerly hopeless prognosis. The enlightening news is that in some of the centers which specialize in childhood cancers, more than half of the children treated since the late 1960s have apparently been cured—and the cure rates are even higher among those presently being treated with the new drugs and combined treatments.

Are children ever born with cancer?

Yes. Wilms tumor is a form of congenital cancer. If detected early during infancy, Wilms tumor can be removed and the child can grow to be a healthy adult.

If my child's leukemia had been diagnosed earlier would there be a better chance for a cure?

Most parents blame themselves or others for any delay in making their child's diagnosis. They feel that if the child had received treatment sooner, he might have been cured or the severity of the disease lessened. This is not so. The long-term response to therapy in childhood leukemia is not significantly affected by how early the disease is diagnosed. Of course, once the diagnosis is confirmed, therapy should be started as soon as possible.

Is leukemia contagious?

Leukemia is not contagious. Other children cannot "catch" leukemia from an affected child. Therefore, children with leukemia can continue to live at home, attend school, and play with their friends.

What causes leukemia?

At the present time, the cause of leukemia is unknown. It does not seem to be related to a child's past health, dietary history, or any of the other factors which appear to affect the onset and course of some other diseases. It is known that persons exposed to near-lethal doses of radiation at the atomic blasts at Hiroshima and Nagasaki developed leukemia. Researchers have also proved that some types of leukemia in animals are caused by virus. However, there is no proven association with viruses in humans. ALL occurs more frequently among children with Down's syndrome (mongolism). It has been found that if an identical (not fraternal) twin is diagnosed with ALL, in 20 percent of cases, the other twin will also develop the disease.

What types of leukemia are usually found in children?

The most common type, accounting for 45 percent of all childhood leukemia, is acute lymphocytic leukemia, known as ALL for the initials of its name. This chapter will be discussing that type of leukemia. It is most likely to occur in children below the age of 6. More information about the other types of leukemia can be found in Chapter 14.

What are the symptoms of childhood leukemia (ALL)?

Early symptoms often appear gradually and include: fatigue, weakness, pallor, low-grade temperature, bleeding gums, frequent nosebleeds, bone or joint pain, enlargement of lymph nodes, liver, or spleen, pinpoint-sized red or deep-purple spots on the skin and/or infection that does not respond well to antibiotics and persists.

What is acute lymphocytic leukemia (ALL)?

This is the most common type of childhood leukemia. Leukemia begins when the bone marrow manufactures an overabundance of abnormal lymphocytic cells that are unable to mature or to function. These abnormal blood cells, called lymphoblasts (commonly referred to as "blasts"), crowd out normal bone-marrow cells. These blasts may leave the marrow, circulate in the bloodstream, and end up in the liver, spleen, lymph nodes, and around the brain. The leukemic cells crowd the bone marrow so that it can no longer produce enough normal cells.

What is the usual treatment for acute lymphocytic leukemia (ALL)?

The child must first be hospitalized. Intensive chemotherapy is usually the preferred treatment. Chemotherapy with radiotherapy is also being used.

Why are the first six months of treatment considered to be the most difficult?

The first six months following diagnosis are a time of intense medical treatment. At the same time, the patient and the family are faced with the emotional crisis of learning to live with leukemia. The outcome is unknown and the whole family must accept and adjust to the many things that must be learned about the disease and its treatment.

What can I expect to happen during the initial treatment period?

This is a very critical time. Treatment, of course, varies with the severity of the symptoms, the treatment plan, the doctor, and the hospital. Generally, however, the child is anemic, susceptible to infections, and often at risk of bleeding. Various supportive measures may be necessary, including the use of blood transfusions to correct the anemia, platelet transfusions to prevent or treat bleeding, antibiotics and, rarely, white-blood-cell transfusions to cope with infections. Once the disease is in remission, these supportive measures will no longer be required.

What happens once remission takes place?

Though there is no single way to treat leukemia, once remission takes place, routine therapy makes life easier for the patient and his family. Radiation treatments are sometimes given daily for several weeks after the child is released from the hospital. Sometimes brain and spinal-cord therapy—in the form of radiation and drugs given through a lumbar puncture—are prescribed as a preventive measure because leukemia can affect the brain and spinal cord. The lumbar puncture, though it sounds traumatic, is similar to a routine blood or bone-marrow test. Routine treatment, with blood tests each week, chemotherapy on a routine basis, bone-marrow tests every few months, and lumbar punctures every four or five months will then continue for several years.

What is a complete remission?

A complete remission means that the bone marrow, blood count, physical examination, and general well-being of the child are all within normal limits. In acute lymphatic leukemia, complete remission usually takes about four weeks and is achieved in about 90 percent of all cases.

How long does a remission last?

Times vary. At least 50 percent of all children with acute lymphatic leukemia should be in remission for at least five years. Many have had remissions that have lasted ten years or more. The chances of a relapse after ten years are considered rare. However, some remissions last a much shorter period of time. When a patient is no longer in remission, he is said to have had a relapse.

What is a relapse?

Relapse occurs when leukemic cells reappear in the bone marrow, blood, central nervous system, or any other site. The symptoms of relapse are usually similar to those at the time the disease was first diagnosed.

Can the same treatment be used to achieve another remission?

With the currently available therapy, children who relapse can usually be reinduced into remission. However, third and subsequent relapses are more difficult to control because the cells become resistant to the chemotherapy.

Is it true that the faster the response to remission-inducing therapy, the more favorable the chances of a long remission?

According to one of the study groups in children's cancer, patients who responded to remission-inducing therapy by the 14th day of treatment had a better prospect of lengthy remission than those whose induction took longer.

What are the chances for a relapse if a child has been in remission for five years?

According to the director of the Sidney Farber Cancer Institute, if a child with acute lymphocytic leukemia remains in complete remission with no relapse for five years, there is only roughly one chance in ten that a relapse will occur in years five to ten. After ten disease-free years, relapse is almost nonexistent.

What kind of reactions can I expect my child to have from the various drugs he will be taking?

These will all be carefully outlined for you by the doctor and nurse when they review the treatment your child will be receiving. However, you should be sure to check Chapter 8 to refresh your memory.

How long does the usual leukemia treatment last?

The chemotherapy treatments usually last for about three years. Usually, the child misses a month or so of school at the start, during which time the disease is brought under control.

Do all cases of leukemia progress in the same way?

No two cases are alike—and exact predictions are impossible to make. Much depends on the type of leukemia, the treatment given, and the way in which the individual body reacts to treatment.

How can I be assured that the latest treatment methods are being used on my child?

To maximize the chance of cure, the first treatment your child receives must be the best available to totally eradicate his leukemia. The cancer centers and major medical institutions have teams that specialize in treating cancer in children.

What does it mean when the doctor talks about "lymphoma presenting as leukemia"?

Sometimes, even if the diagnosis is leukemia, the child responds poorly to the standard leukemia therapy and the doctor finds that using the treatment usually prescribed for lymphoma patients is more successful than treatment with the less intensive leukemia regimens.

Is it dangerous to a child with leukemia to be exposed to chickenpox?

Yes it is. The doctor should be informed immediately if the child has been exposed. ZIG (zoster immune globulin) or ZIP (zoster immune plasma) are "anti-chickenpox vaccines" which can be used to reduce the chances of catching chickenpox. In order to be effective, ZIG or ZIP must be administered within 72 hours after your child has been exposed to chickenpox.

Is it dangerous for my leukemic child to be vaccinated?

Your child should not receive live-virus medicine—such as that used in smallpox and measle vaccinations. Always check with the doctor before allowing any such procedures on your leukemic child.

I've heard a lot about St. Jude Hospital in connection with leukemia. Can you tell me something about it?

St. Jude Hospital was founded by entertainer Danny Thomas. It is a research center to which patients are admitted only by physician referral, and only if their disease is under study. Research studies are underway in the various forms of childhood cancers as well as in severe infectious diseases and malnutrition.

Where can I turn for information about leukemia and how to handle telling my child, dealing with his siblings, and dealing with his disease?

Fortunately, there is a great deal of help available, on many different levels. An unusual amount of helpful, well written literature is available from the National Cancer Institute, the American Cancer Society, and the U.S. Department of Health, Education and Welfare. In some states, the local crippled children associations also offer information and assistance. You can call the 800 number of the Cancer Information Service nearest you and ask any questions you may have and request that they send a supply of all the literature they have available. A book available from W.B. Saunders Co., West Washington Square, Philadelphia, Pa. 19105, ($7.95) entitled *You and Leukemia, a Day at a Time*, by Dr. Lynn S. Baker, is an excellent handbook on childhood leukemia which will provide both children and parents with many insights into the disease and its management. The American Cancer Society publishes a booklet, *Parents' Handbook on Leukemia*, which is a free, useful guide. The Candlelighters is an organization formed to help families cope with living with the disease. For information on the local chapter nearest you, write: Candlelighters, 123 C Street, S.E., Washington, D.C. 20003.

What is Ewing sarcoma?

This tumor occurs in children and young adults and may involve almost any part of the skeleton. It differs from other bone tumors in that it often attacks the shafts, rather than the ends, of the long bones. It is known to metastasize to the lungs and apparently to other bones. Pain, and later swelling, are the initial symptoms.

How is Ewing sarcoma diagnosed?

X-rays are helpful, but diagnosis must be confirmed by biopsy.

What treatment is used for patients with Ewing sarcoma?

The newest treatments use a combination of chemotherapy and radiation. This treatment has changed the statistics in the survival rate of children diagnosed with this disease. It was formerly fatal in more than 90 percent of cases, but today more than half of the children with localized Ewing sarcoma are being saved.

What is osteogenic sarcoma?

This is one of the most common malignant bone tumors. It occurs most often in young persons, many only in their teens. It can occur in the long bones, flat bones, pelvis, and spine. The normal bone is destroyed and replaced by tumor cells. Metastases occur by way of the veins and usually first involve the lungs. The first symptom of osteogenic sarcoma is usually pain, followed by swelling.

How is osteogenic sarcoma diagnosed?

X-rays usually are taken, but final diagnosis is dependent upon biposy.

What treatment is usually used for osteogenic sarcoma?

Amputation, usually through or above the next joint, presently offers the only hope for cure. The tumors do not respond to radiology. Until a few years ago, osteogenic sarcoma was fatal in 80 percent of patients within two years of diagnosis. Powerful chemotherapy treatment following surgery has reversed the percentage so that 60 percent of children are now alive two years after diagnosis, with final results unknown because this treatment has been used only for that length of time.

What is parosteal sarcoma?

This is a less malignant form of bone cancer which involves the surface but not the interior of the bone. This type can often be cured by removing the affected section of bone, or by amputation. In children who have reached puberty, alternatives to amputation (such as bone-replacement grafts) are being investigated in major cancer centers.

What should a child with bone cancer who requires an amputation be told?

It is important to prepare the child ahead of time—and to be very honest. Usually, the surgeon will get to know the child during the workup and will explain exactly what will be done. It is possible, often, for the prosthesis to be applied in the operating room, allowing the surgeon to be able to assure the child that he will be able to use the limb within two or three days.

Are some tumors of the bone not really bone tumors at all?

That is correct. Malignant tumors in other parts of the body sometimes metastasize to the bone. In some cases, the metastases are discovered before the primary tumor is discovered. A biopsy can often give a clue as to the source of the metastasis.

What is neuroblastoma?

This is a cancer of the central nervous system, which is the second most common children's cancer—after leukemia. It is usually found in certain nerve fibers of the body—most commonly in the adrenal gland, abdomen, chest, or eye. It is a disease of infants and young children. More than 75 percent of all cases are diagnosed in children under 3 years of age. More males than females are found to have neuroblastoma. The older the child, the more difficult it is to treat. Neuroblastomas sometimes regress spontaneously and sometimes will revert to a benign state.

What treatment is usually used in neuroblastoma?

If the entire tumor can be removed, surgery is recommended. Radiotherapy is sometimes used, but the doctor must carefully evaluate the use of radiotherapy if it involves radiation to the growth centers of bones and soft tissues. Newest studies show that chemotherapy plus immunotherapy can achieve longer remissions, especially in older children with neuroblastoma.

Are brain tumors often found in children?

Brain tumors account for 12 to 15 percent of childhood cancers. There are a great variety of brain tumors, affecting many different parts of the brain.

What symptoms signal a brain tumor?

Brain tumors are very difficult to diagnose in young children. Symptoms vary a great deal, depending on the location of the tumor. If the tumor is located in a part of the brain that is not near a vital nerve center, it may grow quite large without producing any signs. However, disturbances such as blurred vision, complaints of "seeing double," peripheral-vision problems, changes in muscular coordination, unexplained vomiting, changes in personality, sudden drowsiness, momentary loss of consciousness, convulsions, and persistent headaches are all signs that should not be ignored. Though these signs can be caused by many conditions totally unrelated to brain tumors, the appearance of many of them suggests the need for investigation.

What kinds of tests can be done to detect brain tumors?

Careful studies must be made before any steps are taken. Complete neurologic examination, testing of vision and hearing, electroencephalography, brain scans, and x-rays of skull and chest (to rule out involvement in other parts of the body) must all be completed before any conclusions are reached.

How are brain tumors treated?

Once the tumor has been pinpointed, a decision will be made about whether it can be removed safely with surgery. Sometimes surgery is followed with radiation therapy, or radiation may be used alone. Some tumors are treated with radiation and chemotherapy. Many brain tumors are responsive to treatment and when discovered early are quite curable. (More information on brain tumors can be found in Chapter 19.)

What is retinoblastoma?

This is an eye cancer which affects young children under the age of 4. Usually, the family will notice a change in the appearance of the pupil of one eye, making the size of the two pupils look uneven. The widening of the pupil allows a peculiar white reflection to shine through the pupil of the eye, which is actually the tumor itself. There may also be pain, redness, and vision loss. If allowed to advance, swelling will occur, closing the eye. In one out of every four or five cases, retinoblastoma can affect both eyes.

Does retinoblastoma run in families?

Because so little is known of the genetics of most types of cancer, it is still unknown precisely how the disease is transmitted, but retinoblastoma seems to have a hereditary factor. The fact that multiple cases are found in some families suggests that some cases are due to a dominant gene. However, this occurs in only about 20 percent of all cases. Young children in families where the disease has occurred should be watched carefully and examined frequently for early signs.

Is vision usually lost in patients with retinoblastoma?

No. Even in patients where the disease is quite advanced, partial vision can often be saved. Where discovered early, vision is preserved in 95 percent of cases.

How is retinoblastoma treated?

When discovered in the early stages, radiotherapy is usually the treatment. In more advanced cases—and many cases are far advanced when discovered—surgery or radiotherapy, sometimes in combination with chemotherapy, is the method used. When both eyes are affected, surgery is usually performed on the most severely involved eye and radiation is used on the other in an effort to preserve the greatest amount of sight.

What is Wilms tumor?

Wilms tumor, which is a cancerous tumor, is usually found in children 1 year of age and older. Peak incidence occurs at about 3 years of age. The tumor is uncommon after 8 years of age. More boys than girls are found to have Wilms tumor. Wilms tumor is sometimes referred to as nephroblastoma or cancer of the kidney.

What are the symptoms of Wilms tumor?

In the majority of children, an abdominal mass is discovered by the parents. Symptoms can also include abdominal pain, nausea, vomiting, diarrhea, fever, and blood in the urine.

Do these young children still have to go through all the testing as an adult would before surgery is performed?

Yes. It is important that the disease be properly evaluated before surgery. Therefore, diagnosis for Wilms tumor would probably include a chest x-ray, intravenous pyelogram, liver and bone scans, complete blood count, urinalysis, and bone-marrow examination. These tests are usually done in the hospital prior to surgery.

What is the treatment for Wilms tumor?

Usually surgery is followed by radiotherapy and chemotherapy. Radiotherapy is sometimes used prior to surgery to reduce the size of the tumor if it is very large.

Is there a good chance a child with Wilms tumor can live a normal life?

The outlook for Wilms tumor has changed completely in the last 40 years. Previously considered a fatal disease, today approximately 80–90 percent of children can be cured. If the child remains disease-free for two years following surgery and treatments, he will be considered cured.

What is rhabdomyosarcoma?

This is the most common soft-tissue cancer among children—usually found in the head, neck, eyes, genitourinary area, extremities, chest, and abdominal cavity. It occurs most frequently between the ages of 2 and 6. Symptoms depend upon where the tumor is located—a swelling in the eye, a bloody nasal discharge, a mass in an extremity—grapelike clusters protruding from the vagina, vaginal bleeding, or obstruction of the urinary outlet.

How is rhabdomyosarcoma treated?

Treatment depends upon where the tumor is located and the cell type. Since this cancer is highly malignant, the stage at which it is found is an important factor. Metastases occur early and often spread to distant organs, generally the lung. Biopsy is usually performed to establish the diagnosis.

Are there any new studies being done on rhabdomyosarcoma?

Yes—and they are encouraging, especially for patients with localized nonmetastatic rhabdomyosarcoma. Children with localized rhabdomyosarcoma are potentially curable with intensive chemotherapy and radiotherapy following surgery. The results are much less encouraging if the disease has spread. For information on National Cancer Institute studies see Chapter 23.

Should I tell my child he has cancer?

Openness and honesty are usually the best course to follow— naturally depending upon the age and understanding of the child. The toddler can be told that he is sick and needs to take his medicine to get better. Older children need to know that cancer is a serious but treatable illness. Many of them have the impression from watching television that everyone who has cancer or leukemia dies. They need reassurance that there are successful treatments, that new treatments are being used with very hopeful results. Try not to avoid the subject because you are afraid of saying something wrong. Painful and awkward though you may feel, it is better to deal with the question honestly and to keep communication open between you and the child.

My child gets angry over the inconveniences that the treatments impose. How do I handle his anger?

Anger is a very normal reaction—and you should allow the child to vent some of it. Let him know you share his concerns but that the treatment is necessary for him to be able to lead a normal life.

Should the other children in the family be told when a brother or sister has cancer?

It really is best to do this right at the start. Children are concerned and worried and need to be included and reassured. The age of the child dictates how much needs to be told. A 3- or 4-year old can be told that his brother is sick and needs to go to the hospital and will be taking medicine for a long time. Young children often feel guilty when another member of the family becomes sick and need to be reassured that they are not responsible. Children also worry that they might come down with the same illness. Being aware of these fears and understanding that the special attention the sibling is receiving does not detract from their own specialness will help keep them from becoming resentful about the time you must spend with the sick child. Let them know that anger and guilt feelings are normal and that you understand.

Where can I get more information about childhood cancers?

The Cancer Information Service in your area (listed in Chapter 23) will be able to give you information about the specific disease which has been diagnosed. The volunteers or staff can tell you what hospitals in your local area are participating in the latest treatments. They can also send you a supply of the latest booklets that are available. Some wonderfully helpful and sensitive material has been written by parents who have cared for their children at home to the end. One of the most informative and most poignant, *Coping at Home with Cancer, for Parents, by a Parent*, by Nina Cottrell, may be purchased from Children's Hospital of St. Paul, 311 Pleasant Avenue, St. Paul, Minn. 55102.

Is financial help available for children with cancer?

Some help is available through the American Cancer Society, the Leukemia Society of America, and in some states, through the local associations for crippled children. The Leukemia Society will often help in paying costs of anti-leukemic drugs, transportation to and from treatment centers, and costs of typing and cross-matching of blood, and in some states provides aid to families whose medical costs in the course of a year have gone beyond $20,000.

chapter 21

Coping With Pain

Treatments for Pain

TREATMENT	WHAT IS DONE	COMMENTS
Drugs	Pain medication is given either orally or by injection.	Doctor usually starts with mild drug and moves to stronger medication, (tranquilizers, anti-depressants, and narcotics) depending upon severity of pain. Brompton mixture often used. Continuous medication seems better than medication given only when need arises.
Nerve blocks	Anesthesia or alcohol is injected at a point in the nerve to deaden the nerve fibers.	Local nerve blocks give temporary relief. Sometimes used in combination with steroids. Nerve blocks with alcohol injected into or around spinal cord deaden nerves for longer period of time.
Cordotomy	Precise area in the spinal cord where bundles of nerves are located is cut.	Surgeon must be careful not to destroy nerve fibers that control muscle movement.

Treatments for Pain (continued)

TREATMENT	WHAT IS DONE	COMMENTS
Percutaneous cordotomy	Electric current is used to destroy nerve fiber.	Can be performed on awake patient, has low mortality, can be repeated as required.
Nerve-root clipping	Nerve roots clipped high in neck.	Used for pain problems in upper part of body.
Rhizotomy	Pain nerve is cut where it enters spinal cord.	Dangerous because it can leave organs or limbs useless.
Transcutaneous nerve stimulation	Electrical impulses are sent through pads applied to the skin in the affected area.	Pain is relieved for period longer than application time.
Epidural dorsal column stimulator	Electrodes are surgically implanted over spinal cord. Patient controls electrical impulses.	Needs surgery to implant electrodes.
Acupuncture	Thin needles are put into body at key points.	Opinion of effectiveness varies.
Hypnosis	Person is put in state of intense concentration.	No one knows how hypnosis works to control real pain. Opinion of treatment varies.
Biofeedback	Patient learns how to control inner functions of body through mind control and electronic survey.	Usually used in combination with another method. Opinion of effectiveness varies.

Is it true that most cancer patients do not experience any pain?

That is true. Most people think of cancer as a painful disease. The truth is that most cancers cause no pain in their early stages. Therefore, the people whose cancers are treated early usually have only the pain or discomfort which is part of any operation or treatment. This pain is temporary. It can be easily tolerated and can be controlled with medicine, if necessary.

Is pain more of a problem with advanced cancers?

Yes, pain occurs more often in people with advanced cancers. But even among people with advanced disease, more than half have little or no pain or discomfort. Some of the advanced patients require some light medication. For those who experience severe pain, there are several modern methods of pain relief which can be prescribed.

Is cancer pain different from pain of other illnesses?

Some recent studies seem to indicate that cancer pain has different characteristics, since it may be both severe and of long duration. And since it is a reminder of the disease, the pain of cancer patients is thought to have psychological consequences.

Do some people feel more pain than others?

Some people's nervous systems are naturally more sensitive to pain than others. It depends upon a person's general makeup and how much pain he can take (called tolerance or threshold). The pain also depends upon the type of cancer and whether or not it is located in a place in the body where the nerves are especially sensitive.

Can worry, unhappiness, or fear cause pain?

Studies have shown that fear, worry, or unhappiness can make pain more intense. It doesn't mean that pain is not there physically, it means that if you can take some positive steps to keep yourself from worrying about it, it can be lessened and more easily tolerated.

Are there any cancer patients who do not suffer pain in their terminal illness?

Yes, there are some cancer patients who have little or no pain even in the terminal stages.

Can pulse and blood pressure indicate how much pain a person is in?

No. Pulse and blood pressure are not reliable measures of the amount of pain a person is experiencing.

What are the main causes of pain for advanced-cancer patients?

There are several main causes of pain for people who have cancer:

- A nerve which is being compressed or destroyed
- Some organ or tube in the body which is blocked
- Swollen blood vessels which are pressing on nearby nerves
- Cancer cells which have spread to the bone and are causing pressure
- Emotional responses to the disease (both guilt and anxiety can cause and intensify pain)

What kinds of things should I tell my doctor about my pain?

You need to be as specific as you can when you are describing pain to your doctor. Try to tell him:

- How long your pain lasts, and what time of the day it comes. Does it come and go every few minutes? Every hour? Does it appear every morning for a half hour? In the afternoon?
- How much it hurts. More than the last time you saw him? How much more? Try to be as specific as possible.
- Where the pain is. It is best to show the doctor rather than tell him. Point to the place with your finger.
- Whether or not the pain moves and whether it is continuous.
- Relationship to events. Does it come after your treatment? After you have eaten? When you have visitors?

Who decides on which method of pain management should be used?

The doctors (oncologist, radiologist, neurosurgeon, chemotherapist) and the patient are the main decision-makers although sometimes social workers, nurses, the clergy, and the family are also involved. In deciding which method is best, one must look at the site and type of the cancer, the general health of the patient, where the pain is, the type and how severe it is, the life expectancy of the patient, the temperament and psychological state of the patient, the occupational, domestic and economic background of the patient, and the availability and practicality of the various methods of pain relief. The management of pain is a complex problem.

What can be done about the pain of cancer patients?

There are two main avenues to take in trying to manage the pain of the cancer patient. The first is to remove the cause of the pain. This is done by using palliative operations, radiation therapy, sex hormones, or chemotherapy drugs or other substances to decrease the size of the tumors or to completely eliminate them. The second way is to control the pain by drugs, neurosurgical operations, nerve blocks, or psychologic techniques such as hypnosis, biofeedback, or acupuncture. The first methods are described in the chapters on each subject. We will concentrate on the other means of relieving pain in this chapter.

What kinds of drugs are usually prescribed as painkillers for cancer patients?

It varies greatly depending upon the kind of cancer, the patient, the doctor, and the type of pain. Usually the doctor will start with the usual kinds of pain medications such as aspirin or Tylenol, Darvon, or aspirin combined with codeine. Low doses of major tranquilizers and antidepressants can be used. The doctor can order these in increasing doses to the maximum and then go on to stronger narcotics. Methadone and morphine are usually used to control severe pain.

Is it true that in England, stronger medications, including heroin, are being used to treat the pain of cancer patients?

There has been much work done in England in the area of controlling physical pain for cancer patients. The leader in the field is St. Christopher's Hospice in England, which in the past has included heroin in its pain treatments. St. Christopher's Hospice was founded by Dr. Cicely Saunders in 1967 as a research, treatment, and teaching facility devoted to meeting the needs of the dying and the long-term sick. One of its aims is the control of physical pain. Dr. Saunders believes that patients who have constant pain need constant control. The drugs are given to the patient regularly rather than when the need arises.

What is the benefit of prescribing pain medicine regularly rather than only when the need arises? Won't that lead to addiction?

Dr. Saunders has found that by prescribing the medicine

regularly the patient is reassured. He will not have to worry about when he will feel the pain next and how long it will take the medicine to work again. It has been found that fear and anxiety help to intensify pain. The medication is not given as needed (PRN) but instead is given before it is needed to prevent pain and fear of pain as well as to prevent feelings of dependency in patients who have to ask for relief. Some doctors using this method in the United States have found that less of the narcotic substance is required when medicine is given in this manner than if the patient has to ask for it.

What is Brompton cocktail?

Brompton cocktail, or Brompton mixture as it is also called, is a mixture of drugs in liquid form (varying doses of morphine, heroin, cocaine, alcohol, syrup, and chloroform water) which was first used at St. Christopher's Hospice to treat pain in cancer patients. The physicians at this hospital use the medication regularly, increase the doses of the narcotic as necessary to overcome the body's tolerance to it, and carefully adjust the dose to the needs of the patient. St. Christopher's claims that this medication has relieved pain in 95 percent of its patients.

Is Brompton mixture being used in the United States?

Mixtures similar to Brompton cocktail with methadone or morphine (instead of heroin) are being used in many places in the United States. The dosages are carefully worked out with the patient so that the drugs are given before the pain begins. Brompton mixture is usually used in conjunction with other kinds of pain-control treatments.

Are there any side effects from Brompton mixture?

The side effects from the Brompton mixture can be similar to side effects from any narcotic drug, including lowering of activity, sleepiness, and grogginess; nausea and vomiting (an antinausea drug is usually given along with the mixture); and constipation.

If the patient is always on pain medicine, isn't he groggy?

No. The doctors using this method aim to have the patients free from pain but also alert. The medicine is usually taken in liquid or pill form so that the patient can be independent.

Doesn't the patient get addicted to the drugs?

The doctors using this method find that the patient's need for pain-control drugs disappears when the pain goes away. They have found that when the dosage has to be increased it is due to additional pain rather than to addiction to the drug. They feel that the possibility of drug addiction in terminally ill patients or those with chronic pain should not be of major concern.

Why has Brompton mixture caught on as a pain-control method?

It is being used more often for several reasons. Unlike many other methods for controlling severe pain it can be taken by mouth. It seems to give the patient a balance between tolerable pain and some degree of mental alertness—apparently the cocaine counteracts the consciousness-depressing effects of the morphine.

Is it true that it takes longer for a drug to work if the pain is very severe?

Generally, that is true. If you wait too long for relief from pain the pain may become more severe and more difficult to take care of. It might take twice as much medicine to control the pain adequately. That is why it is important to ask for painkillers before the pain becomes too severe. You should also know that drugs vary as to how long it takes them to become effective.

Do drugs taken orally or drugs given by needle take longer to take effect?

Drugs taken orally generally take longer to work than those that are injected. Most injected drugs reach their peak in about an hour. The peak effect of oral drugs takes longer. On the other hand, oral drugs are effective for a longer time than injected drugs. It usually takes a smaller amount of an injected drug than an oral drug to give relief.

Does the same amount of drug give the same results for each patient?

Different people react differently to drugs. That is why it is important to tell the doctor and/or the nurse about your experience with the pain medication being given to you. They can give you a greater dose if the original dosage does not work for you, or cut the dosage if it is too strong. It is important not to change the dose yourself without telling the doctor and not to stop taking the drug without talking to someone on the medical team.

Is it true that heroin is being tested for pain relief in the United States?

There are presently some controlled studies being conducted on this subject under the auspices of the National Institute on Drug Abuse. Heroin is being compared with morphine and other substances in scientific studies for the management of pain in incurably ill patients. Since heroin is presently classified as a Schedule I drug under the 1970 Controlled Substance Act, which prohibits its general use for medical purposes, the institutions (Georgetown University's Vincent T. Lombardi Cancer Research Center and Sloane-Kettering Institute for Cancer Research) have been granted special exemptions for the clinical trials.

Are there any tests presently being conducted regarding the use of marijuana in pain control?

There are tests being conducted, but marijuana itself is not being used. The drug tetrahydrocannabinol (THC), which is the principal active substance in marijuana, is used. There is some evidence that marijuana can combat nausea and vomiting in patients receiving chemotherapy. The controlled trials are comparing THC with other antinausea drugs.

What kinds of procedures on nerves are used to control pain?

There are several procedures—surgical or injections of substances—which interrupt the nerve pathways and may be used effectively to control pain in patients. These procedures all try to do the same thing—interrupt the nerves that carry pain messages to the brain. The nerves can be interrupted anywhere between the brain and the cancer—along the nerve to the cancerous organ, in the nerve roots of the spinal cord, and within the spinal cord proper. The procedure of injecting substances into the nerve pathways is called a nerve block. The other procedures are all considered surgery.

How are nerve blocks used for pain control?

After medication, nerve blocks are the second most used method of cancer pain control. Chemicals that will destroy nerve fibers— such as anesthetic or alcohol—are injected at a point in the nerve. Local-anesthetic nerve blocks are usually only temporarily effective in relieving pain, but they can give several hours of relief. They break up the cycle and enable patients to have a few hours of sleep. Sometimes local nerve blocks are used in combination with steroid preparations to decrease the swelling of nerves which are trapped. At other times, nerve blocks are performed with alcohol injected into or around the spinal cord, which destroys nerves for long periods of time. In addition to the nerves leading to the spinal cord and upward to the brain, certain nerve centers called ganglia are located in various parts of the body. Sometimes pain can be relieved by injecting one of these ganglia with chemicals.

What kind of surgery can be performed for pain control?

There are several surgical procedures which can be used for pain control. They include cordotomy, percutaneous cordotomy, nerve-root clipping, and rhizotomy.

How are these operations usually performed?

The doctor first determines the location of the painful tumor. He then figures out which nerve carries the pain sensations from the area of the tumor to the spinal cord and from there to the brain. When he has found the correct nerve, he performs a delicate neurosurgical operation to destroy the pain-carrying nerve at some point along the path—either before or after it enters the spinal cord. Because the nerve has been cut, it cannot carry sensations to the brain. Therefore, the patient will not feel the pain.

What is a cordotomy?

A cordotomy cuts the precise areas in the spinal cord where bundles of nerves are located. The surgeon removes bone from the spinal column, making a hole in the bony back wall of the spinal-cord tunnel. The operation is performed either under local anesthesia (there will be some pain if it is done in this manner) or under general anesthesia. The surgeon must be careful to clip the pain-nerve bundles without destroying those nerve fibers that control muscle movements.

What is percutaneous cordotomy?

It is a technique for selectively destroying the nerve fibers. The doctor uses an x-ray for guidance. He inserts the tip of a hollow needle directly through the skin into the pain-nerve bundle along the front and side of the spinal cord. The nerve bundle is destroyed by an electric current passed through the needle. The operation is usually performed high in the back of the neck. Local anesthesia is used. Some of the advantages of the percutaneous cordotomy are that it can be performed while the patient is conscious, it has low mortality, and it can be repeated as required.

Does a person sometimes have to have more than one percutaneous cordotomy?

Sometimes, yes. It is not uncommon if the cordotomy was performed on one side to have the pain or the awareness of the pain move to the originally pain-free side. Apparently, the pain on the side where the cordotomy was performed was intense enough to mask pain on the original pain-free side. If this happens, a second cordotomy may be necessary.

Do I have to take any special precautions after having a cordotomy?

You will usually be up and around and able to eat anything you wish after one or two days. Some patients complain of headaches, but these are usually easily taken care of with mild medication. You must be careful because you will not feel pain or temperature on the side where the cordotomy has been done, so you should avoid doing things that might cause burns, scratches, and bruises.

What is rhizotomy?

In performing a rhizotomy the surgeon cuts the pain nerve where it enters the spinal cord. This procedure can eliminate pain, for example in the arm or leg, but it also leaves the arm or leg without sensation so that it is not usable. A rhizotomy can also be used to relieve abdominal and chest pain, but there may be loss of bladder and bowel control. Chemical rhizotomies are now being performed with alcohol or phenobarbital injected into the spaces around the spinal cord. This type of rhizotomy may relieve pain for a period of time without many of the unpleasant aftereffects of the surgical rhizotomy.

Under what circumstances would a physician use a nerve-root clipping operation?

Nerve-root clipping is usually done for pain problems in the upper part of the body. Nerve roots are clipped high in the neck. Individual head nerves—cranial nerves which lead out from openings in the skull bones—also can be clipped.

How are electrical signals used to relieve pain?

There are two devices which use painless electrical impulses to control pain—the transcutaneous nerve stimulator and the epidural dorsal-column stimulator. Both work on the theory that nerves can transmit only one sensation at a time and that there is a gate in the spinal cord through which messages are sent to the brain. If the nerves are stimulated artificially, pain impulses apparently cannot get through the gate.

What is transcutaneous nerve stimulation?

This method uses an electrical device in which pads are applied to the skin in the affected area. Electrical impulses are sent through from a small, battery-operated activating box. The impulses jam up incoming pain sensations so that pain is relieved, and the relief continues for a period after the application.

What is an epidural dorsal column stimulator?

This is another device for controlling pain by using electrical signals. In the epidural dorsal-column stimulator, electrodes are implanted surgically over the spinal cord. They are connected to receivers usually put on the patient's left side under his arm. When the person feels a small pain, he connects the antenna to a small transmitting box. This box is placed over the receiver and the patient turns on the transmitter. Electrical impulses are sent to the electrodes, which stimulate the nerves to relieve pain.

What other methods are used to control pain?

Acupuncture, biofeedback, and hypnosis are being used. There is a great deal of controversy regarding the use of these three methods in the cancer field. There is little scientific evidence that any of these three methods is valuable in long-term control. That is, there is little validation or proof that can convince the medical scientist that these methods actually work. On the other hand, the classic double-blind technique (when neither the investigator nor the patient knows what is being given) which has been successfully used in the drug field cannot be used with these since the techniques are such that both the patient and investigator know when they are being used. However, there are several places in the country where these techniques are being used in the treatment of pain in cancer patients. Studies are being done to prove the effectiveness of these pain treatments in the field of cancer.

How is acupuncture done?

A specialist in this method puts thin needles into the body at key points. The patient is given no painkiller and usually feels no pain from the insertion of the needles. Usually the treatments are given in a series—sometimes every day for a week or more. There are no side effects to this pain-treatment method.

What is hypnosis?

There is little agreement on what hypnosis is or why or how it accomplishes what it does. Hypnosis is usually defined as intensive concentration, a state in which the person is open to suggestions on which he will then or later act, often without realizing why. It is total concentration on a thought or object so that the person is out of touch with the world.

Has hypnosis ever been used to manage cancer pain?

Yes, in several places in the country, hypnosis is being used in an attempt to relieve cancer pain.

Are there any benefits to hypnosis over other kinds of pain management?

Hypnosis seems to offer many benefits and few drawbacks, mainly because hypnosis does not usually have any unpleasant side effects. Some doctors have found that hypnosis is so effective that patients are able to give up painkilling drugs.

How does hypnosis work on cancer pain?

It depends upon the techniques being used. Hypnosis has been used to block awareness of pain, to substitute another feeling for the pain, to move the pain to a smaller or less significant area of the body, to change the sensation to one that is not painful, and in extreme cases to dissociate the body from the awareness of the patient. Although no one knows exactly how hypnosis works to control real physical pain, there are cancer patients who feel they have been helped by this treatment.

Is hypnosis dangerous?

Hypnosis can be dangerous if it is not being done by a trained professional. A trained hypnotist will not usually attempt to remove pain unless the cause has been fully probed and definitely known, because hypnosis can also succeed in concealing real pain and thus concealing the underlying condition.

Can hypnosis be used with other remedies?

Sometimes it is used alone. In other cases it can be used in combination with other techniques, painkilling drugs, blocks, and biofeedback, for instance.

How many hypnosis sessions are necessary to work in the pain-control area?

Hypnotists maintain that it takes only a few sessions to teach a person to become hypnotized. Thereafter, the person can hypnotize himself when necessary. It is this self-hypnosis that is found to be most useful in pain control.

What is biofeedback?

Biofeedback is a system by which you can monitor the signals coming from the various organs of your body—heart, brain, muscles, stomach, etc. Using electronics, biofeedback tunes in on body functions and transposes them into a visible or audible signal that an individual can actually hear or see so he can be aware of what is going on in his own body. Biofeedback has been shown to be useful in slowing or speeding up heart rates, and in relaxing tense muscles. In learning how to relax muscles which produce tension headaches, for example, patients are hooked up to a machine which picks up the electrical current produced by a muscle when it contracts. The machine converts this signal to a tone which the patient can hear. The person can reduce the tone by relaxing the muscle. With practice he learns to relax his muscles and keep them relaxed and thus eliminates his headaches.

Is biofeedback being used for cancer patients?

It is not in widespread use. It is felt that it may be useful if the pain is caused by a bodily function which if brought under more direct control by the individual might at least partially reduce the factors causing the pain. Sometimes it is used if the patient cannot take other kinds of medications or use other pain-reducing techniques. Biofeedback has usually been used in combination with other methods. Certainly if the pain being suffered by the cancer patient is due to causes other than the cancer itself—such as tension headaches or hypertension—then biofeedback can be used to control this kind of pain. It can also be used to lessen tension which might be increasing the patient's pain.

I am a cancer patient and my doctor told me not to take aspirin for any reason, including pain. Why is this?

Aspirin is known to cause bleeding, particularly in patients with gastrointestinal problems. Therefore doctors usually prescribe another pain reliever, such as Tylenol or Datril, instead of aspirin.

I had radiation as part of my treatment. Can I use a heating pad for relieving pain?

No. Patients who have received radiotherapy should not apply heat (whether with a warm cloth or a heating pad) directly on the part of the body that was treated. Radiotherapy can lessen nerve activities and so the body becomes less sensitive to heat and the patient is more susceptible to burns.

When I get a pain, I worry about how long it is going to last. Am I unusual?

No, you certainly are not. It is common for people in pain to worry whether or not the pain will last. They also are concerned about what is causing it, whether or not it will get worse, and whether or not they will be able to stand it, all of which seems to help intensify the pain.

Is this whole subject of pain medication a new subject?

The subject itself is not new. Medications and treatments for pain have been in use since the practice of medicine first started. What is new is that the subject is now receiving much more attention and major studies of it are being undertaken. For example, the National Cancer Institute is supporting research programs concerned with pain control, with some investigators studying the nature of the pain and others investigating specific ways to cope with it. However, the study of cancer pain in the United States is still in the early stages, and most methods, especially those such as acupuncture and hypnosis, are considered highly experimental by the physicians. See Chapter 23.

Can relaxation exercises help?

Some people have found that passive relaxation exercises that can be done lying in bed can help relieve pain. Such simple devices as tensing up the muscles of the hands and then releasing them, doing the same thing with the muscles of the legs and feet, the back, the head and neck, etc., repeating until the body feels loose and relaxed, have been used by patients with success. Simple deep breathing also is a wonderful relaxant. Concentrate, with eyes closed, on inhaling and filling the lungs completely and deeply, then exhaling, slowly and fully. Do this in a rhythmic fashion. There are many methods of using exercise of this type to relax and relieve pain. Your local library is a good source for more information on this subject.

Are there any ordinary things which can be done to help a person in pain?

Since some people's pain is caused by anxiety, talking can be useful. Good mouth care, a back rub or massage, putting on clean bed linen, offering special foods, giving the person something else to think about (watching television, doing a crossword puzzle, needlework or model construction, reading a book), listening to music, talking to friends and relatives on the phone, applying compresses of warm heat to the affected areas—all these sometimes help.

When a person is in bed, little things like changing the angle of the bed, or sometimes just adding an extra pillow can make a lot of difference. If the person is not in bed, keeping busy is important. When we are busy we don't have as much time to dwell on our problems.

chapter 22

Living With Cancer

We have called this chapter "Living with Cancer" because it deals with many of the practical aspects as well as with the difficult emotions which are encountered in living with cancer on a day-to-day basis. It covers a wide range of information—some of it applies to all patients, some to only a few. The information on health insurance and wills should be of interest to the healthy as well as to those who are ill, since they are subjects best considered before the need arises. Since dying is a part of living, this chapter deals frankly with that subject and includes information on caring for the patient at home, euthanasia, the hospice movement, dying, death, and autopsies.

Types of Health Insurance

KIND OF POLICY	COVERAGE
Hospital	Covers costs during hospital stays as a result of illness or accident. Policies usually include payment in whole or part for room, drugs, general nursing, operating and recovery room, laboratory tests.
Surgical	Covers whole or partial cost of operation. Preset schedule of allowable fees.

Types of Health Insurance (continued)

KIND OF POLICY	COVERAGE
Medical	Covers doctor's services other than surgery, such as home, office, and hospital visits. Check to see if this covers diagnostic examinations and checkups.
Major medical	Covers major illness and accidents. Usually a deductible amount before payment starts. Covers hospital, surgical, drug, and medical. Usually there is a maximum amount. Some pay 75 to 80 percent of covered expenses.
Medicare, Plan A	Covers inpatient hospital care, skilled-nursing-facility care, part-time skilled nursing care at home. Not covered: prescription drugs.
Medicare, Plan B	Covers x-ray treatments, lab services, services of physician, emergency-room and clinic services, physical therapy, lab and diagnostic tests, x-ray, radiology, rental or purchase of medical equipment, ambulance services. Not covered: prescription drugs.

Things to Check Your Policy For

ITEM OR FEATURE	COMMENTS
Number of days of hospitalization	The very least should be 30 days. Many have special provisions for over 90 days.
Outpatient services	Check carefully, since vital cancer treatments such as chemotherapy and radiation are usually given on an outpatient basis.
In-hospital services	Check to see if nursing care, anesthesia, x-rays, laboratory tests, drugs, CT scans, etc., are covered.
Home health benefits	Check to see if your plan offers some payment for services of homemakers and visiting nurses.
Deductibles	Often the first $100, $500, or $1,000 may not be covered. *Often policies with the higher deductible figures give better long-range coverage.* For long illnesses, such as some cancer illnesses, this type gives better protection, since it gives long-range help.

Things to Check Your Policy For (continued)

ITEM OR FEATURE	COMMENTS
Who is covered	Check especially if you have stepchildren or foster children, or expect more children.
Retirement benefits	Check limitations relating to age or place of employment. Can benefits be converted from group to individual policy upon termination or retirement?
Cancellation	Under what terms can the policy be canceled? Check to be sure you will be covered even if health deteriorates or you have severe or repeated need for treatment.
Maximums or benefit limits	Check to see what the maximum figure refers to. Is it paid in full for each illness or all illnesses in the course of a year? Is it paid only once in the life of the policy?
Preexisting conditions	If there is an exclusion against coverage of preexisting conditions, it should never go back longer than one year.
Waiting period	In buying a new policy, check to see if there is a waiting period longer than 30 or 60 days during which new illnesses will not be covered. You should know this in making your plans. The shorter the waiting period the better.
Guaranteed renewable	This means that the policy stays in effect up to a specified age as long as the premium is paid promptly. The premium rate cannot be raised for any one individual but only for all policyholders with the same type of benefits.
Noncancellable— guaranteed renewable	This is the safest type. It cannot be canceled and the premium rate cannot be changed.

Questions to Ask About Your Health/Surgical/Medical Insurance

- What kind of hospital room will my insurance allow?
- What percentage of daily rate is paid?
- How many days are covered? (Can vary from 30 days to a year.)

- What is the current cost of hospital room in my locality?
- What is the current cost of a nurse for one shift?
- What is the current cost of a doctor's visit—office, hospital, home?
- What in-hospital procedures are covered? General nursing care? Anesthesia? Operating room? X-rays? Laboratory tests? Drugs? Surgical supplies? Doctors' fees? Radiation therapy? Chemotherapy?
- Is there a limitation on the amount paid for these hospital services?
- Is there a deductible toward hospital expenses before benefits start?
- What provisions exist for renewing the policy?
- What exclusions or limitations are contained in the policy?
- Are surgical fees paid in line with surgeons' fees in my community?
- What kind of limitations are placed on surgical fees?
- Is hospitalization for diagnostic purposes covered?
- How much does the policy pay for each time my doctor visits me in the hospital?
- How many visits are allowed per confinement?
- How much is allowed for a house call or office visit?
- Is there a deductible, either a dollar amount or number of visits not covered before benefits start?
- Is there a waiting period before any conditions are covered?
- What is the maximum lifetime amount my policy will pay?
- What maximum yearly amount per family member will the policy pay?
- How much must I pay before insurance benefits start (deductible amount)?
- Is there a deductible for each claim for a different illness or injury?
- Is the deductible on a calendar-year basis with one deductible in a given year charged against total bills? Or is it on a per-illness basis?
- What percent of the total cost above the deductible does the policy pay?
- Is the policy renewable?
- What top benefit limits, if any, exist for such expenses as hospital room and board, surgery, consultations, treatments?

Questions to Ask About Your Disability Insurance

- Is there a waiting period before benefits begin?
- Does the waiting period vary depending on whether sickness or an accident is involved?
- How is total disability defined?
- Are there any benefits for partial disability?
- What is the amount of weekly or monthly benefits? (Between 50 and 75 percent of gross income should be covered.)
- How long do regular payments continue?
- Are lifetime payments available?
- What provisions exist for renewing the policy?

General Questions to Ask About Insurance

- Can benefits be converted from group to individual policy?
- What benefits will be continued after retirement?
- Can the policy be changed or canceled?

What types of health insurance are available?

Sometimes several types are combined in one policy, such as hospital/surgical and medical. *Hospital insurance* pays certain costs during hospital stays. *Surgical insurance* covers whole or partial cost of operations within a schedule of allowable fees. *Medical insurance* covers the doctors' services such as home, office, and hospital visits. *Major-medical insurance* usually covers expenses above an established deductible amount with a maximum limit. *Disability or loss-of-income insurance* pays monthly income benefits to offset the loss of income because of total disability resulting from an accident or sickness.

Medicare, Part A, covers most of the hospital costs for those 65 and over. *Medicare, Part B,* is similar to a major-medical plan, paying 80 percent of doctors' bills, plus extras such as outpatient hospital services, home health services, and medical supplies.

Where can I get information about the types of health policies available?

The Health Insurance Institute (277 Park Avenue, New York, N.Y. 10017) has information available to help guide you in purchasing your health-insurance policies. Your place of business has information on the group insurances available to you. If you are not eligible for group insurance or wish to seek insurance in addition to the group plan, you should contact an insurance agent for information about the various policies available. Be sure that he is a licensed representative of the company issuing the policy or a reputable insurance broker in the community. You might also check out your library for a copy of *Best's Insurance Reports* or *Timesaver for Health Insurance,* published by the National Underwriter Co.

Is there some way I can check out my health insurance company?

Yes. The leading authority on the financial strength of insurance companies is the rating it receives in *Best's Insurance Reports.* Copies of this report are sometimes available in the reference room of the public library.

Is there some way I can compare health insurances?

Since there is no standard of comparison, comparing health insurances is not an easy job. However, one comparison that can be made is by looking at the loss ratios of different companies. This can be tricky, because different policies within the same company may have different loss ratios. However, it is a starting point. The loss ratio is the percentage of premiums which a company pays back to its policyholders in benefits. A high loss ratio means a good value for the buyer. For instance, a company which returns 60 percent of its premiums to its policyholders gives a better value than one which returns only 30 percent. Some companies return as much as 95 percent. Some Blue Cross/ Blue Shield groups return better than 100 percent. Others return as low as 30 percent. Steer clear of any company which returns less than 50 percent. Check *Best's Insurance Reports* for ratings. *Timesaver for Health Insurance,* available through the National Underwriter Co., (420 East Fourth Street, Cincinnati, Ohio 45202), lists descriptions of various policies.

If I have the opportunity to get group insurance, should I take it?

Group insurance is usually offered by employers, labor unions, and professional organizations. These policies, because of the large number of persons covered and the subsequent pooling of risks, will usually have lower premiums than individual policies. In addition, the employer or group policyholder often pays part or all of the premium. Individuals are eligible for protection regardless of physical condition. For these reasons group insurance is usually desirable.

Are individual policies better than group policies?

Health policies written individually represent the very poorest form of health care financing. They should be considered only as carefully planned supplements to group coverage or as last-resort attempts to gain some security when nothing else is available. Most individual and family hospital and surgical policies available are totally inadequate in terms of modern price tags. If you are not eligible for a group policy, your best bet is probably the Blue Cross and Blue Shield policies, which are recognized by most hospitals and generally offer better benefits than individual policies.

Do all health policies cost the same for the same kind of protection?

No, they do not. Nor are the benefits for all policies the same. If you're not in a group and must buy an individual policy, the coverage, value, and claims practices vary widely from company to company. First, consider Blue Cross and Blue Shield. Almost every state has a Blue Cross and Blue Shield plan, and most provide comprehensive benefits at a fair value. Since they are nonprofit companies, almost every dollar they receive in premiums is returned to the policyholder in benefits. The cost of the total package, however, is high. If you can't afford Blue Cross and Blue Shield premiums, then look at other health policies. The premiums charged will usually be lower, but so will the benefits. Check them carefully against the questions asked so that you know exactly what is being provided.

I always get Medicare and Medicaid mixed up. What is the difference?

Medicare is the federally sponsored program for people who are 65 and over. Medicaid is a public assistance program for people of all ages run by the state which pays hospital bills and doctors' fees and covers additional services as well. Benefits for Medicare are the same in all states. Those for Medicaid vary from state to state.

What is Medicare?

Medicare is the health-insurance program of the federal government provided through Social Security or Railroad Retirement for people 65 and older and some people under 65 who are disabled. The program is available in two parts—A and B. Benefits automatically go into effect when you reach age 65, though it is wise to apply to your Social Security office for your Medicare card a few months before you reach 65 to be sure you are covered.

What does regular Medicare cover?

Medicare Hospital Insurance, Part A, covers room and board in a semiprivate room, nursing care, supplies and equipment, x-ray, radiology, operating room, drugs, medical supplies, and lab tests. The patient assumes $104 of the bill for any part of the first 60 days. From the 61st to the 90th day, the patient pays $26 per day. After the 90th day, the patient has only a lifetime reserve of 60 additional days for which the patient must assume a payment of $52 a day. In addition, the patient may be eligible for care in a skilled nursing facility or convalescent home which is a participant of Medicare. Admission must be made within 14 days of discharge from the hospital. At that point the patient can stay in the nursing home for the first 20 days without charge; from the 21st to the 100th day, the patient pays $13 per day. Medicare will also cover care at home, provided the patient has been hospitalized for three days and arrangements are made within 14 days of discharge from hospital to nursing home. A total of 100 visits of part-time public-health skilled nursing care—including physical, occupational, or speech therapy or skilled home health aides—are allowed within one calendar year. It is important to know that further coverage, known as Medical Insurance, Part B, is available.

What do Medicare Supplementary Benefits (Part B) cover?

This part of Medicare insurance, known as Medical Insurance, Part B, is available to all those age 65 and over and some people

under 65 who are disabled. However, you must apply for these
benefits and agree to pay half the premium cost, currently $6.70
a month, deducted from your Social Security payments. Under
this plan, the first $60 in medical bills must be paid by the
patient. Thereafter, Medicare will assume 80 percent of the
allowable charge. Covered items include medical and surgical
services of physician, in hospital, nursing home, office, clinic, or
patient's home. They include radiology and pathology costs as
well as services prescribed by the physician in connection with
his diagnosis or treatment. X-ray treatments, lab services, and
physician's services in a convalescent home are also covered.
Additionally, emergency-room and clinic services, physical
therapy, lab tests, diagnostic tests, x-rays, radiology services,
surgical dressings and casts, and rental or purchase of medical
equipment such as oxygen, wheelchair, prosthetic devices to
replace internal organs, and colostomy equipment are covered.
Medicare will also help pay for transportation by an approved
ambulance service to a hospital or skilled nursing facility if used
to avoid endangering the patient's health.

What is Medicaid?

Medicaid is a federally sponsored plan which is administered by
the states—and therefore each state sets its own rules for
eligibility and coverage. Contact your city or county government
Social Services office for information on eligibility. Medicaid in
some states helps with hospital bills and bills for inpatient
physician services when those costs exceed 25 percent of annual
net income. Medicaid also may cover the following: recipients of
old-age assistance, persons with income or resources sufficient to
meet general living expenses but not enough to meet the cost of
medical care, those receiving Medicare but whose medical needs
are not fully met under that program, recipients of aid to the
disabled and blind, and persons under 21 whose resources are
insufficient to meet the cost of medical care. Those receiving
Medicare benefits can check with their local Medicaid or Social
Security offices to see if they are eligible.

Is insurance to supplement the Medicare A and B plans available?

Yes. Some companies offer plans with an annual premium based on age, sex, and number in the family. Most of these are guaranteed renewable and offer hospital payments. One plan, offered by the New York Life Insurance Company, offers $144 per day for the 1st to 60th days, $36 a day for the 61st to 90th day, $72 a day for the 91st to 150th day, and $144 a day for the 151st to 365th day. These are in addition to the Medicare benefits. The cost of this insurance ranges between $10 and $12 per month.

If I have Medicare do I need any other insurance?

As good as Medicare is, it was never meant to cover all the health-care expenses of older people. Medicare Plan B helps to cover major-medical expenses. However, with Medicare, as with most health insurance, there are deductible amounts and percentages of charges for various services which you must pay before you become eligible for payment. Whatever type of basic health insurance you have—Medicare or other—adding some supplemental protection can be a wise idea. Some companies offer a special Medicare supplement insurance. Some Blue Cross/Blue Shield companies have a "65-Special" which will fill most of the gaps in Medicare A and Medicare B for slightly over $5 a month.

What Social Security disability benefits are available?

Workers who become disabled before they are 65 as well as certain family members may be eligible for income benefits under Social Security starting with the seventh full month of disability. Persons disabled in childhood who continue disabled are covered, as are disabled widows, dependent widowers, and disabled surviving divorced wives. Claims for benefits are made by contacting the local Social Security office.

Is cancer insurance available?

Cancer insurance, as a supplement to existing health insurance, is available in all states except Connecticut, New York, and New Jersey where sale of this type of insurance is banned. Many of the benefits offered are similar to those available through a hospital, surgical, or major-medical plan which also covers the family in other medical emergencies and usually gives more economical coverage. The prospective buyer is asked to sign a pledge that he does not have cancer and never had it before being accepted. The cost of a family policy such as is available from Family Life Assurance Company of Columbus, Ga., costs between $4.80 and $6.25 per month. The policy covers hospitalization costs ($60 daily for the first 12 days, $40 daily thereafter, and 100 percent after the 91st day of hospitalization up to $6,000 per month) as well as $750 per operation without limit on operations, up to $1,500 for radiotherapy and chemotherapy, and costs of physician and nursing care, anesthesia, transfusions, ambulances, etc. These payments are made in addition to claims paid by basic health insurance. Several other companies, such as Reserve Life Insurance of Dallas, Texas, and Constitutional Life Insurance Co. of Chicago, Ill., have similar plans. Some of the policies specifically state that they do not cover diagnostic x-ray and laboratory examinations. Most insurance experts feel that good general medical and surgical policies are a better investment than specialized cancer insurance.

How can I be sure I'm getting all the benefits to which I am entitled?

Take the time to read through your insurance policies. Check to see that you have the necessary insurance forms. Keep all your medical bills and information together in one spot. Accept the help of a friend who has some knowledge of insurance or hire a tax accountant to go over your bills with you to be certain you are getting all the benefits available to you. The social service department of your hospital can also be helpful.

Are mail-order policies a good buy?

As with every other type of product, there are good and poor buys in mail-order policies, but in every case you should check the company and the policy carefully before buying. The buyer should bear in mind that any omission of pertinent health information will be held against him when he tries to collect. At claim time, some companies have been known to find some preexisting condition to justify nonpayment of claims. Furthermore, the benefits in many of the mail-order health-insurance policies are based on the number of days you spend hospitalized.

Usually they are advertised as having a maximum payment of $400, $800, or $1,000 a month. The payment is usually a cash payment made directly to you. $1,000 a month breaks down to $33.33 a day—far less than daily hospital costs and far less coverage than most people need. The average hospital stay is usually eight days, and 14 days for people over 65. As you can well understand, this type of policy is a very inadequate one as a basic protection plan.

What is an HMO (Health Maintenance Organization)?

HMOs are medical supermarkets in which a group of doctors join together to provide almost all your health-care needs. Instead of operating on a fee-for-service basis, the way most doctors and hospitals do, they work on a prepaid basis much as an insurance company does. You pay one premium—sometimes as much as $700 a year for a family—and your coverage includes all your medical expenses. Since the doctors' incomes are fixed in advance, their incentive is to keep you healthy and out of the hospital to keep costs down. They emphasize preventive medicine—keeping you well rather than treating you after you are sick. Your state insurance department can tell you if there are any health maintenance organizations in your area.

Do health-insurance companies ever turn down claims?

Indeed they do. The most standardized policy provisions are subject to widely different interpretations from company to company. If you have a complaint or feel you have been treated unfairly by your insurance company, agent, or broker, be sure to report it to your state insurance department. Send a copy of your letter to your state representative or senator.

Are health-insurance premiums an allowable tax deduction?

The government allows the deduction of one-half of the cost of premiums paid for medical insurance, up to $150. If your total health insurance cost is over $300, the balance may be added to your other medical expenses and is subject to the 3 percent limitation. Amounts paid as premiums under Part B of Medicare are deductible as medical expenses.

What kinds of medical expenses are deductible for income-tax purposes?

A wide variety of medical expenses are deductible. However, the deductions only apply to those medical expenses that were not covered by medical insurance and if they exceed 3 percent of the taxpayer's adjusted gross income. These include such items as:

- Expenses paid for transportation primarily for, and essential to, the rendition of medical care
- Transportation to and from the physician's office, such as taxi fare
- Amounts paid for bus, train, or plane fares or ambulance hire, actual substantiated expenditures for parking fees, tolls, gasoline (or a flat fee of 7 cents per mile)
- Social Security taxes on wages of private nurses providing medical care
- Hospital services, nursing services (including nurses' board when paid by the taxpayer), medical, laboratory, surgical, and diagnostic services, x-rays, artificial teeth and limbs, hearing aids, eyeglasses, therapy and special equipment such as wheelchairs, special beds and oxygen equipment
- Medicines and drugs (exceeding 1 percent of adjusted gross income)

Do I have to pay state sales taxes for medical devices?

In some states, sales tax is not charged on such items as ostomy equipment, mastectomy prosthesis and bra, braces, supports, artificial electrolarynx and batteries, crutches, wheelchairs, oxygen, etc. Be sure to check your local laws so that you will know whether or not you are eligible for these deductions.

How can I possibly keep track of all the bills?

Bills and insurance forms are part of all our lives—but they are especially important when they involve hospitalization and medications. It is helpful from the start to keep all of your medical records in one spot, so that they are available to you or to your accountant when tax time rolls around. Keep a running record—just a sheet of paper will do—with date, check number, who the bill is from, total charge, and any other information such as how much was reimbursed by the insurance company. Records of mileage driven (or cab fares paid) to appointments, treatments, hospitals, and pharmacies should all be kept.

Whom can I turn to for help in solving my financial problems due to prolonged cancer treatment?

The social service department of your hospital should be able to give you advice about financial help which is available in your locality. The American Cancer Society also offers information about local programs.

The drugs I am taking for cancer are so expensive. Is there any program that can help me pay for them?

Check your insurance coverage carefully. If you have a major-medical policy other than Blue Cross/Blue Shield (which does not usually at this time pay for chemotherapy drugs except those taken in the hospital) it may pay for drugs and medicines dispensed by a licensed pharmacist or given in a doctor's office.

Can the American Cancer Society or the Leukemia Society provide financial help?

The ability of these organizations to provide financial help in any great amount is limited—and such aid may be determined by a means test. However, these organizations may be able to help provide transportation to and from treatment centers, baby-sitting services, and special equipment and dressings for home care. If you get in touch with them early in your illness, they can sometimes intervene in your behalf in the area of doctor and medical bills. Don't wait to call them for help. Have someone talk with them while you are still in the hospital so they can help investigate financial help possibilities before the bills begin to come in.

What other local organizations can I contact for help?

Services are sometimes available from the Red Cross, Salvation Army, labor unions to which any family member belongs, churches, and fraternal or social organizations. In time of need, do not hesitate to reach out for help. These organizations exist to perform many services. Be sure to contact them and let them know you need help.

What help is available through the Veterans Administration hospital or state veteran's hospitals?

Bonafide veterans of the United States services are eligible to receive full benefits from the various veterans hospitals across the country. Hospital care may be authorized for the veteran if Veterans Administration or state veterans hospital facilities are unavailable or if conditions warrant admission to another hospital.

Are there any special places to turn for help in rehabilitation?

Yes. Many states have a department of vocational rehabilitation or department of health which provides assistance for the rehabilitation of cancer patients, including prostheses and ambulatory training. It may even help pay for college education of recovering cancer patients.

What sorts of specialized organizations are available?

Reach to Recovery programs are available in most states for mastectomy patients. Candlelighters organizations have been formed to help families of children stricken with cancer. Ostomy patients can turn to the Ostomy Association, and laryngectomees have the support of New Voice Clubs. Many American Cancer Society units are also running support groups for cancer patients and their families. The American Cancer Society or the Cancer Information Office in your locality can give you the names and phone numbers of local chapters for these organizations (see Chapter 23).

Should I be thinking about writing a will?

Everyone should have a will, and this is probably as good a time as any to think about it. You would be wise to consider having a lawyer draw one up for you. A lawyer can help you with all the intricacies of your own special situation. If you do not have a lawyer, you can find one by checking the yellow pages for "Attorneys" or "Lawyer Referral Services." Lawyer Referral Services is run by bar associations in many cities and counties and allows lawyers to register, often indicating whether they specialize in wills, divorce, criminal law, etc. For a small set fee— usually about $10—you may have an initial 30-minute office consultation to review your problem, discuss fees, and determine whether you will choose him as your lawyer. If Lawyer Referral Services is not listed in your phone book, you can write to the American Bar Association (1155 East 60th Street, Chicago, Ill. 60637) for a free copy of the *Directory of Lawyer Referral Services.* If your will is a simple one, it can be drawn up for between $50 and $100—sometimes less. If you wish, you can call the lawyer, outline the sort of will you feel you need, explaining your property worth, and ask about the charge for such a will. Of course, the more complicated your situation, the higher the cost.

Can I write my own will?

If there are any complicated trust or tax situations, this can be risky. However, in every state, you can buy a standard will form from a stationery store.

Many people have a legally drawn up will and a handwritten will for their personal possessions. Some states will accept an unwitnessed will in the form of a letter or note written entirely in your own handwriting. However, most states require at least two witnesses, while some require three. You might benefit by reading *How to Avoid Probate,* by Norman Dacey (Crown Publishers, N.Y.) for background information.

How can I make arrangements to donate my body?

A uniform anatomical gift act or similar law has been passed in all 50 states. Persons can become donors by signing a card in the presence of two witnesses. The card allows the person to specify what donation is desired. He may contribute any needed organs or parts, restrict donation to certain organs or parts, or give the entire body for anatomical study. More information can be obtained by writing to: Living Bank, P.O. Box 6725, Houston, Texas 77005 or by calling 713-528-2971.

Is it normal to be depressed following cancer surgery?

Yes, it is the most normal reaction in the world. Fear and anger are very normal reactions and you should allow yourself to express them. Once expressed and understood by those around you, your depression will be easier to deal with and will soon lessen.

What do I do if I feel that the treatment is worse than the disease?

In the midst of treatments, many patients feel this way, and you would be wise to talk through your feelings with your doctor or nurse. Don't discontinue taking your treatments without discussion with your doctor—it is unfair to yourself to do this. He can explain the alternatives to you and you can then make the decision about how you will proceed.

Why is it important to eat well when a person has cancer?

There are several reasons:
- A balanced diet can help maintain strength, prevent body tissues from breaking down, and rebuild normal tissues which have been affected by the treatments.
- Patients who eat well during treatment periods—especially foods high in protein and calories—are better able to stand the side effects of treatments, whether the treatment is chemotherapy, radiation therapy, immunotherapy, or surgery. It may even be possible for the patient to withstand a higher dose of certain treatments.
- Patients with good eating habits tend to have fewer infections and are often able to be up and about more.
- When a person eats less, for whatever reason, the body uses its own stored-up fat, protein, and other nutrients, such as iron.

What exactly is meant by the term "eating well"?

"Eating well" means using a variety of foods to provide the vitamins, minerals, protein, and other elements necessary to keep the body working normally. It means:
- Having a diet that is high enough in calories to keep up a normal weight.
- Eating foods which are high in protein needed to build and repair the skin, hair, muscles and organs in the body (people who have had surgery or are ill need extra protein and other nutrients for repair of body tissues—protein can be used for repair if the body is also getting enough calories. If it is not, the body will use the protein for energy instead of for repair).
- Eating a mixed diet, including the basic four groups of food—

four servings a day of salads, cooked vegetables, raw or cooked fruits; three servings a day of meats, fish, poultry, eggs, or cheese; four servings a day of grains and cereals; two servings a day of milk or other dairy products.

Are there any general hints for cancer patients who are having difficulty in eating?

There are a few:

- Remember that what sounds unappealing today may sound good tomorrow.
- When feeling well, take advantage of it by eating well and by preparing meals which you can freeze for the "down" days. On good days, eat when you feel hungry, even if it is not mealtime. Eat food with good nutritional value, as many nutrients can be stored in your body for later use.
- Talk to your doctors and your health team about your eating problems. Many hospitals and Visiting Nurse Associations have dietitians and nutritionists on their staffs who can help you with these problems. Before you try home remedies, be sure that your problems are not symptoms needing medical attention.
- Take advantage of time-saving foods and appliances, such as foods which can be prepared as a meal-in-a-dish, with little preparing and cooking.
- Make your eating atmosphere pleasant, with an attractively set table, varying the place in your home where you eat, or eating with friends. A glass of wine or beer before meals (with your doctor's approval) helps to relax you and can help to make you hungry.

I am not hungry. Is that a common problem among cancer patients?

This seems to be a common complaint. Loss of appetite (anorexia, in medical terms) sometimes is caused by treatments, such as radiation or chemotherapy. But it also happens to people who are not having treatments. No one really knows whether the loss of appetite is due to illness, fatigue, pain, stress, or depression—or to a combination of all of these. Some people's appetites come and go. Others rarely feel hungry. Among patients' complaints are that food doesn't taste right (especially meat), that they have a bitter metal taste in their mouths or on their tongues, and that they simply get full too soon.

Are there any hints for increasing one's appetite?

There are several things you can try:

- Eat small meals more often. Keep snacks handy for nibbling. Try eating a good snack before going to bed in addition to your regular meals.
- Mix ice cream with ginger ale or a favorite carbonated beverage. Drink milk shakes. Eat frozen yogurt.
- Tart food may enhance flavors (for people who have no problems with their mouths and throats). Pickles, lemonade, and orange juice may help. Use vinegar and lemon juice for flavorings.
- Add bacon bits, sliced almonds, ham strips, or pieces of onion to vegetables for added flavor and nourishment. Chicken and fish can be added to cream soups for flavor and protein.
- Wine, beer, or mayonnaise added to soups and sauces makes them taste better.
- Marinate meat, chicken, or fish in sweet fruit juices, sweet wines, Italian or French dressing, or sweet-sour sauce for more taste. Use more and stronger seasonings in your cooking, such as basil, oregano, rosemary, tarragon, lemon juice, or mint.
- If meat doesn't taste right, cook chicken, turkey, or fish instead (choose fish that does not have a strong flavor and cook it on a barbecue, if possible). Use eggs and dairy products as substitutes.
- If you have a strange taste in your mouth, try taking it away by drinking more liquids (water, tea, or ginger ale) or by eating foods which leave their own taste in your mouth (fresh fruit or hard candy).
- If you feel you are full when you've only eaten a little, chew your food more slowly to prevent your stomach from becoming too full too quickly, don't drink liquids with your meals (take them 30 to 60 minutes before meals to reduce the volume of material in your stomach), and make sure that the liquids have nutritional content (such as juices, milkshakes, or milk).

- Try to add protein to your foods without increasing the amount of food you eat.

How can I add protein to my food without increasing the amount of food I eat?

- Skim-milk powder adds protein. Try adding two tablespoons of dry skim-milk powder to the regular amount of milk in recipes. Add milk powder to hot or cold cereals, scrambled eggs, soups, gravies, ground meat (for patties, meat balls, meatloaf), casserole dishes, desserts, and in baking.
- Use milk or half-and-half instead of water when making soup, cereals, instant cocoa, puddings, and canned soups. Soy formulas may also be used.
- Add diced or ground meat to soups and to casseroles.
- Add grated cheese or chunks of cheese to sauces, vegetables, soups, and casseroles.
- Add peanut butter to butter on hot bread.
- Choose dessert recipes which contain eggs such as sponge cake, angel-food cake, egg custard, bread pudding, or rice pudding.
- Add peanut butter to sauces and use it on crackers, waffles, or celery sticks.

I have trouble eating enough food to keep up my weight. What should I do?

If you are having trouble eating enough food to keep up your weight, you could add some high-fat or high-carbohydrate foods to your diet. For instance:

- Spread peanut butter on fruit (such as an apple, banana, or pear) or stuff celery with it. Add it to a sandwich with mayonnaise or cream cheese. Peanut butter is high in both calories and protein.
- Spread honey on toast, use it as a sweetener in coffee or tea, or add it to cereal in the morning.
- Mix butter or margarine into hot foods such as soups, vegetables, mashed potatoes, cooked cereal, and rice. Serve butter on hot bread (more butter is used when it melts into hot bread).
- Use mayonnaise (it has 100 calories per tablespoon, which is

about twice as much as salad dressing) in salads, in eggs, or with lettuce on sandwiches.

- Add sour cream and yogurt to vegetables (potatoes, beans, carrots, squash), to gravies, or as a salad dressing for fruit.
- Use sour cream as a dip for fresh vegetables. Scoop it on fresh fruit and add brown sugar for a quick dessert.
- Add whipped cream to pies, fruit, puddings, hot chocolate, Jell-o, and other desserts (it has 60 calories in a tablespoon).
- Snack with foods such as nuts, dried fruits, candy, popcorn, crackers and cheese, granola, ice cream, and popsicles. Add marshmallows to fruit and to hot chocolate.
- Add powdered coffee creamers to gravy, soup, milkshakes, and hot cereals. Creamers add calories without volume.
- Bread meat, chicken or fish before cooking.
- Add raisins, dates or chopped nuts, and brown sugar to hot or cold cereals for a snack.

I am bothered by nausea and vomiting because of my treatment. What can I eat to help this problem?

There are several things you can try. You will need to experiment to see which ones will work for you.

- Eat smaller portions of food that is low in fat (be sure to eat more often to make up for your calorie and protein needs if you are eating foods low in fat).
- Take whatever liquids you feel you can handle, such as clear soups, flavored gelatin, carbonated beverages (ginger ale), popsicles, and ice cubes made of any favorite kind of liquid. Sip liquids slowly through a straw.
- Eat dry foods such as toast and crackers, especially soon after getting up in the morning.
- Avoid liquids at mealtimes. Take them 30 to 60 minutes before eating.
- If you have been vomiting, eat salty foods. Don't eat overly sweet ones.
- If the smell of food makes you feel nauseated, let someone else do the cooking while you sit in another room or take a walk. Use prepared foods from the freezer that can be warmed at a low temperature or eat a meal of food that does not need to be cooked.
- Do not lie down flat for at least two hours after eating. You

might want to rest after eating, since activity can slow down digestion and increase your discomfort. If you wish to rest, sit down. If you do lie down, make sure your head is at least 4 inches higher than your feet.

- If your problems with nausea or vomiting are severe, ask your doctor for anti-nausea medicine. If you are bloated, have pain, or have a swollen stomach before nausea and vomiting occur (and if these problems are relieved by vomiting), call the doctor.

What are some of the foods which are low in fat?

Foods which are low in fat include:
- Crab, white fish, shrimp, light tuna (packed in water)
- Veal, chicken and turkey breast, and lean cuts of other meats which are braised, roasted or cooked without adding fats
- Broth-type soups
- Spaghetti with plain sauces
- Fruits and fruit juices, vegetables and vegetable juices
- Hot and cold cereals except granola-type cereals
- Low-fat yogurt, low-fat cottage cheese, 1-percent buttermilk, 1-percent low-fat milk
- Plain bread, soda crackers, pretzels, toast with jelly or honey (no butter)
- Popsicles, sherbet, gelatin ices
- Angel food cake, danish pudding and fruit-pie fillings; sauces, Junket, pudding, or shakes made with skim milk
- Hard and jelly candies

My mouth and throat are sore, which makes it very hard for me to eat. Do you have any suggestions?

Yes. The linings of the mouth and throat are among the most sensitive areas of the body. Cancer patients, especially those receiving chemotherapy or radiation treatments, often complain of soreness in these areas. There are a few important things to remember:
- If you have sores under your dentures, do not wear dentures when you do not need them for eating.
- Drink lots of fluids and eat well, because part of the healing in these sensitive areas depends upon your having good food and liquids for your body.

- If you have mouth or throat problems, be sure your doctor examines the area to see whether or not you need special medication.
- Make sure you see your dentist for special care of your teeth during this period.
- If your mouth is dry, ask the doctor whether the medicines you are taking are causing the dryness.
- Cold foods can sometimes be soothing. Add ice to milk and milkshakes for extra coldness. Eat ice cream or yogurt and make popsicles with milk or milk substitutes.
- Use gravies and sauces on meats and vegetables. Cook stews and casseroles, adding more liquids to make them softer.
- Cut your meats up in small pieces. Use a blender (cook your food first and then put it in the blender to make it easy to eat).
- Choose soft foods such as mashed potatoes, yogurt, scrambled or poached eggs, egg custards, ricotta cheese, milkshakes, puddings, gelatins, creamy cereals, and macaroni and cheese.
- Stay away from foods that sting or burn such as citrus-fruit juices and tomatoes. Fruits low in acid (bananas, canned pears) and nectars (peach, pear, apricot) are easier to swallow. Use a little sugar to tone down acid or salty foods.
- Soak foods in coffee, tea, milk, cocoa, or warm beverages. Try taking a swallow of liquid with each bite of food.
- Eat food lukewarm or cold rather than hot. Do not use hot spices such as pepper, chili powder, nutmeg, and cloves. Avoid rough or coarse foods such as raw vegetables and bran. Don't eat dry foods like toast or hard bread unless you soak them (they can scratch delicate tissues).
- If you smoke or drink, talk to your doctor about it. Certain alcoholic beverages can irritate your mouth and throat as does any smoking.
- If your house is heated with dry heat, a humidifier or a steam kettle in the bedroom may help.
- Rinse your mouth whenever you feel you need it—to remove debris, to stimulate your gums, to lubricate your mouth, or to put a fresh taste in your mouth. You can make a mouthwash from 1 teaspoon of salt to 1 quart of water (or 1 teaspoon of baking soda to 1 quart of water). A mixture of equal parts of glycerin and warm water is also effective. Do not use a commercial mouthwash without your doctor's permission. Do

not use hot water; let it cool before using. Rinsing with club soda can relieve dry mouth or thick saliva. Oragel, available at the pharmacy, can help deaden the pain.
- Stay away from strong fumes such as cleaning solutions and paints.
- If your problem is severe, talk to your doctor about medicine to numb your gums and tongue. If you need it, artificial saliva is also available.

I feel too tired to eat. What should I do?

Try resting first and then eating later on. Many times you will feel more like eating after you have napped or rested. In addition:
- Rely on meals you have frozen when you felt well or on convenience foods that are easy to prepare.
- If your tired feeling is related to your recovery from surgery or from other treatments and you are gradually building up your strength, start by eating smaller portions of easily digested foods and slowly work back to normal.
- Accept the offers of friends to help you. Tell them what you need. People like to do things for others. Do not be embarrassed to ask for help and to accept and direct your friends' aid.
- If you live alone, you might wish to arrange for "Meals on Wheels" to prepare your meals. Many communities offer this service. Contact your doctor, Visiting Nurse Association or American Cancer Society for information on this service.
- If you feel tired when you wake up or if you are not sleeping at night talk with your doctor. Do not take sleeping pills without the doctor's permission.

I have diarrhea. Is this a common problem with cancer patients?

Some patients with some kinds of cancers (such as tumors in the pancreas) and on some kinds of treatment (radiation and chemotherapy) have problems with diarrhea, excessive gas, or a bloated feeling.

What can I do about these problems?

There are several suggestions:
- Drink liquids between meals instead of with them. Make sure

you drink plenty of liquids, since diarrhea causes you to lose fluids and salts which you must replace.

- Eat smaller amounts of food more often. Eat foods which help control diarrhea, such as applesauce, bananas, boiled white rice, tapioca, and plain tea. Stay away from fatty foods and foods which are highly spiced.

- Use less fiber (roughage) in your diet. If your intestines are irritated, the normal amount of fiber may be too much for them. Use only cooked fruits and vegetables, omitting those with seeds and tough skins, beans, broccoli, corn, onions, garlic, breads, grains and nuts.

- Potassium, an important element to your body, is lost in great quantities when you have diarrhea. If you are lacking potassium, you can feel very weak. Make sure you eat some foods that are high in potassium but won't worsen the diarrhea, such as bananas, apricot or peach nectar, fish, potatoes, and meat. If you cannot eat these foods, talk to your doctor about taking potassium supplements.

- If you have cramps, stay away from foods that may encourage gas or cramping such as carbonated drinks, beer, beans, cabbage, broccoli, cauliflower, highly spiced foods, too many sweets, and chewing gum.

- Do not skip meals. Try to chew with your mouth closed. Talking while you chew may cause you to swallow too much air, which can cause gassiness or cramps.

- If your diarrhea is persistent or has blood in it or if you start to lose weight, be sure to tell the doctor.

What can I do about constipation?

Constipation can be a problem for people with cancer. It may result from treatment with some drugs.

- Make sure your regular diet includes whatever has helped you move your bowels before, such as a variety of fruits and vegetables, breads, cereals, bran, dried fruits (raisins, prunes or apricots), and nuts to add more fiber. If you cannot chew or swallow these, try grating them or putting them in a blender.

- Drink plenty of liquids (eight or ten glasses each day are needed). You can drink prune juice to stimulate bowel activity.

- Add one or two tablespoons of bran to your foods to keep you regular. Try it in cooked cereals, casseroles, eggs, or baked goods or eat it as a raw cereal.
- Eat high-fiber snack foods such as sesame bread sticks, date-nut bread, oatmeal cookies, fig newtons, date or raisin bars, granola, prune bread, or corn chips.
- Do some light exercise. Set aside 10 to 20 minutes a day to sit quietly on the commode.
- If you are undergoing treatment, check with the doctor or nurse before taking a laxative or a stool softener.

What suggestions do you have if I need to eat soft foods?

- Use tender cuts and ground meat. Use moist-heat cookery such as braising, simmering, and poaching.
- Use only cooked eggs. Make omelets or scrambled, poached, or soft-boiled eggs.
- Choose soft breads, hot or soaked cereals, and cooked grains such as rice or macaroni.
- Use cooked vegetables, removing seeds and tough skins.
- Choose fruits which are well ripened, canned, or cooked. Remove seeds and tough skins.
- Warm meats, vegetables, or potatoes before putting in the blender.
- Cut meat finely. Blend with liquids such as broth or gravy.
- Strain liquid meals if you want to avoid particles.
- Include pancakes, pudding, gelatin, custard, and similar foods which can be served without blending.
- If you need tube or gastrostomy feeding, ask for a consultation with the nutritionist or dietitian at the hospital to determine the contents, method of preparation, and feeding techniques.

How much protein and how many calories do I need?

The needs will differ for each person. However, there are several basic facts which can help you:

- Protein and calorie needs are greater during illness, treatment, and recovery than they normally are.
- Maintaining your weight is a good indication that you are getting enough calories each day.
- Protein needs are more rigid than calorie needs. Therefore, your diet should emphasize protein.

- Daily needs for proteins and calories for healthy adults (U.S. Recommended Dietary Allowances) are 2,700 calories and 56 grams of protein for men; 2,000 calories and 45 grams of protein for women. During illness treatment and recovery, 90 grams of protein for men and 80 grams of protein for women plus an additional 200 to 300 calories are usually recommended.
- You can get simple calorie guides in most department or discount stores or you can ask the dietary staff at your own hospital for help.

Can therapy really help to make me feel better?

Whether your disabilities are permanent or only temporary, and whether they are caused by the cancer or its treatment, there is therapy available which can help you to cope with your daily tasks. One of the most common problems is loss of strength or paralysis. It is amazing what simple exercises designed to strengthen muscles or improve balance and coordination can do to help make normal movement return.

What is a physical therapist, and where can I find one to help me?

The role of the physical therapist is to help maintain and increase normal body function, to prevent loss of function where possible, to help teach a patient to substitute when loss occurs, and to help the patient become as independent as possible. Special exercises needed by the patient are determined by testing. Then a plan of activity is prescribed to suit the needs and limitations of the patient. This kind of help can mean the difference between a helpless invalid and someone who is able to care for himself. Physical therapists can be recommended by your doctor or are available through cancer rehabilitation hospital services and visiting nurse associations. There is a listing in the phone book, usually under "Physical Therapists."

I've heard of homemaker services. What do they do?

Homemaker services provide well-trained, adaptable, mature women to help keep the household running. Homemaker service may be available in your area through a community health or welfare agency, a church, a club, or some other organization.

What can visiting nurses do to help?

Visiting nurse associations or city health departments provide part-time nursing help to patients at home and offer advice and guidance in the care of the patient. She will give health instruction and referrals to other agencies that may be of help. You can contact the visiting nurse either directly or through the doctor. If you have health insurance which covers nursing care, the charges (which are adjusted to the patient's ability to pay) may be payable under the policy. Medicare covers some part-time public health nursing in the home. Many public-health nursing organizations use practical nurses, who attend to all general health needs of the patient and work under the direction of the professional nurse.

How can I possibly deal with the idea that I might be dying?

There are no simple answers to that question except to try to put into perspective the whole idea of death and dying. Simplistic as it may sound, everyone is one day closer to dying every day of his life. If at all possible, try to talk about your fears and the possibility of dying. As Orville Kelly, founder of Make Today Count, says: "We don't have to like death, but we don't have to be terrified of it, either." He has learned to "live with cancer, not die from it."

What is Make Today Count?

Make Today Count was founded by Orville Kelly, a cancer patient who felt the need for patients and their families to have group support of their problems. An organization was formed and there are now over 100 chapters across the country. Meetings and workshops are conducted and a newsletter is published. The organization's address is: MTC, Box 303, Burlington, Iowa 42601.

Does the fear that cancer will recur ever disappear?

Usually the fear remains in the back of the mind. This is a normal reaction—one that is shared by every patient who has ever had cancer. However, if you learn to face the fact that you have cancer and know as much as you can about your own case, you can lay many of these fears to rest in the knowledge that you have been treated with the best methods known to date.

What should I tell relatives, friends, neighbors, and others?

Knowing what to tell others, and how much, is something that each patient or family must come to grips with. Experience indicates that it is better to discuss the subject than to try to hide it. However, the way in which this is done depends upon your own life-style—whether you prefer to share your problems with those around you fully or whether you prefer to keep discussions of problems at a low level. In the case of children with cancer, it is wise to inform schoolteachers, administrators, and nurses, as they can be most helpful when they understand the situation. It might be helpful to contact the American Cancer Society to see if there are support groups or discussion sessions being held in your locality. Talking with others who are dealing with the same problems as you are often helps to put your own feelings into perspective.

I want to talk about my feelings about my having cancer but I can't because I'm trying to protect other people's feelings. What can I do?

Cancer is a very stressful disease, and even the most well-adjusted people sometimes need help in dealing with all the complicated feelings that go with it. You might try discussing your problem with your doctor or with the nurses where you are getting treatment. If you would like to become involved in group discussion, the American Cancer Society has been active in helping to bring people together and can tell you where support groups are meeting. These groups, offered in many areas to cancer patients and their families, give reassurance that there are many others who are going through what you are going through, others who share your concerns, your anger and your problems. Some patients and family members have found seeing a psychologist or a social worker helpful.

I notice my friends don't discuss the nature of my illness with me. Should I bring up the subject?

You can help communication with your friends if you initiate the discussion and use the word "cancer" in discussing your illness. Many people are afraid and inhibited at the thought of cancer— and this is misinterpreted by the patient as a lack of empathy and concern at a time when it is most needed. Often a patient wonders if the lack of conversation about his illness means that his family knows something they aren't telling him. It's up to the patient to lead the way in discussing his illness.

Shouldn't children be protected from knowing that a parent has cancer?

It really is best not to try to protect children—you'll find that they intuitively know what is going on. It is frightening and confusing to them not to understand what is happening. Children need support and reassurance that whatever happens, they will continue to live, to be loved and to grow. Better to tell them as much as they are able to understand and give them a chance to share and help. It is also sometimes helpful to tell a child's teacher when there is serious illness in the family.

I think the doctor is avoiding me because he thinks I'm dying. What do I do about the situation?

You may not be dying at all. You should talk to your doctor quite frankly. Difficult as it may sound, your best bet is to confront your doctor with your feelings. Many physicians, because their training has been in "curing" patients, find it difficult to accept long-term disease. The fact is, however, that there are many treatment alternatives available to you as a patient, and you should be sure that the doctor understands that you expect to continue to have his support or, if he is unwilling to give you that kind of care, the support and care of some other health professional. As a consumer, you are entitled to personalized care. You are entitled to be informed about what is happening to you. You have a right to be included in the decisions affecting your treatment. You should feel free to be able to talk about your situation fully and frankly with your doctor. The question is still: How does one go about confronting a doctor with so basic a problem? Perhaps you do not feel you can do this alone. You could ask someone in your family, someone you trust, to talk with the doctor alone or in your presence about the situation. If at all possible, you should try to voice your own feelings to the doctor. It will help him in understanding you and will make it easier for him to deliver the kind of care you expect and deserve.

As a patient who has a visitor but just doesn't feel like talking, what can I say?

Just clue your visitor in on how you're feeling, emotionally as well as physically. You might say: "It's nice just to have you sitting there, even though I don't feel much like talking."

Is it unusual for friends to stop coming to visit when they think someone is dying of cancer?

The fact that a person may be dying of cancer seems to have a profound effect on his relationships with others. The fault lies with society's uncomfortableness with the whole area of dying—which has been a taboo subject for so long. Coupled with what has always been thought of as the dread disease, "cancer," makes it difficult for people to handle the situation comfortably—and so they just withdraw. Even doctors and nurses have a difficult time, and this leaves the patient without the emotional support so desperately needed. The patient and his family can help the situation by encouraging people to visit, by letting friends know when is the best time for a visit, by discussing the illness, and by letting others share the concern and the needs.

Is it possible for me to choose not to prolong dying?

There is a document called the Living Will which is not legally binding at the present time, though legislation is in progress in many parts of the country to make it so. Issued by an organization called Concern for Dying, it reads: "To my family, my physician, my lawyer and all others whom it may concern: Death is as much a reality as birth, growth, maturity and old age—it is the one certainty of life. If the time comes when I can no longer take part in decisions for my own future, let this statement stand as an expression of my wishes and directions, while I am still of sound mind. If at such a time the situation should arise in which there is no reasonable expectation of my recovery from extreme physical or mental disability, I direct that I be allowed to die and not be kept alive by medications, artificial means or 'heroic measures.' I do, however, ask that medication be mercifully administered to me to alleviate suffering even though this may shorten my remaining life. This statement is made after careful consideration and is in accordance with my strong convictions and beliefs. I want the wishes and directions here expressed carried out to the extent permitted by law. Insofar as they are not legally enforceable, I hope that those to whom this Will is addressed will regard themselves as morally bound by these provisions." (The will should be signed, dated, and witnessed by two persons.)

If this reflects your feelings, your family, your close friends and your regular physician should be informed of this will and be given a copy of it. If the physician is unwilling to comply, another more sympathetic physician should probably be sought. A copy should also be submitted to the hospital to be entered with your charts. There is some excellent reading material presently available, including:

VEATCH, ROBERT M. *Death, Dying, and the Biological Revolution, Our Last Quest for Responsibility.* New Haven, Ct.: Yale University Press.

KOHL, MARVIN, ed. *Beneficent Euthanasia.* Buffalo, N.Y.: Prometheus Books.

KUBLER-ROSS, ELISABETH. *On Death and Dying.* New York: Macmillan.

Material, including copies of the Living Will, is available from Concern for Dying, 250 West 57th St., New York, N.Y. 10019.

Will I be allowed to make a decision about whether I plan to die at home or in the hospital?

It is important for you to let your feelings be known to your doctor so that he can do everything possible to see your wishes are followed. For those who prefer to spend their last days at home, some forward-looking hospitals, and the program known as Hospice, have instituted home-care programs, with medical supervision in the home under trained medical staff. Hospice emphasizes the management of pain and other symptoms, providing help for the family as well as the patient. Hospice makes the family the unit of care, centering much of the caring process in the home, and seeks to enable the patient to carry on an alert and pain-free existence. The decision of how your illness will be managed depends on many different factors—but if you feel strongly about your desire to die at home, be certain that you tell your doctor and discuss it with your family so that when the time comes, your wishes can be carried out.

What is a hospice?

This is a new concept in the United States for care of terminally ill patients. Hospice programs have been in operation in Britain for some time. A key element in most is encouraging families to care for a dying person at home whenever possible. Some hospices have buildings where patients may be admitted for short periods of treatment, but home care is the heart of the program. The concept is the management of terminal disease to make it possible for the patient to live until he dies, with the family being involved to the end. Some provide help for the family for a year after the patient dies. Home-care teams, involving doctors, nurses, and social workers as well as volunteers, help in practical ways to make it possible for the whole family to help the dying person really "live" his last days.

What is the National Hospice Organization?

The National Hospice Organization is a specialized home health-care program, involving groups, presently in various stages of planning and development in 33 states and the District of Columbia. The goals of Hospice are to help the patient to live as fully as possible, to support the family as the unit of care, to keep the patient at home as long as appropriate, to educate health professionals and lay people, to supplement rather than duplicate existing services, and to keep costs down. Following the precept that pain is nearly always manageable, its goal is to enable patients to carry on an alert and pain-free existence through the administration of drugs and other types of therapy. Care of the family continues through the period of bereavement. Members of Hospice make regular visits and are on call 24 hours a day, seven days a week to make house calls on patients.

How can I find out about hospices in my area?

For information on hospices, contact the National Hospice Organization (765 Prospect Street, New Haven, Conn. 06511; telephone 203-787-5871). Hospice Action, a group recently formed to act as friends of the National Hospice Organization, has as its objective public education and securing political and financial support for the National Hospice Organization. It can be contacted at P.O. Box 32331, Washington, D.C. 20007.

Where can I get more information on questions of death and dying?

This whole subject has been covered most beautifully and

practically by Elisabeth Kubler-Ross in her books *On Death and Dying, Questions and Answers on Death and Dying,* and *On Children and Death,* all published by Macmillan. The first two are presently available in paperback. We especially recommend *Questions and Answers on Death and Dying* ($1.75), which consists of the questions most frequently asked of Dr. Kubler-Ross.

As a friend I want to be able to talk freely about cancer. What kinds of needs do cancer patients have that I should understand?

Most people feel first and foremost that they want to maintain control over their situation. In some cases this is difficult—but it is important for family and friends to allow it as much as possible. Further, they need to be able to share with friends and family the feeling of being robbed of the ability to function and of life itself by something which they are unable to control. Try to be sensitive to how your friend is feeling. Try to plan simple outings—visiting a friend, going for a ride, going out to lunch or for an ice-cream soda, doing an errand—on those days when your friend feels up to doing these things. Keep in close touch by telephone. Just a quick call at a set time every day, every other day, or once a week lets your friend know you're thinking of him or her.

When someone close to me who has cancer starts to talk about the disease, should I change the subject?

Please try not to. If the person feels he can talk with you about this difficult subject, help to keep that communication going. Be honest about how difficult it is for you to talk about it. But try to give realistic support and reassurance. Help to maintain hope. Don't brush off conversation with a comment like, "Don't worry about it," or "Don't be silly, you're not going to die." Help bolster hope by reminding the person that he's not a statistic, that every case is different, that he's responding to this drug and there are others that can be tried in the future—but discuss it. A reminder that hope survives in the thought of being able to go home, get outdoors, resume old interests and hobbies can be helpful.

Isn't it better if everyone just pretends that the patient isn't dying?

When death is imminent and inevitable, pretending that a patient isn't dying is very difficult both for the patient and for his family and friends. It puts a tremendous burden on the patient, often plunging him into depression. Accepting the fact that the patient is going to die opens the way for the patient to dissipate his loneliness and depression by allowing him to verbalize some of his feelings. Naturally, if stoicism is the family's way of life, they can deal with this in their accustomed ways. But stoicism is not denial, and pretense really does not make it easier for the patient.

Is it normal for me to feel angry that my husband/wife/child has had such a long illness?

This is a perfectly natural response that has nothing to do with your feelings about the person—so don't punish yourself by feeling guilty.

How can I respond or find out if my friend wants to talk about the cancer?

Many comments will lead you to an opening where you can ask a question which leads into whatever that friend wants to tell you. Just say, "Do you feel like talking about it?"

Where can I look for information on the different kinds of health services available in my community?

Many communities, even quite small ones, have a directory of health agencies available in the community. Ask at the public library—you'll be amazed to find agencies you never knew existed. Look also in the yellow pages, ask your doctor, call the social services department at your hospital, the American Cancer Society, or the Visiting Nurses Association.

What kinds of help are available in the community which might make it possible for me to care for a patient at home?

The American Cancer Society is a good place to turn for information, counseling, transportation help, nursing care, medications, blood, prostheses, loans of such items as wheelchairs, beds, walkers, bedpans, etc. The United States

Department of Health, Education and Welfare and state, city, and county health departments as well as family service agencies can be contacted for advice and guidance. The important thing to remember is that you must let others know you need help—and you must not be shy about asking for it. There are many skilled professionals and volunteers out there who want to be of help, but you have to let them know your needs.

Where can I get some information about caring for a patient at home?

The American Red Cross offers a course which teaches home-nursing skills as well as first aid. Learning the basics and following the guidance of available health personnel can make it possible for you to care for the patient at home—bringing comfort and peace to convalescence. There is a great deal of helpful written material on the subject of home nursing available either through your library or other resources. One of the most comprehensive is *Home Care*, by Jane Henry Stolten, R.N. (New York: Little, Brown). Inexpensive pamphlets are available through the U.S. Department of Health, Education and Welfare, Washington, D.C.; your local state, county, and city health departments; such companies as the Metropolitan Life Insurance Company (1 Madison Avenue, New York, N.Y. 10010); and Public Affairs Pamphlets (381 Park Avenue South, New York, N.Y. 10016). Copies of the National Directory of Medicare Home Health Agencies may be obtained by writing the Social Security Admnistration, 6401 Security Blvd., GM1 E. Low Rise Building, Baltimore, Md. 21235. Ask for SSA-PUB-10018. The National League of Nursing also has free booklets on home health care. Copies are available from National League of Nursing, 10 Columbus Circle, New York, N.Y. 10019.

How can I create a restful atmosphere for convalescence?

The best way is to be aware. To someone who is ill, little things create problems—a noisy TV, loud music, heavy footsteps, a rattling window, incessant telephone, constant chattering. Being alert to such patience-triers and resolving them before they become problems can help to make convalescence easier. Turning down the bell sound on the telephone, wearing rubber-soled shoes, and in other small ways giving consideration to the patient's needs can make life easier for everyone.

What suggestions do you have for setting up the sickroom?

- Make sure the room is near a bathroom.
- Give the patient a handbell so you can be called when needed. A small transistorized walkie-talkie set might be used for this purpose.
- A hospital bed is helpful if the patient will spend much time in bed. A low bed is best for a patient who is able to move from bed. Be sure such a bed is firmly anchored and will not slip when the patient uses it to support himself.
- Mattresses can be protected with a waterproof pad. Placing a drawsheet on the bed under the patient's hips provides added protection. Disposable waterproof bed pads are a great innovation.
- A visitor's chair encourages relaxed visiting.
- A bedside table with space for tissues, drinking water, a radio, extension telephone, and reading and writing materials should be provided.
- A good light, firmly attached and within easy reach, is a must.
- A pull-up device can be made to help some patients in rising from bed or in changing position. A strong rope, tied to the end of the bed, knotted at intervals, is very useful.
- Other special items such as bathtub handrails, bed tables, and such items available at surgical supply houses should be considered.
- Whenever possible, help the patient to enjoy a change of scenery by making it possible for him—through the use of a wheelchair or walker if necessary—to spend part of the day sitting up or resting in the family living room or kitchen, where he can join the rest of the family and not feel so isolated.

What is a normal temperature?

Depending on where the temperature is taken—mouth, rectum, or under the armpit—the temperature varies slightly. When the thermometer is placed under the tongue and held there for three minutes with the mouth firmly closed, the normal oral temperature is 98.6° Fahrenheit or 37° Centigrade. When taken rectally—and this method is usually used when the patient is having difficulty breathing, is confused, or is a small child—the normal temperature is 99.6° Fahrenheit or 37.5° Centigrade. A rectal thermometer has a fat bulblike silver tip and should be lubricated before being inserted. An oral thermometer has a long slender silver tip. Either an oral or a rectal thermometer may be used to take the armpit (axillary) temperature. The silver tip should be placed well inside the armpit and the arm held tight against the body. The thermometer is left in place for ten minutes. Normal armpit (axillary) temperature is 97.6° Fahrenheit or 36° Centigrade.

How is a sterile dressing applied?

A sterile dressing is one which is free of germs, and it is used to protect a wound from infection or to absorb a discharge. Usually the doctor or nurse will instruct you in how a dressing should be applied. If medication is to be used, the object which will be used to apply the medication must be sterilized. You can use a spoon, a round-edged silver knife, or a wooden tongue depressor. Sterilize by placing in a pan, completely covered with water, and boiling for 10 minutes. Holding cover in place, drain off water, leaving articles in the covered pan. After removing the soiled dressing, carefully unwrap the sterile dressing, apply medication to the inside of the dressing with the sterile knife, spoon, or wooden blade, and apply dressing to the wound. Be careful not to touch anything but the edges of the dressing (or better yet, wear sterilized gloves). If you touch any part being placed on the patient's wound, you will contaminate the dressing and it will no longer be sterile.

Is it a good idea to get a hospital bed for use at home?

Hospital beds are a wonderful help and may be purchased or rented (the monthly fee may be covered by your medical insurance or Medicare) or they may be borrowed from the American Cancer Society, visiting nurses, or various voluntary health agencies.

How can I help prevent bedsores?

It is important to change the position of the patient frequently. Pillows of various sizes, both hard and soft, are a help, and it is a good idea to have a variety of them on hand to help make the patient comfortable. Rolled-up pillows can also be used to help keep the weight of bedclothes off the toes, knees, or other parts of the body. Covered cardboard cartons placed under the upper sheet at the foot of the bed to protect the toes or next to the thigh or abdomen will help keep the weight of bedclothes away from the body. Also available are bedpads of real or synthetic sheepskin which form a soft, comfortable surface for the frail patient.

What can I do about leg cramps when I'm in bed?

Leg cramps can be a problem when lying in bed for long periods of time. One simple exercise which is effective in relieving leg cramps is pumping the toes. This can be done with the legs extended or with the knees bent. All that is needed is to flex the toes toward the sole of the foot, then straighten them out flat. Doing this regularly, several times a day, can help prevent leg cramps.

How do you give a back rub?

Warm body lotion or alcohol by placing the bottle in a pan of warm water. Then, starting at the patient's neck, move gently with long, firm strokes down to the lower spine and buttocks and up again to the neck. Repeat several times. Circular motions can also be used. Back rubs are a wonderful way to help the patient to relax, and they help to stimulate circulation.

Can I learn how to give a bed bath?

This is one of the techniques which the visiting nurse can teach. Briefly, these are the things to remember:
- Always follow the same order starting with the eyes, face, neck, ears, chest and abdomen, far arm, near arm, hands, far leg, near leg, feet, back, buttocks, genitals. You'll notice this order is designed to use the cleanest water on the most sensitive areas. Another method used recommends: face, arms and trunk to hips, back and buttocks, legs, feet, and genitals. Bath water can be changed before the back, buttocks, and genitals are washed. Hands and feet can be washed in the basin. Allow the patient to wash the genitals if he or she is able to do so.

- Prepare washbasin, warm water, washcloths, towels, soap, and toilet articles beforehand. An extra cotton blanket or large bathtowel will be needed to cover the patient when you remove the gown or pajamas. Expose only the part of the body to be washed. Place a towel under each part as you wash it, dry thoroughly, and cover. Remember to support the patient's arms and legs directly under the joints during the bath.
- Allow the patient to do as much for himself or herself as is safely possible.

How do you give a patient a shower?

A shower is less strain on a patient than a tub bath and is often recommended by the doctor. A shower chair—a small straight chair on locking wheels—is most useful. Some have a cut-out seat for easier bathing of genitals. Soap on a string around the patient's neck is another convenience. A ramp so that the shower chair can be wheeled into the shower will help simplify the procedure. Be sure to test the strength, direction, and temperature of the water before the patient enters. Aim the spray to reach below shoulder level. Lock brakes on the shower chair. Never leave the patient alone in the shower.

What is the best way to help clean the teeth and mouth and to shave a patient?

If the patient needs help in doing these tasks, place a towel under his or her chin and across the chest and clean the teeth and gums gently with toothpaste and toothbrush or large cotton swabs and mouthwash. Have the patient turn the head to the side and hold the basin snugly under the chin so he or she can rinse when you have finished. If the patient wears dentures, they should be put on before attempting to shave. Soften the whiskers by leaving a towel wrung out in hot water on the face for a few minutes. Stretch the patient's skin tight at all times to prevent cutting skin. Shave by stroking upward and returning downward over the same area.

How can I cope with home-care problems like incontinence and bedsores?

There are numerous ways of dealing with these problems, which often loom as barriers to providing home care for a patient. The doctor and visiting nurse will be most helpful in the decision as to how the patient can be handled best. Incontinence is an embarrassment to the patient—and comes often as such a shock that the patient becomes depressed, cries, and even may insist he or she wants to die rather than be a bother. Organizing the changing process so that it is done quickly and simply helps to alleviate guilt feelings. The use of adult toss-away diapers, sanitary napkins, and bed pads can be helpful. In the case of the male patient, a plastic bag, filled with absorbent toweling or tissues, secured to the patient with masking tape can sometimes help solve much of the problem. The visiting nurse can be most helpful in teaching you specific techniques for handling this difficult job.

How can I keep track of the medicines that need to be taken?

It is a good idea to keep a daily written record of the type and amount of medicine and the time it was given, along with a record of the patient's temperature and pulse, etc., as recommended by the doctor—especially when more than one person is helping care for the patient. Remember that you must give only the medicines prescribed by the physician at the times and in the amounts specified. One helpful idea for pills is to set out the amount needed for the day when the first pill is taken. This makes it easy to check to see that all medications are taken each day.

What do the abbreviations mean on prescriptions?

The typical prescription gives the dosage strength in milligrams (mg.), usually notes the type of medicine such as capsule or tablet, how many times a day it should be taken, and how much of the medicine you can get from the prescription. If the prescription can be refilled, it is also noted on the prescription blank. Some of the terms commonly used include:

- a.c. (ante cibos): before meals
- ad lib. (ad libitum): at pleasure, at discretion, take drug freely as needed
- d (die): day
- dur. dolor (durante dolor): while the pain lasts
- g.: gram

- h. (hora): hour
- h.d. or h.s. (hora somni): at bedtime
- mg.: milligrams
- omn. hor. or omn. noct.: every hour or every night
- p.c. (post cibos): after meals
- p.o. (per os): by mouth
- p.r.n.(pro re note): whenever necessary
- q. (quaque): every
- q.2.h. (quaque 2 hora): every two hours (number in middle changes)
- q.d. (quaque die): every day

What is parenteral feeding?

This form of feeding is used for patients who, as a consequence of surgical or radiation treatment, are unable to eat normally or patients who need to be built up nutritionally before surgery, chemotherapy, or radiation treatments. A hollow plastic tube is inserted surgically into a central vein. The parenteral fluids—a mixture of amino acids, fat, sugar, vitamins, and other essential nutrients—are slowly infused into the tube by means of a small pump which the patient operates. It takes 10 to 14 hours to infuse a full day's nourishment but the patient can usually rest or sleep while the food is being injected. Any patient who requires long-term parenteral feeding and who does not otherwise require being in a hospital can be cared for at home.

What should I tell the doctor when I call him to tell about a change in the patient's condition?

Always start by giving your name and the patient's name, address, and telephone number. Explain that you are calling because of changes in the patient's condition. Before calling, write down all the pertinent information such as:

- What has happened to prompt you to call the doctor—heavy breathing, weak pulse, rise in temperature, etc.
- The time when the changes took place and how the patient's condition has changed

If you want the doctor to visit the patient, be sure to say so. Listen carefully and write down any instructions you are given.

Should I feel guilty about not being able to care for my child/ parent/spouse at the end?

Many people who have been able to take part in care during the course of the illness find it impossible to cope with the final stages of the illness. This is a very painful time, and each family must find its own answers. If the patient is hospitalized, arrangements can usually be made for some member of the family to stay at the hospital, helping as much or as little as he or she chooses.

How can the patient be helped to die in comfort?

When it is determined that the patient is dying and there is no reasonable hope that he will recover, the family and his doctor can make plans to help the patient die comfortably. Either at home or in the hospital, all testing and transfusions, etc., can cease. This means that temperature no longer needs to be taken at the usual intervals, and the measuring of intake and output and the obtaining of blood samples can all be curtailed so that the patient will not be disturbed. Glucose and water can be given intravenously if the patient cannot eat or drink and complains of thirst. Morphine, or whatever drugs are most effective, should be prescribed to be given according to need. Oxygen may be used if there is shortness of breath. A catheter can be inserted in the bladder for comfort. The important thing for everyone to keep in mind is that any measures that are taken should be only for the purpose of maintaining the patient's comfort.

What kind of care must be given to the dying patient?

Being with the patient as much as possible is the most important consideration. Remember that even if the patient does not seem to be able to hear what is happening, his awareness may be very acute. The patient may want to talk about dying, and we should help him to do so. He may be in physical distress and frightened, restless, gasping for breath and disoriented. Keep the patient warm. Most important, keep the mouth moist. Special oiled swabs which can be used to remove mucus from inside the mouth and which help keep the mouth and lips moist are most helpful. Placing the patient on his side helps drain mucus from mouth and nose. Every effort must be made to reduce irritating conditions. and provide an atmosphere that is peaceful and comfortable.

What can the family do when the hospital wants to continue to prolong life but the patient and his family do not want heroic measures used?

This is not an uncommon situation—and it is a difficult one for the patient, family, doctor, and hospital. The hospital is geared to prolonging life and health-care personnel often find it difficult to deal with death. Ideally, the question should be discussed with the doctor early in the illness so that he understands the family's viewpoint from the outset. But ideal conditions do not always prevail and the doctor's views may not always coincide with the feelings of the family and his patient. Several avenues can be considered. Asking for a consultation with another doctor is a possibility. The patient can be transferred to another facility, or better still, brought home. Though it may be frightening to think of caring for the patient at home, most families are able to handle the patient very well in the home with the support of some outside help—such as the visiting nurses and an understanding physician.

What is the final stage in the life of most cancer patients?

Every case is different, so there is no certainty regarding the pattern the disease will follow. Most cancer patients die of something other than cancer itself. If there is extensive involvement of cancer with various body systems, a great strain is placed on the heart and respiratory system. The patient often lapses into a coma or intermittent unconsciousness. It is at this time that decisions regarding life-prolonging measures must be made—and they should be made in accordance with the patient's wishes if they have been made known. When it is no longer possible to communicate with the patient, it is the patient's known feelings and the family's wishes that will help to guide the physician to what course must be taken whether to continue to keep the patient alive (and this can be done, these days, almost indefinitely, if that is desired) or to allow the patient to die naturally.

What are the specific signs of impending death?

People in the health-care field who see death almost every day tell us that although many people think of death as being a traumatic time for the patient, in reality, most people die very peacefully, in their sleep or while at rest. The signs of death will vary from patient to patient. It is very important to note changes in the patient's normal status. Some of the significant changes to be aware of include:

- Marked changes in breathing: labored, spasmodic heavy breathing, followed by quiet or shallow breathing or a decreased number of breaths per minute (sometimes referred to as Cheyne-Stokes respiration)
- Heartbeat rate either faster or slower than usual
- Change in skin texture and temperature; though the patient feels cold to the touch, he may perspire profusely.
- Lapsing in and out of consciousness, being confused, or going into a coma
- Loss of sensation, power of motion, and/or reflexes first in legs, then in arms
- A tendency to turn the head toward the light as a result of failing sight and hearing

When the patient dies, be sure the body is laid flat on the back with one pillow under the head. Close the eyes and mouth. If necessary, clean the patient. Put any dentures or artificial parts in place. Fold the hands on the chest.

Why are autopsies necessary after someone has suffered so much?

This final examination, made so the physician may see the effects of the disease and gather new information for use in the future, is sometimes requested. By comparing clinical findings, treatment for others with the same disease may be improved in the future.

The medical profession treats an autopsy as a surgical procedure with full respect of the individual.

My husband's/child's/parent's illness was so prolonged that I felt only relief when the end came, and this makes me feel so guilty.

When the illness is prolonged, often the grieving process is completed before the actual death. It is not uncommon for the family to feel relief that the pain, suffering, and uncertainty have ended. Some people may misinterpret this acceptance and think that you are hard-hearted and unfeeling. You must not feel guilty, for this has been found to be a perfectly normal reaction. People experience grief in different ways, and often the deepest grief is felt by those who do not show grief outwardly.

I'd like to make a contribution in memory of a friend who died of cancer. How can I do this?

There are several ways. The American Cancer Society, listed in the white pages of the telephone directory, accepts contributions for research. Contributions can be earmarked for the specific type of cancer in which you are interested. On a more personal level, you can send contributions to the oncology department of your local hospital or to one of the cancer centers listed in Chapter 23. Hospice, St. Jude's, and other such organizations accept contributions in the name of someone who has died of cancer. Be certain that you include with your contribution the name of the deceased, the name and address of the person to whom you wish the acknowledgment sent, and your own name and address.

Do you have suggestions on ways I can express my sympathy?

Most of us say, "If there's anything I can do, let me know"—and feel terribly helpless and disappointed if our friends do not ask for help. Better to look for an immediate need and try to fill it— helping with baby sitting, or providing food, being there when needed, taking charge of some routine task such as telephoning those who need to be notified, quietly returning the rented hospital bed or wheelchair, meeting an incoming train or plane, offering a spare room to an overnight visitor, or providing transportation for necessary errands. When bringing food, it is wisest to use a container that can be discarded. If you bring food in your own dish, be sure to mark your name on the bottom, and stop by to pick up the dish so the family won't have to think about returning it. A little note with a personal reference, recalling some special quality you will remember about the deceased, or referring to some event that was shared, makes it easy to write something meaningful and comforting. The important time to be aware is after the funeral is over and all the relatives have departed. Stay in touch, suggest an outing, include your friend in your family plans, and help your friend to get involved in outside activities.

chapter 23

Where to Get Help

Although the information given in this chapter is as up to date as possible, the situation in cancer research and treatment is constantly changing. You should expect to find that some of your inquiries will be routed to different organizations or individuals, and you should not limit your investigations to the organizations listed here.

Where is the best place to start to get help?

There are two major sources of information: the Cancer Information Service and the American Cancer Society.

What is the Cancer Information Service?

The Cancer Information Service (CIS) is a nationwide telephone service funded by the National Cancer Institute. A trained staff answers (or will find answers) to questions for the general public (in layman's language) and for health professionals. The staff can give you information on causes of cancer, how to help prevent it, methods of detection, how cancer is diagnosed, ways of treatment, rehabilitation assistance, medical facilities, home-care assistance programs, financial aids, emotional counseling services, and patient referrals. It can provide support, understanding, and rapid access to the latest information on cancer and local resources. It can tell you where in the country investigational treatment is being conducted, and what hospitals and doctors in your area are involved in which kinds of investigational treatment. If, for instance, your relative lives in a different part of the country, the staff can get information from the appropriate CIS office for you. The Cancer Information Offices are affiliated with comprehensive cancer centers (specialized research and treatment centers recognized by the National Cancer Institute) and the American Cancer Society.

What kind of questions should I ask when I call the Cancer Information Service?

The more specific you can be with your questions, the better the information you will receive. It is wise to think through what you want to know and to write down the questions you want to have answered before you call. You can call as many times as you wish. You do not have to give your name if you do not want to. All calls are kept confidential.

Can the Cancer Information Service send me written information about cancer?

The Cancer Information Offices are supplied with a wealth of printed information about cancer. All of them have brochures which are supplied by the National Cancer Institute. Some also have available brochures from the American Cancer Society. The material will be sent to you free of charge.

How can I call the Cancer Information Service?

More than half the country's population is within the areas directly served by regional Cancer Information Service offices which maintain toll-free lines for use by residents in the areas they serve. The rest of the country is served by the Cancer Information Service Office at the National Cancer Institute.

The phone numbers are:

ALASKA:	1-800-638-6070
CALIFORNIA:	southern part—area codes 213, 714, 805: 1-800-252-9066 rest of state: 213-226-2374
COLORADO:	1-800-332-1850
CONNECTICUT:	1-800-922-0824
DELAWARE:	1-800-523-3586

FLORIDA:	1-800-432-5953 in Dade County: 305-547-6920 for Spanish-speaking callers: 1-800-432-5955 for Spanish-speaking callers in Dade County: 305-547-6960
HAWAII:	Oahu—524-1234 (neighboring islands—ask operator for Enterprise 6702)
ILLINOIS:	800-972-0586
KENTUCKY:	800-432-9321
MAINE:	800-225-7034
MARYLAND:	800-492-1444
MASSACHUSETTS:	1-800-952-7420
MINNESOTA:	1-800-582-5262
MONTANA:	1-800-525-0231
NEW HAMPSHIRE:	1-800-225-7034
NEW JERSEY:	800-523-3586
NEW MEXICO:	1-800-525-0231
NEW YORK STATE:	1-800-462-7255
NEW YORK CITY:	212-794-7982
NORTH CAROLINA:	1-800-672-0943
OHIO:	800-282-6522
PENNSYLVANIA:	1-800-822-3963
PUERTO RICO:	1-800-638-6070
TEXAS:	1-800-392-2040
VERMONT:	1-800-225-7034
VIRGIN ISLANDS:	1-800-638-6070
WASHINGTON, D.C. metropolitan area:	202-232-2833
WASHINGTON STATE:	1-800-552-7212
WISCONSIN:	800-362-8038
WYOMING:	1-800-525-0231
ALL OTHER AREAS:	800-638-6694

What is the American Cancer Society?

The American Cancer Society (ACS), a voluntary organization of some 2.5 million Americans, is a national organization fighting cancer through research, education, patient service and rehabilitation programs. It is composed of a national society with 58 chartered divisions and nearly 3,000 local units. The national society administers programs of research, medical grants, and clinical fellowships and is charged with carrying out public and professional education at the national level. The divisions are in all states, in addition to six metropolitan areas, the District of Columbia, and Puerto Rico. The units are organized to cover the counties in the United States. Some units have branches which cover smaller geographic areas.

What kind of help can I get through the American Cancer Society?

The units of the American Cancer Society conduct basic service programs, including information and counseling service for the cancer patient and the patient's family (information and guidance concerning ACS services, community health services and other resources), equipment loans (sickroom supplies and special comfort items to assist in caring for the homebound patient, such as hospital beds, walkers, aspirators, blenders, bedpans, urinals, pressure pillows, incontinent pads, and wheelchairs, etc.), surgical dressings prepared by volunteers, and transportation to and from a doctor's office, clinic, or hospital for treatment. Some units also provide home health care, blood programs, assistance with employment problems, social-work assistance, and medications. Rehabilitation programs, primarily directed toward laryngectomy, mastectomy, and ostomy patients, are an important part of the service offered. These include Lost Cord clubs, Reach-to-Recovery volunteers, ostomy clubs, and Candlelighters as well as support groups for patients and their families.

How can I reach the American Cancer Society?

You can reach local units in most areas of the country by telephone. Look in the white pages under "American Cancer Society." Ask for the person in charge of patient services. The American Cancer Society can also answer many questions by telephone and offers printed material on cancer free of charge.

Will I have to visit the offices of the American Cancer Society in order to get help?

It depends upon what you are looking for. If you want counseling help or are looking for guidance in finding resources for financial aid, you will probably need to visit the office to discuss your problems. If you are looking for loan equipment, you will have to make arrangements to pick it up. If you have a simple question, it will probably be answered immediately on the phone. Your first step in all cases, however, is to make a telephone call.

What is the mailing address for the American Cancer Society?

The address for the national office is American Cancer Society, 777 Third Avenue, New York, N.Y. 10017. The addresses for the divisions are:

Alabama Division, Inc.
2926 Central Avenue
Birmingham, Ala. 35209
205-897-2242

Alaska Division, Inc.
1343 G Street
Anchorage, Alaska 99501
907-277-8696

Arizona Division, Inc.
634 West Indian School Road
P.O. Box 33187
Phoenix, Ariz. 85067
602-264-5861

Arkansas Division, Inc.
5520 West Markham Street
P.O. Box 3822
Little Rock, Ark. 72203
501-664-3480-1-2

California Division, Inc.
731 Market Street
San Francisco, Calif. 94103
415-777-1800

Colorado Division, Inc.
1809 East 18th Avenue
P.O. Box 18268
Denver, Colo. 80218
303-321-2464

Connecticut Division, Inc.
Barnes Park South
14 Village Lane
Wallingford, Conn. 06492
203-265-7161

Delaware Division, Inc.
Academy of Medicine Bldg.
1925 Lovering Avenue
Wilmington, Del. 19806
302-654-6267

District of Columbia Division, Inc.
Universal Building, South
1825 Connecticut Avenue, N.W.
Washington, D.C. 20009
202-483-2600

Florida Division, Inc.
1001 South MacDill Avenue
Tampa, Fla. 33609
813-253-0541

Georgia Division, Inc.
2025 Peachtree Road, N.E.
Suite 14
Atlanta, Ga. 30309
404-351-3650-1-2

Hawaii Division, Inc.
Community Services Center Bldg.
200 North Vineyard Boulevard
Honolulu, Hawaii 96817
808-531-1662-3-4-5

Idaho Division, Inc.
1609 Abbs Street
P.O. Box 5386
Boise, Ida. 83705
208-343-4609

Illinois Division, Inc.
37 South Wabash Avenue
Chicago, Ill. 60603
312-372-0472

Indiana Division, Inc.
2702 East 55th Place
Indianapolis, Ind. 46220
317-257-5326

Iowa Division, Inc.
Highway No. 18 West
P.O. Box 980
Mason City, Iowa 50401
515-423-0712

Kansas Division, Inc.
3003 Van Buren Street
Topeka, Kan. 66611
913-267-0131

Kentucky Division, Inc.
Medical Arts Bldg.
1169 Eastern Parkway
Louisville, Ky. 40217
502-459-1867

Louisiana Division, Inc.
Masonic Temple Bldg., Room 810
333 St. Charles Avenue
New Orleans, La, 70130
504-523-2029

Maine Division, Inc.
Federal and Green Streets
Brunswick, Me. 04011
207-729-3339

Maryland Division, Inc.
200 East Joppa Road
Towson, Md. 21204
301-828-8890

Massachusetts Division, Inc.
247 Commonwealth Avenue
Boston, Mass. 02116
617-267-2650

Michigan Division, Inc.
1205 East Saginaw Street
Lansing, Mich. 48906
517-371-2920

Minnesota Division, Inc.
2750 Park Avenue
Minneapolis, Minn. 55407
612-871-2111

Mississippi Division, Inc.
345 North Mart Plaza
Jackson, Miss. 39206
601-362-8874

Missouri Division, Inc.
715 Jefferson Street
P.O. Box 1066
Jefferson City, Mo. 65101
314-636-3195

Montana Division, Inc.
2820 First Avenue South
Billings, Mont. 59101
406-252-7111

Nebraska Division, Inc.
Overland Wolfe Centre
6910 Pacific Street, Suite 210
Omaha, Neb. 68106
402-551-2422

Nevada Division, Inc.
953-35B East Sahara
Suite 101 S. T. & P. Bldg.
Las Vegas, Nev. 89104
702-733-7272

New Hampshire Division, Inc.
22 Bridge Street
Manchester, N.H. 03101
603-669-3270

New Jersey Division, Inc.
2700 Route 22, P.O. Box 1220
Union, N.J. 07083
201-687-2100

New Mexico Division, Inc.
525 San Pedro, N.E.
Albuquerque, N.M. 87108
505-262-1727

New York State Division, Inc.
6725 Lyons Street
P.O. Box 7
East Syracuse, N.Y. 13057
315-437-7025

> **Long Island Division, Inc.**
> 535 Broad Hollow Road
> (Route 110)
> Melville, N.Y. 11746
> 516-420-1111

> **New York City Division, Inc.**
> 19 West 56th Street
> New York, N.Y. 10019
> 212-586-8700

> **Queens Division, Inc.**
> 111-15 Queens Boulevard
> Forest Hills, N.Y. 11375
> 212-263-2224

> **Westchester Division, Inc.**
> 246 North Central Avenue
> Hartsdale, N.Y. 10530
> 914-949-4800

North Carolina Division, Inc.
222 North Person Street
P.O. Box 27624
Raleigh, N.C. 27611
919-834-8463

North Dakota Division, Inc.
Hotel Graver Annex Bldg.
115 Roberts Street
P.O. Box 426
Fargo, N.D. 58102
701-232-1385

Ohio Division, Inc.
453 Lincoln Bldg.
1367 East Sixth Street
Cleveland, Ohio 44114
216-771-6700

Oklahoma Division, Inc.
1312 Northwest 24th Street
Oklahoma City, Okla. 73106
405-525-3515

Oregon Division, Inc.
910 N.E. Union Avenue
Portland, Ore. 97232
503-231-5100

Pennsylvania Division, Inc.
3309 Spring Street
P.O. Box 4175
Harrisburg, Penn. 17111
717-545-4215

> **Philadelphia Division, Inc.**
> 21 South 12th Street
> Philadelphia, Penn. 19107
> 215-567-0559

Puerto Rico Division, Inc.
(Avenue Domenech 273
   Hato Rey, P.R.)
GPO Box 6004
San Juan, P.R. 00936
809-764-2295

Rhode Island Division, Inc.
345 Blackstone Blvd.
Providence, R.I. 02906
401-831-6970

South Carolina Division, Inc.
2442 Devine Street
Columbia, S.C. 29205
803-787-5623

South Dakota Division, Inc.
700 South 4th Avenue
Sioux Falls, S.D. 57104
605-336-0897

Tennessee Division, Inc.
2519 White Avenue
Nashville, Tenn. 37204
615-383-1710

Texas Division, Inc.
3834 Spicewood Springs Road
P.O. Box 9863
Austin, Texas 78766
512-345-4560

Utah Division, Inc.
610 East South Temple
Salt Lake City, Utah 84102
801-322-0431

Vermont Division, Inc.
13 Loomis Street, Drawer C
Montpelier, Vt. 05602
802-223-2348

Virginia Division, Inc.
3218 West Cary Street
P.O. Box 7288
Richmond, Va. 23221
804-359-0208

Washington Division, Inc.
323 First Avenue West
Seattle, Wash. 98119
206-284-8390

West Virginia Division, Inc.
Suite 100
240 Capitol Street
Charleston, W. Va. 25301
304-344-3611

Wisconsin Division, Inc.
611 North Sherman Avenue
P.O. Box 1626
Madison, Wis. 53701
608-249-0487

Milwaukee Division, Inc.
6401 West Capitol Drive
Milwaukee, Wis. 53216
414-461-1100

Wyoming Division, Inc.
Indian Hills Center
506 Shoshoni
Cheyenne, Wyo. 82001
307-638-3331

**Affiliate of the
American Cancer Society**
Canal Zone Cancer Committee
Drawer A
Balboa Heights, Canal Zone

What are other organizations which give direct help to cancer patients and their families?

There are several.

ASK A FRIEND TO EXPLAIN RECONSTRUCTION (AFTER)
99 Park Avenue
New York, N.Y. 10016
212-986-9099

Volunteer group. Puts you in touch with a woman who has had breast-reconstruction surgery. Also sends out pamphlet on subject.

CANDLELIGHTERS
123 C Street, S.W.
Washington, D.C. 20003
202-483-9100

Organization of parents of young cancer patients. Helps other families of cancer patients cope with living with disease. Regular meetings held to discuss problems and exchange ideas. Nationally, supports programs for cancer research with Congress. About 100 active groups in 43 states. Call the American Cancer Society or the Cancer Information Service to get information about groups in your area.

ENCORE
YWCA

For postoperative breast-cancer patients. Exercise plan (usually includes some swimming) plus discussion group. Call your local YWCA branch.

DES ACTION
Long Island Jewish Hillside Medical Center
New Hyde Park, N.Y. 11040
212-343-9222

Grass-roots, self-help support organization of volunteers. Active in public
education and legislation related to the DES problem. Serves as a resource for
mothers and daughters confronted with the DES problems. Maintains a
telephone hotline. Chapters in California, Connecticut, Massachusetts, Michigan,
New Jersey, Oregon, Pennsylvania, and Washington, D.C.

HOSPICE
NATIONAL HOSPICE ORGANIZATION
765 Prospect Street
New Haven, Conn. 06511

Hospice concept is modeled after St. Christopher's Hospice in England. Can
include both home care and inpatient services. Focuses on quality of survival
rather than length of survival. To be admitted in most cases, patient must be
referred by physician, and live in area served by hospice. For home care, must
have a family member, friend, or other helper available on around-the-clock
basis. Over 100 groups now exist in 33 states in various stages of development.
The national organization, formed in 1978, aims at realizing the goal of hospice as
individual programs and as a nationwide method of delivering health care. It is
publishing a directory listing institutions giving service.

INTERNATIONAL ASSOCIATION OF LARYNGECTOMEES (IAL)
219 East 42nd Street
New York, N.Y. 10017
212-867-3700

Voluntary organization composed of 190 member clubs. Also called Lost Cord,
Anamilo, or New Voice Clubs. Assists people who have lost their voices as a result
of cancer, provides education in skills needed by laryngectomees, and works
toward total rehabilitation of patient. Maintains registry of postlaryngectomy
speech instructors, publishes educational materials, sponsors meetings and other
activities. Sponsored by American Cancer Society. Look in phone book for local
chapter or call local cancer society office.

INTERNATIONAL UNION AGAINST CANCER (UNION INTERNATIONALE
CONTRE LE CANCER)
Rue Conseil-General 3
1205 Geneva
Switzerland
Tel: 20 18 11

Nongovernmental, voluntary organization devoted solely to promoting
throughout the world the campaign against cancer in its research, therapeutic,
and preventive aspects. Worldwide association with member organizations in 78
countries. Facilitates exchange of information between national cancer organizations. Published, with NCI support, "International Directory of Specialized
Cancer Research and Treatment Establishments," first edition 1976.

LEUKEMIA SOCIETY OF AMERICA, INC.
211 East 43rd Street
New York, N.Y. 10017

National voluntary health agency which provides supplementary financial assistance to patients with leukemia, the lymphomas and Hodgkin disease as well as referral services to other sources of help in the community. Program is administered through society chapters located throughout the United States. Payment can be made for drugs used in care, treatment and/or control of disease, transfusing of blood, transportation to and from a doctor's office, hospital or treatment center, and x-ray treatment. There are chapters in Alabama, Arizona, California, Colorado, Connecticut, Delaware, District of Columbia, Florida, Georgia, Illinois, Kansas, Louisiana, Maryland, Massachusetts, Missouri, New Jersey, New York, Ohio, Pennsylvania, Rhode Island, Texas, Virginia, and Wisconsin. Look in your local directory or write to the address above.

MAKE TODAY COUNT, INC.
P.O. Box 202
Burlington, Iowa 52601
319-754-7266 during business hours
319-754-8977 other times

Provides psychological assistance to patients with advanced cancer and to their families. Helps people live each day as fully and happily as possible. Group meetings, home visit programs, newsletters, and material distribution. Founded by Orville E. Kelly, a cancer patient. About 135 chapters in some 20 states. Look in local directory or write to address above.

REACH TO RECOVERY
American Cancer Society
777 Third Avenue
New York, N.Y. 10017
202-371-2900

Offers assistance to breast-cancer patients. Trained volunteers who have had breast cancer lend emotional support and furnish information. In most places, must have physician referral. Look in phone book for number of local American Cancer Society office.

UNITED OSTOMY ASSOCIATION (UAC)
1111 Wilshire Boulevard
Los Angeles, Calif. 90016
213-481-2811

Organized and administered by ostomates. Helps ostomy patients return to normal life through mutual aid and moral support. Has nearly 500 local chapters. Provides information to patients and public and contributes to improvement of ostomy and supplies. Publishes *Ostomy Quarterly* and other educational materials. American Cancer Society also furnishes services to ostomates through its ostomy rehabilitation program. Helps ostomates adjust to everyday experiences of work, travel, and recreation. Offers ostomy therapy training. Call the American Cancer Society for information about local chapters.

What is the National Cancer Institute?

The National Cancer Institute (NCI) is a branch of the U.S. Department of Health, Education and Welfare. It is responsible for establishing a structure for a coherent and systematic attack on cancer throughout the United States through a network of shared information, funding for research, and standards for research facilities and treatment centers. Its director is Arthur C. Upton, M.D. The address is National Cancer Institute, National Institutes of Health, Bethesda, Md. 20014.

Where are the comprehensive cancer centers located?

There are 21 comprehensive cancer centers designated by the National Cancer Institute. These medical research centers investigate new methods of diagnosis and treatment of cancer patients and provide new scientific knowledge to doctors who are treating cancer patients. They must meet 10 specific criteria, which include basic and clinical research and patient care. This listing includes the physician director and the director of public and professional information.

ALABAMA:

John R. Durant, M.D., Director
Comprehensive Cancer Center
University of Alabama in Birmingham
University Station
Birmingham, Ala. 35294
205-934-5077

Ms. Gail Bayer, Coordinator,
Cancer Communication Office
205-934-2651

CALIFORNIA:

G. Denman Hammond, M.D., Director
Los Angeles County-University of Southern California Comprehensive Cancer Center
2025 Zonal Avenue
Los Angeles, Calif. 90033
213-226-2008

Gordon Cohn, Director
Office of Cancer Communications
213-226-2371

CALIFORNIA (continued)

Richard J. Steckel, M.D., Director
UCLA-Jonsson Comprehensive Cancer Center
UCLA School of Medicine
924 Westwood Boulevard, Suite 940
Los Angeles, Calif. 90024
213-825-5268

Mrs. Devra Breslow, Editor, Bulletin
213-825-5412

COLORADO:

Steven G. Silverberg, M.D.
Executive Director
Colorado Regional Cancer Center, Inc.
165 Cook Street
Denver, Colo. 80206
303-320-5921

Ms. Judy Spolum, Project Supervisor
303-320-5921

CONNECTICUT:

Jack W. Cole, M.D., Director
Yale University Comprehensive
  Cancer Center
333 Cedar Street
New Haven, Conn. 06510
203-432-4122

Ms. Marion Morra, Communications
  Program Manager
203-436-3779

DISTRICT OF COLUMBIA:

Georgetown University/Howard
  University Comprehensive Cancer
  Center
John F. Potter, M.D., Director
Vincent T. Lombardi Cancer Research
  Center
Georgetown University
3800 Reservoir Road, N.W.
Washington, D.C. 20007
202-625-7066
and
Jack E. White, M.D., Director
Howard University Cancer Research
  Center
Department of Oncology
2041 Georgia Avenue, N.W.
Washington, D.C. 20060
202-745-1406

Mr. Godfrey Jacobs, Executive Director
Cancer Coordinating
Council for Metropolitan Washington
202-797-8876

FLORIDA:

C. Gordon Zubrod, M.D., Director
Comprehensive Cancer Center for the
  State of Florida
University of Miami School of
  Medicine/Jackson Memorial Medi-
  cal Center

FLORIDA (continued)

Centre House, Roof Garden
1400 N.W. 10th Ave.
Miami, Fla. 33136
305-547-6758

Ms. Beth H. Strunk, Coordinator,
  Cancer Information Service
305-547-6678

ILLINOIS:

Jan W. Steiner, M.D., Director
Illinois Cancer Council (includes
  Northwestern University Cancer
  Center, University of Chicago
  Cancer Research Center, Rush-
  Presbyterian-St. Luke's Medical
  Center, University of Illinois and
  several other health organizations)
37 S. Wabash Avenue
Chicago, Ill. 60603
312-346-9813

Carol Gibson, Coordinator, Cancer Information Service
312-346-9813

MARYLAND:

Albert H. Owens, Jr., M.D., Director
Johns Hopkins Comprehensive Cancer
  Center
600 N. Wolfe Street
Baltimore, Md. 21205
301-955-3300

Ms. Donna Cox, Communications Director
301-955-3636

MASSACHUSETTS:

Emil Frei III, M.D., Director
Sidney Farber Cancer Institute
44 Binney Street
Boston, Mass. 02115
617-732-3555

Ms. Martha Wood, Communications
  Officer
617-732-3150

MICHIGAN:

Michael J. Brennan, M.D., Director
Comprehensive Cancer Center of
  Metropolitan Detroit (includes the
  Michigan Cancer Foundation and
  Wayne State University)
110 East Warren Street
Detroit, Mich. 48201
313-833-0710

Ley Chilton, Cancer Information Service Coordinator

MINNESOTA:

Charles G. Moertel, M.D., Director
Mayo Comprehensive Cancer Center
200 First Street, S.W.
Rochester, Minn. 55901
507-282-3261

Ms. Kristin Gunderson Ritts, Communications Specialist
507-284-8285

NEW YORK:

Paul A. Marks, M.D., and Richard A.
  Rifkind, M.D., Directors
Columbia University Cancer Center
Institute of Cancer Research
Hammer Health Sciences Center
701 West 168th Street
New York, N.Y. 10032
212-694-3807

Mrs. Mae Rudolph, Public Information
212-694-4161

Lewis Thomas, M.D., President
Memorial Sloan-Kettering Cancer
  Center
1275 York Avenue
New York, N.Y. 10021
212-794-7646

Ms. Miriam Adams, Director, Office of
  Cancer Communications
212-794-7982

NEW YORK (continued)

Gerald P. Murphy, M.D., Institute
  Director
Roswell Park Memorial Institute
666 Elm Street
Buffalo, N.Y. 14203
716-845-5770

Mr. Russell Sciandra, Cancer Control
  Communications Officer
716-845-4402

NORTH CAROLINA:

William W. Shingleton, M.D., Director
Duke University Comprehensive
  Cancer Center
P.O. Box 3814
Durham, N.C. 27710
919-684-2282

Diane McGrath, Ph.D.
Director, Cancer Control Program
919-286-2214

OHIO:

David S. Yohn, Ph.D., Director
The Ohio State University Comprehensive Cancer Center
357 McCampbell Hall
1580 Cannon Drive
Columbus, Ohio 43210
614-422-5022

Ms. Nancy Kesselring Brant, Communications Director
614-422-5022

PENNSYLVANIA:

Timothy R. Talbot, M.D., President
Fox Chase/University of Pennsylvania
  Comprehensive Cancer Center
7701 Burholme Avenue
Philadelphia, Pa. 19111
215-728-2717

Ms. Christine Wilson, Communications
  Coordinator
215-728-2700

TEXAS:

Charles LeMaistre, President
The University of Texas System Cancer
  Center
M.D. Anderson Hospital and Tumor
  Institute
6723 Bertner Avenue
Houston, Texas 77030
713-792-3000

Ms. Sandy Pinto, Cancer Information
  Service Program Administrator
713-792-3363

WASHINGTON:

William B. Hutchinson, M.D., Director
Fred Hutchinson Cancer Research
  Center
1124 Columbia Street
Seattle, Wash. 98104
206-292-2930

Mr. David Docter, Communications
  Officer
206-292-6301

WISCONSIN:

Paul P. Carbone, M.D., Director
The University of Wisconsin Clinical
  Cancer Center
Clinical Science Center
600 Highland Avenue
Madison, Wisc. 53705
608-263-5404

Ms. Pixie Hoopes, Public Affairs Coordinator
608-262-0046

Where are clinical and nonclinical cancer centers?

Clinical and nonclinical cancer centers are medical centers
which have support from the National Cancer Institute for
clinical programs to investigate promising new methods of cancer
treatment or for nonclinical research programs.

CALIFORNIA:

Dr. Steven K. Carter*
Director, Northern California
Cancer Program
770 Welch Road, Suite 190
Palo Alto, Calif. 94304
415-497-5353

Dr. Henry S. Kaplan**
Maureen Lyles D'Ambrogio Professor
  of Radiology
Director, Cancer Biology Research
  Laboratory

Stanford University Medical Center
Stanford, Calif. 94305
415-497-7313
415-497-5055

Dr. C. Arthur Knight**
Chairman, Department of Molecular
  Biology
Director, Virus Laboratory
University of California
Berkeley, Calif. 94720
415-642-7057

  *Clinical Cancer Center
 **Non-Clinical Cancer Center

Dr. Gordon H. Sato°°
University of California
P.O. Box 109
La Jolla, Calif. 92037
714-452-3095

Dr. F.M. Huennekens°°
Chairman, Department of Biochemistry
Director, Specialized Cancer Center
Scripps Clinic and Research Foundation
10666 N. Torrey Pines Road
La Jolla, Calif. 92037
714-455-9100, ext. 338

Dr. William R. Clark°°
Associate Professor in Biology
Department of Biology
University of California
Los Angeles, Calif. 90024
213-825-7684

Dr. Walter Eckhart°°
Associate Research Professor
Armand Hammer Center for Cancer
Biology
The Salk Institute
P.O. Box 1809
San Diego, Calif. 92112
714-453-4100, ext. 386

GEORGIA:

Dr. Charles H. Huguley, Jr., Director°
Emory University Cancer Center
Rm. 606F, Emory University Hospital
Atlanta, Ga. 30322
404-329-7016

HAWAII:

Dr. Lawrence H. Piette, Director°
Cancer Center of Hawaii
University of Hawaii at Manoa
1997 East-West Road
Honolulu, Hawaii 96822
808-948-7173
808-948-7246

IDAHO:

Dr. Charles E. Smith°
Medical Director
Mountain States Tumor Institute
151 East Bannock
Boise, Ida. 83702
208-345-1780

KANSAS:

Dr. James T. Lowman, Director°
Mid-America Cancer Center Program
The University of Kansas Medical
Center
College of Health Sciences & Hospital
Rainbow Boulevard at 39th
Kansas City, Kans. 66103
913-588-5700

MASSACHUSETTS:

Dr. Sidney R. Cooperband, Director°
Boston University Cancer Research
Center
80 East Concord Street
Boston, Mass. 02118
617-247-6075

Dr. Mahlon B. Hoagland°°
President and Scientific Director
Worcester Foundation for Experimental Biology, Inc.
222 Maple Avenue
Shrewsbury, Mass. 01545
617-842-8921

MISSOURI:

Missouri Cancer Programs, Inc.°
115 Business Loop 70 West
Columbia, Mo. 65201
314-449-3945

Dr. Samuel B. Guze°°
Director of Cancer Centers
Washington University School of
Medicine
660 South Euclid Avenue
St. Louis, Mo. 63110
314-454-3013

°Clinical Cancer Center
°°Non-Clinical Cancer Center

NEW JERSEY:

Dr. Jacques R. Fresco, Director°°
Basic Science Cancer Center
Princeton University
Frick Chemical Laboratory
Princeton, N.J. 08540
609-452-3927

NEW MEXICO

Dr. Morton M. Kligerman, Director°
Cancer Research and Treatment
  Center
University of New Mexico
Albuquerque, N.M. 87131
505-277-2151

NEW YORK:

Dr. Leonard Weiss, Director°
Department of Experimental
  Pathology
Roswell Park Memorial Institute
Cancer Cell Center
666 Elm Street
Buffalo, N.Y. 14203
716-845-3311

Dr. Harry Eagle, Director°
Cancer Research Center
Albert Einstein College of Medicine
1300 Morris Park Avenue
Bronx, N.Y. 10461
212-430-2302
212-792-2233

Dr. Vincent P. Hollander, Director°
Research Institute for Skeletomuscular
  Diseases
Hospital for Joint Diseases and Medi-
  cal Center
1919 Madison Avenue
New York, N.Y. 10035
212-876-7222

NEW YORK (continued)

Dr. Paul A. Marks, Director°
Columbia University Cancer Research
  Center
College of Physicians & Surgeons
701 West 168th Street
New York, N.Y. 10032
212-694-3807
212-694-4138

Dr. H. Sherwood Lawrence°
Professor & Head, Infectious Disease
  & Immunology Division
Department of Medicine
New York University Medical Center
550 First Avenue
New York, N.Y. 10016
212-679-3200

Dr. Robert A. Cooper, Jr., Director°
University of Rochester Cancer Center
601 Elmwood Avenue
Rochester, N.Y. 14642
716-275-4865

Dr. Norton Nelson°°
Professor and Chairman
Department of Environmental
  Medicine
New York University Medical Center
550 First Avenue
New York, N.Y. 10016
212-679-3200, ext. 2881

Dr. Ernst L. Wynder°°
President and Medical Director
American Health Foundation
1370 Avenue of the Americas
New York, N.Y. 10019
212-489-8700

°Clinical Cancer Center
°°Non-Clinical Cancer Center

NORTH CAROLINA:

Dr. Joseph S. Pagano, Director°
Cancer Research Center
University of North Carolina
Box 3, Swing Building 217H
Chapel Hill, N.C. 27514
919-966-1183
919-966-3036

Dr. Charles L. Spurr°
Director, Oncology Research Center
Bowman Gray School of Medicine
300 South Hawthorne Road
Winston-Salem, N.C. 27103
919-727-4464

OHIO:

Dr. Arthur Flynn, Director°
The Cancer Center, Inc.
11000 Cedar Avenue
Cleveland, Ohio 44106
216-421-7300

Dr. Earle C. Gregg°°
Professor of Radiology (Physics)
University Hospitals
2065 Adelbert Road
Cleveland, Ohio 44106
216-444-3522

OKLAHOMA:

Dr. G. Bennett Humphrey, Director°
Oklahoma Cancer Center
University of Oklahoma Health
  Sciences Center
P.O. Box 26901
Oklahoma City, Okla. 73190
405-271-4485

PENNSYLVANIA:

Dr. Fred Rapp, Professor and Chairman°°
Department of Microbiology
The Pennsylvania State University College of Medicine
Hershey, Pa. 17033
717-534-8253

PENNSYLVANIA (continued)

Dr. Hilary Koprowski, Director°°
The Wistar Institute of Anatomy and
  Biology
36th Street at Spruce
Philadelphia, Pa. 19104
215-387-6700, ext. 201

Dr. Peter N. Magee, Director°°
Fels Research Institute
Temple University Medical School
3420 N. Broad Street
Philadelphia, Pa. 19140
215-221-4312

PUERTO RICO:

Dr. Enrique Perez-Santiago°
Director, Puerto Rico Cancer Center
University of Puerto Rico
Medical Sciences Campus
G.P.O. Box 5067
San Juan, P.R. 00936
809-763-2443
809-765-2363

RHODE ISLAND:

Dr. Paul Calabresi°
Physician-in-Chief
Roger Williams General Hospital
825 Chalkstone Avenue
Providence, R.I. 02908
401-456-2070

TENNESSEE:

Dr. James J. Nickson, Director°
Memphis Regional Cancer Center
800 Madison Avenue
Memphis, Tenn. 38163
901-528-5739

Dr. Alvin M. Mauer, Medical Director°
St. Jude Children's Research Hospital
332 North Lauderdale
Memphis, Tenn. 38101
901-525-8381, ext. 271
°clinical
°°non-clinical

TEXAS:

Dr. Eugene P. Frenkel*
Director, Cancer Center
University of Texas Health Science
    Center
5323 Harry Hines Boulevard
Dallas, Texas 75235
214-688-2182

Dr. William C. Levin, President*
The University of Texas Medical
    Branch
Administration Building, Suite 646
Galveston, Texas 77550
713-765-1902

WISCONSIN:

Dr. Donald Pinkel*
Professor & Chairman
Department of Pediatrics
Medical College of Wisconsin
1700 West Wisconsin Avenue
Milwaukee, Wis. 53233
414-344-7100, ext. 374

  *Clinical Cancer Center
**Non-Clinical Cancer Center

VIRGINIA:

Dr. Walter Lawrence, Jr.*
MCV/VCU Cancer Center
Box 37 MCV Station
Medical College of Virginia
Virginia Commonwealth University
Richmond, Va. 23298
804-770-7682
804-770-7476

How can I tell which types of cancer are being studied by the various National Cancer Institute groups?

Each group with a set of initials after its name is doing studies in various areas. If you check the disease in which you are interested, you will be able to determine which group is studying that disease. Your doctor can then contact the chairman of the group to see if you will be eligible to become involved in the study or to get information about the new treatments being used. You can also call the Cancer Information Service to find out if any doctors in your area are part of the group.

BTSG	Brain Tumor Chemotherapy Study Group
CALB	Cancer and Leukemia Cooperative Group B
CCG	Children's Cancer Study Group

EORTC	European Organization for Research on Treatment of Cancer
EST	Eastern Cooperative Oncology Group
GTSG	Gastrointestinal Tumor Study Group
GOG	Gynecologic Oncology Group
HNCP	Head and Neck Contracts Program
LCSG	Lung Cancer Study Group
NSABBP	National Surgical Adjuvant Project for Breast and Bowel Cancers
NWTS	National Wilms Tumor Study Group
NCOG	Northern California Oncology Group
OCSG	Ovarian Cancer Study Group
PVSG	Polycythemia Vera Study Group
RTOG	Radiation Therapy Oncology Group
RHDG	Radiotherapy Hodgkin Disease Group
SEG	Southeastern Cancer Study Group
SWOG	Southwest Oncology Group
UORG	Uro-Oncology Research Group
VALCSG	Veterans Administration Lung Cancer Study Group
VASAG	Veterans Administration Surgical Adjuvant Cancer Chemotherapy Study Group

BREAST

EORTC
CALB
EST
NSABBP
RTOG
SEG
SWOG

BRAIN &
SPINAL CORD

EORTC
BTSG
CCG
EST
RTOG
SWOG

GASTROINTESTINAL

Esophagus	Stomach	Hepatoma	Pancreas	Colon/ Rectum
EORTC	EORTC	CCG	EST	EORTC
EST	EST	EST	GTSG	CALB
RTOG	GTSG	SEG	SWOG	GTSG
SWOG	NCOG	SWOG	VASAG	NSABBP
VASAG	SWOG			EST
	VASAG			SEG
				RTOG
				SWOG
				VASAG

GENITOURINARY

General	Bladder	Ureter	Kidney	Prostate	Testes
EORTC	EORTC	EST	EORTC	EORTC	EST
CCG	CCG	SWOG	EST	EST	SEG
EST	EST		SWOG	RTOG	SWOG
NCOG	NCOG			SEG	
RTOG	RTOG			SWOG	
SEG	SEG			UORG	
SWOG	SWOG				
UORG	UORG				

GYNECOLOGIC

General	Cervical	Ovary	Uterus	Vulva/ Vagina
EORTC	GOG	EORTC	EST	GOG
CCG	NCOG	CCG	GOG	
EST	SEG	EST	RTOG	
GOG		GOG		
NCOG		NCOG		
SEG		OCSG		
SWOG		RTOG		
		SEG		

HEAD
& NECK
_____

EORTC
CALB
EST
HNCP
NCOG
SWOG
VASAG
RTOG

LUNG
Small
Cell   *Other*
_____

EORTC	EORTC
CALB	CALB
EST	EST
NCOG	LCSG (Surg. & Adj. Chemo)
RTOG	SEG
SEG	SWOG
SWOG	VASAG
	VALCSG

MELANOMA
_____

EORTC
EST
SEG
SWOG

LEUKEMIA
(CHILDREN)
_____

CALB
CCG
SWOG

LEUKEMIA
(ADULTS)

EORTC
CALB
EST
NCOG
SEG
SWOG

LYMPHOMAS
(*Both Hodgkin &*
non-Hodgkin)

EORTC
CALB
CCG
EST
SEG
SWOG

OTHER
HEMATOLOGIC
(*Myeloma, Histiocytosis,*
Polycythemia Vera,
Mycosis Fungoides, Other)

EORTC
CALB
CCG
EST
PVSG
SEG
SWOG

PEDIATRIC SOLID TUMORS

Wilms	*Neuro-blastoma*	*Retino-blastoma*	*Rhabdomyo-sarcoma*	*Ewing*
CALB	CALB	CCG	CALB	CALB
CCG	CCG	SWOG	CCG	CCG
NWTS	SWOG		SWOG	SWOG
SWOG				

EORTC also studies Pediatric Solid Tumors

SARCOMA

General	Osteogenic	Soft Tissue
EORTC	CALB	EORTC
CCG	CCG	CALB
EST	EST	EST
RTOG	SWOG	RTOG
SEG		SWOG
SWOG		

Where are clinical cooperative groups located?

Clinical cooperative groups, which are funded by the National Cancer Institute to investigate promising new methods of cancer treatment, are located in many of the medical institutions in the United States and abroad. Some 440 institutes in the United States and abroad are involved, including 3,300 cancer researchers. Following laboratory research, the treatment is evaluated in cancer patients. Clinical cooperative groups are working on anticancer drugs, radiotherapy, immunotherapy, and surgery, alone or in various combinations.

Listed are the various clinical trials groups and institutional projects funded by the National Cancer Institute, and the names of the chairmen of the groups, operations office and statistical office. Your doctor can call doctors on the list to get information about new forms of treatment or to ask about the possibility of entering a patient in a study. If you wish to know whether a doctor or an institution in your area is participating in any of the groups, call the Cancer Information Service number in your area.

BRAIN TUMOR CHEMOTHERAPY STUDY GROUP (BTSG)

Michael D. Walker, M.D., Chairman
Building 31, Room 4B32
National Cancer Institute, NIH
Bethesda, Md. 20014
301-496-6361

Operations and Statistical Office:

Thomas A. Strike, Ph.D., Administra-
tor
Landow Building, Room 8C19
National Cancer Institute, NIH
Bethesda, Md. 20014
301-496-5297

CANCER AND LEUKEMIA COOPERATIVE GROUP B (CALB)

James F. Holland, M.D., Chairman
Department of Neoplastic Disease
Mt. Sinai School of Medicine
100th Street and Fifth Avenue
New York, N.Y. 10029
212-650-6364

Operations Office:

Cathy White, Administrator
Two Overhill Road, Suite 208
Scarsdale, N.Y. 10583
914-472-0710

Statistical Office:

Oliver Glidewell
Two Overhill Road, Suite 208
Scarsdale, N.Y. 10583
914-472-0710

CHILDREN'S CANCER STUDY GROUP

Denman Hammond, M.D., Chairman
University of Southern California
2025 Zonal Avenue
Keith Administration Building
Room 509
Los Angeles, Calif. 90033
213-226-2008

Operations Office:

Richard Honour, Ph.D., Administrator
University of Southern California
School of Medicine
1721 Griffin Avenue
Los Angeles, Calif. 90031
213-223-1373

Statistical Office:

John Weiner, Ph.D.
University of Southern California
School of Medicine
Barracks A
2025 Zonal Avenue
Los Angeles, Calif. 90033
213-226-4051

CLINICAL TRIALS for BREAST, GASTROINTESTINAL, and BRAIN TUMORS

Umberto Veronesi, M.D., Principal
  Investigator
Gianni Bonadonna, M.D., Co-Principal
  Investigator
Istituto Nazionale per lo Studio e la
  Cura dei Tumori
Via Venezia 1
20133 Milano, Italy

COORDINATING CENTER for CLINICAL STUDY of MELANOMA

Umberto Veronesi, M.D., Principal
  Investigator
Gianni Bonadonna, M.D., Co-Principal
  Investigator
Istituto Nazionale per lo Studio e la
  Cura dei Tumori
Via Venezia 1
20133 Milano, Italy

EASTERN COOPERATIVE ONCOLOGY GROUP (EST)

Paul Carbone, M.D., Chairman
Wisconsin Clinical Cancer Center
701-C University Hospital
1300 University Avenue
Madison, Wisc. 53706
608-262-9703

Operations Office:

905 University Avenue
Suite 415
Madison, Wisc. 53715
608-263-6650

Statistical Office:

Marvin Zelen, Ph.D.
Kenneth Stanley, Ph.D.
Sidney Farber Cancer Institute
44 Binney Street
Boston, Mass. 02115
617-732-3012

GASTROINTESTINAL CANCER RESEARCH PROGRAM

Philip Schein, M.D., Principal
  Investigator
Georgetown University School of
  Medicine
37th and O Streets, NW
Washington, D.C. 20057
202-625-7081

GASTROINTESTINAL TUMOR STUDY GROUP (GTSG)

Charles Moertel, M.D., Co-Chairman
Mayo Clinic
Rochester, Minn. 55901
507-282-2511 x3261

Philip Schein, M.D., Co-Chairman
Georgetown University Medical
  Center
3800 Reservoir Road, NW
Washington, D.C. 20007
202-625-7081

Operations Office:

Philomena Grifone, Administrator
850 Sligo Avenue, Suite 601
Silver Spring, Md. 20910
301-585-4844

Statistical Office:

Philip Lavin, Ph.D.
John McIntyre, Ph.D.
44 Binney Street
Boston, Mass. 02115
617-732-3012

GYNECOLOGIC ONCOLOGY GROUP (GOG)

George C. Lewis, Jr., M.D., Chairman
Gynecologic Group Headquarters
P.O. Box 60
Philadelphia, Pa. 19105
215-928-6030

Operations Office:

Kathleen Dierks, Administrator
P.O. Box 60
Philadelphia, Pa. 19105
215-928-6030

Statistical Office:

John Blessing, Ph.D.
Roswell Park Memorial Institute
Kress Building
666 Elm Street
Buffalo, N.Y. 14203
716-845-5702

HEAD AND NECK CONTRACTS PROGRAM (HNCP)

William McGuire, M.D., Project
  Officer
Landow Bldg., Room 8C04
National Cancer Institute, NIH
Bethesda, Md. 20014
301-496-2522

Operations Office:

Philomena Grifone, Administrator
850 Sligo Avenue, Suite 601
Silver Spring, Md. 20910
301-585-4844

Statistical Office:

Richard Simon, Ph.D.
Building 10, Room 3B16
National Cancer Institute, NIH
Bethesda, Md. 20014
301-496-4504

LUNG CANCER STUDY GROUP (LCSG)

William McGuire, M.D., Project
  Officer
Landow Building, Room 8C04
National Cancer Institute, NIH
Bethesda, Md. 20014
301-496-2522

Operations Office:

Philomena Grifone, Administrator
850 Sligo Avenue, Suite 601
Silver Spring, Md. 20910
301-585-4844

Statistical Office:

David Byar, Ph.D.
Landow Building, Room 5C09
National Institutes of Health
Bethesda, Md. 20014
301-496-4208

NATIONAL SURGICAL ADJUVANT PROJECT FOR BREAST AND BOWEL CANCERS (NSABBP)

Bernard Fisher, M.D., Chairman
914 Scaife Hall
3550 Terrace Street
Pittsburgh, Pa. 15261
412-624-2671

Operations Office:

Lisa Marino, Administrator
914 Scaife Hall
3550 Terrace Street
Pittsburgh, Pa. 15261
412-624-2671

Statistical Office:

Carol Redmond, Ph.D.
914 Scaife Hall
3550 Terrace Street
Pittsburgh, Pa. 15261
412-624-3027

NATIONAL WILMS TUMOR STUDY GROUP (NWTS)

Giulio D'Angio, M.D., Chairman
Children's Hospital of Philadelphia
One Children's Center
3400 Civic Center Boulevard
Philadelphia, Pa. 19104
215-387-5518

Operations Office:

Patricia Wolverton, Administrator
Children's Hospital of Philadelphia
One Children's Center
3400 Civic Center Boulevard
Philadelphia, Pa. 19104
215-387-5518

Statistical Office:

Norman Breslow, Ph.D.
Fred Hutchinson Cancer Research
  Center
1102 Columbia Street
Seattle, Wash. 98104
206-292-2226

NORTHERN CALIFORNIA ONCOLOGY GROUP (NCOG)

Stephen K. Carter, M.D., Chairman
1801 Page Mill Road
Building B, Suite 200
Palo Alto, Calif. 94304
415-497-7431

Operations Office:

Martha Kaplan, Administrator
1801 Page Mill Road
Building B, Suite 200
Palo Alto, Calif. 94304
415-497-7512

Statistical Office:

Byron W. Brown, Jr., Ph.D.
Department of Biostatics
Stanford University Medical Center
Stanford, Calif. 94305
415-497-5687

OVARIAN CANCER STUDY GROUP (OCSG)

William McGuire, M.D., Project
  Officer
Landow Bldg., Room 8C04
National Cancer Institute, NIH
Bethesda, Md. 20014
301-496-2522

Operations and Statistical Office:

Richard M. Simon, Ph.D.
Building 10, Room 3B16
National Institutes of Health
Bethesda, Md. 20014
301-496-4504

PHASE I STUDIES OF NEW ANTICANCER DRUGS

Vincent Bono, M.D., Project Officer
Cancer Therapy Evaluation Program
Building 37, Room 6E22
National Institutes of Health
Bethesda, Md. 20014
301-496-5223

PHASE II/III STUDIES IN PATIENTS WITH DISSEMINATED SOLID TUMORS

William McGuire, M.D., Coordinator
Landow Building, Room 8C04
National Cancer Institute, NIH
Bethesda, Md. 20014
301-496-2522

PHASE II TRIALS IN GASTROINTESTINAL CARCINOMA

Edward Cooper, M.D., Principal
  Investigator
University of Leeds School of Medicine
Leeds LS2, 9NL, England

POLYCYTHEMIA VERA STUDY GROUP (PVSG)

Louis R. Wasserman, M.D., Chairman
Department of Hematology
Mt. Sinai Hospital
11 E. 100th Street
New York, N.Y. 10029
212-876-2734

Operations Office:

Helen Walton, Administrator
19 E. 98th Street
New York, N.Y. 10029
212-876-2734

Statistical Office:

Judith Goldberg, Ph.D.
New York University Medical School
550 First Avenue
New York, N.Y. 10016
212-650-5851

RADIATION THERAPY ONCOLOGY GROUP (RTOG)

Simon Kramer, M.D., Chairman
Thomas Jefferson University Hospital
1025 Walnut Street
Philadelphia, Pa. 19107
215-829-6702

Operations Office:

Meg Kaiser, Administrator
925 Chestnut Street
Philadelphia, Pa. 19107
215-574-3150

Statistical Office:

Marvin Zelen, Ph.D.
Richard Gelber, Ph.D.
Sidney Farber Cancer Institute
44 Binney Street
Boston, Mass. 02115
617-732-3012

RADIOTHERAPY HODGKIN DISEASE GROUP (RHDG)

George B. Hutchison, M.D., Chairman
Harvard University
School of Public Health
Dept. of Epidemiology
677 Huntington Avenue
Boston, Mass. 02115
617-732-1050

Statistical and Operations Office:

George Hutchison, M.D., Administra-
    tor
Harvard University
School of Public Health
677 Huntington Avenue
Boston, Mass. 02115
617-732-1050

SOUTHEASTERN CANCER STUDY GROUP (SEG)

John R. Durant, M.D., Chairman
Comprehensive Cancer Center
University of Alabama
Tumor Institute, Room 214
Birmingham, Ala. 35294
205-934-5077

Operations Office:

Virginia Suppers, Administrator
Tumor Institute, Room 225
University of Alabama
University Station
Birmingham, Ala. 35294
205-934-5270

Statistical Office:

Alfred Bartolucci, Ph.D.
Tumor Institute, Room 225
University of Alabama
University Station
Birmingham, Ala. 35294
205-934-5270

SOUTHWEST ONCOLOGY GROUP (SWOG)

Barth Hoogstraten, M.D., Chairman
University of Kansas Medical Center
Kansas City, Kans. 66103
913-588-5996

Operations Office:

Cherri Stadelman, Administrator
3500 Rainbow Boulevard, Suite 100
Kansas City, Kans. 66103
913-588-5996

Statistical Office:

Edmund Gehan, Ph.D.
M.D. Anderson Hospital & Tumor
   Institute
6723 Bertner Drive
Houston, Texas 77030
713-792-3320

URO-ONCOLOGY RESEARCH GROUP (UORG)

David F. Paulson, M.D., Chairman
P.O. Box 2977
Duke University Medical Center
Durham, N.C. 27710
919-684-5057

Operations Office:

Judy Smith, Administrator
VA Hospital
508 Fulton Street
Durham, N.C. 27705
919-286-0411 x6784

Statistical Office:

W. Kenneth Poole, Ph.D.
P.O. Box 12194
Research Triangle Park, N.C. 27709
919-541-6394

VETERANS ADMINISTRATION GROUPS

Thomas Newcomb, M.D., Coordinator
VA Central Office
810 Vermont Avenue, NW
Washington, D.C. 20420
202-389-2616

Carol Richard, Administrative Assistant
VA Hospital
50 Irving Street, NW
Washington, D.C. 20422
202-389-7529

VETERANS ADMINISTRATION SURGICAL ADJUVANT CANCER CHEMOTHERAPY STUDY GROUP (VASAG)

George A. Higgins, M.D., Chairman
Chief, Surgical Service
VA Hospital
50 Irving Street, N.W.
Washington, D.C. 20422
202-389-7266

Operations Office:

Kathleen Fink, Administrator
VA Hospital
50 Irving Street, N.W.
Washington, D.C. 20422
202-389-7266

Statistical Office:

Robert J. Keehn, MFVA/JH616
National Research Council
2101 Constitution Avenue
Washington, D.C. 20418
202-389-6467

Are there clinical cooperative groups in Canada?

There are groups in Canada which are studying various treatments, some in collaboration with U.S. scientists, researchers and doctors. Information is available from:

Dr. Peter Scholefield
National Cancer Institute of Canada
77 Bloor Street West, Suite 401
Toronto, Ontario, Canada M582 V7
416-961-7223

There is also a Cancer Society in Canada:

The Canadian Cancer Society
77 Bloor Street West
Toronto, Ontario, Canada M582 V7
416-961-7223

Are there clinical cooperative groups in Europe?

There are numerous groups in Europe which are studying various treatments and working in collaboration with U.S. scientists, researchers, and doctors. They are known as the European Organization for Research on Treatment of Cancer (EORTC). The address of the chairman for each group is given below.

EUROPEAN ORGANIZATION FOR RESEARCH ON TREATMENT OF CANCER (EORTC)

Institut Jules Bordet
1000 Brussels (Belgium)
Henri J. Tagnon, M.D., President
Maurice J. Staquet, M.D., Director
Coordinating and Data Center

Screening and Pharmacology

L.M. van Putten
Radiobiological Institute TNO
Lange Kleiweg 151
Rijswijk (ZH) (The Netherlands)

Clinical Screening

E. Pommatau
Centre Léon Bérard
28, rue Laénnec
69373 Lyon Cedex 2 (France)

Leukemia and Hematosarcoma

H.O. Klein
Medizinische Universitätsklinik
Josef-Stelzmann-Strasse 9
Köln-Lindenthal (W. Germany)

Bronchial Carcinoma

O. Monod
8, rue Aubriot
75004 Paris (France)

Breast Cancer

E. Engelsman
Antoni van Leeuwenhoekhuis
Plesmanlaan 121
Amsterdam (The Netherlands)

Gastrointestinal Tract Cancer

J. Loygue
Service de Chirurgie
Hôpital Saint-Antoine
184, rue du Faubourg-St.-Antoine
75012 Paris (France)

Thyroid Cancer

P. Dor
Institut Jules Bordet
rue Héger-Bordet, 1
1000 Bruxelles (Belgium)

Genitourinary Tract Cancer

Ph. H. Smith
Consultant in Urology
St. James's Hospital
Leeds LS9 7TF (England)

Melanoma

E. Macher
Hautklinik, Westfal. Wilhelm Universität
von-Esmarch-Strasse 56
44 Munster (W. Germany)

Radiochemotherapy

M. Burgers
Wilhelmina Gasthuis
Eerste Helmersstraat 104
Amsterdam-Oud-West (The Netherlands)

Radiotherapy

A. Laugier
Hôpital Tenon
4, rue de la Chine
75020 Paris (France)

Head and Neck Cancer

R. Molinari
Istituto Nazionale per lo Studio e la
 Cura dei Tumori
 Via Venezia 1
20133 Milano (Italy)

Brain Tumors

J. Brihaye
Institut Jules Bordet
rue Héger-Bordet 1
1000 Bruxelles (Belgium)

Early Clinical Trials

H. Hansen
Chief, Chemotherapy Department
Finseninstitutet
Strandboulevarden 49
2100 Copenhagen (Denmark)

Cancer of the Ovary

A. Maskens (Secretary)
Clinique Saint Michel
rue L. de Lantsheere, 19
1040 Bruxelles (Belgium)

Soft Tissue Sarcoma

G. Bonadonna
Istituto Nazionale dei Tumori
Via Venezia 1
20133 Milano (Italy)

E.O.R.T.C. PROJECT GROUPS

Gnotobiotic

D. van der Waaij
Department for Medical Microbiology
University Hospital
Groningen (The Netherlands)

Tumor Immunology

R.W. Baldwin
Cancer Research Campaign Labs
University Park
Nottingham NG7 2RD (England)

Antimicrobial Therapy

H. Gaya
Department of Bacteriology
Wright-Fleming Institute
St. Mary's Hospital Medical School
London W2 1PG (England)

Metastases

K. Hellmann
Imperial Cancer Research Fund
Cancer Chemotherapy Department
P.O. Box 123
Lincoln's Inn Fields
London WC2A 3PX (England)

Cell Surface

P. Strauli
Department of Cancer Research
Aussenstation der Universität
Birchstrasse 95
8050 Zürich (Switzerland)

Fast Neutron Therapy

K. Breur
Wilhelmina Gasthuis
Eerste Helmersstraat 104
Amsterdam-Oud-West (The Nether-
 lands)

E.O.R.T.C. CLUBS
Choriocarcinoma

K.D. Bagshawe
Charing Cross Hospital
London W6 8RF (England)

Tissue Culture

L. Morasca
Istituto di Ricerche Farmacologiche
"Mario Negri"
62, Via Eritrea
20157 Milano (Italy)

GI²C (Groupe d'Immunologie et d'Immunothérapie du Cancer)

G. Meyer
Centre Antincancereux
232, boulevard de Ste. Marguerite
13273 Marseille Cedex 2 (France)

Breast Cancer

A. Zwaveling
Academisch Ziekenhuis
Leiden (The Netherlands)

E.O.R.T.C. WORKING PARTIES
Cancer of the Ovary

B. Jamain
Maternité de l'Hôpital Bichat
170 Boulevard Ney
75018 Paris (France)

Osteosarcomas

A. Trifaud
Hôpital de la Conception
144, rue Saint Pierre
13005 Marseille (France)

Hemopathies

P. Stryckmans (Secretary)
Institut Jules Bordet
rue Héger-Bordet 1
1000 Bruxelles (Belgium)

E.O.R.T.C. TASK FORCES
Breast Cancer

J.C. Heuson
Institut Jules Bordet
rue Héger-Bordet 1
1000 Bruxelles (Belgium)

E. Engelsman (Vice-Chairman)
Antoni van Leeuwenhoek Ziekenhuis
Plesmanlaan 121
Amsterdam (The Netherlands)

Gastrointestinal Tract Cancer

A. Gerard
Institut Jules Bordet
rue Héger-Bordet 1
1000 Bruxelles (Belgium)

What are the National Cancer Institute organ site programs?
For four sites of cancer—large bowel, bladder, prostate, and pancreas—the National Cancer Institute is funding separate interdisciplinary research programs. Your doctor may contact the project director for information about current clinical research or the possibility of entering a patient in the treatment study.

LARGE BOWEL

Dr. Murray M. Copeland
Project Director for the National Large Bowel Cancer Project
M.D. Anderson Hospital and Tumor Institute
Prudential Building
Houston, Texas 77025

BLADDER

Dr. Gilbert Friedell
Project Director for the National Bladder Cancer Project
St. Vincent Hospital
25 Winthrop Avenue
Worcester, Mass. 01610

PROSTATE

Dr. Gerald P. Murphy
Project Director of the National Prostatic Cancer Project
Roswell Park Memorial Institute
666 Elm Street
Buffalo, N.Y. 14203

PANCREAS

Dr. Isidore Cohn, Jr.
Project Director for the National Pancreatic Cancer Project
Louisiana State University School of Medicine
1542 Tulane Avenue
New Orleans, La. 70112

What are the National Cancer Institute's clinical treatment programs?

The National Cancer Institute conducts research clinical programs in three facilities: the National Institutes of Health Clinical Center in Bethesda, Md., the Baltimore Cancer Research Center at the University of Maryland in Baltimore, Md., and the Veterans Administration Hospital in Washington, D.C. Doctors who are engaged in studies of particular types of cancer will accept limited numbers of patients for treatment. Nursing and medical care are provided to study patients without charge. You must be referred by your doctor, who must furnish full medical reports on the patient. The telephone number of the Patient Referral Service is (301) 496-4891. The various branches and kinds of cancer being treated are listed.

CLINICAL ONCOLOGY BRANCH
Baltimore Cancer Research Program

Chief: Peter H. Wiernik, M.D.

Selected adult patients with untreated acute and chronic leukemia, and lymphoma are acceptable for study. Patients with metastatic testicular carcinoma, breast cancer, colon cancer, oat cell carcinoma of the lung, and metastatic sarcoma are acceptable for study provided they have received no prior chemotherapy.

DERMATOLOGY BRANCH

Chief: Marvin A. Lutzner, M.D.

Selected patients with the following diseases will be admitted for study:

Ataxia Telangiectasia
Progeria
Werner's Syndrome

Selected patients with the following diseases will be admitted for treatment and study:

Basal Cell Nevus Syndrome
Benign Mucosal Pemphigoid (ocular pemphigoid)
Bullous Pemphigoid
Cystic Acne
Darier's Disease (keratosis follicularis)
Dermatitis Herpetiformis
Epidermodysplasia Verruciformis (genetic predisposition for flat warts and squamous cell carcinoma)
Erythema Elevatum Diutinum
Fanconi's Anemia (with or without dyskeratosis congenita)
Ichtyosis
Keratosis Palmaris et Plantaris
Multiple Basal Cell Carcinoma
Multiple Warts
Pemphigus Vulgaris
Pityriasis Rubra Pilaris
Rothmund-Thompson Syndrome
Sezary Syndrome
Toxic Epidermal Necrolysis
Skin Cancer—Selected patients with extensive cutaneous basal cell carcinoma will be admitted for study and investigative therapy.
Xeroderma Pigmentosum—Selected patients will be admitted for treatment, study, and long-term follow-up.

IMMUNOLOGY BRANCH

Chief: William D. Terry, M.D.

Immunotherapy and Immunobiology of Neoplastic Diseases—The role of adjuvant immunotherapy is being evaluated in patients between the ages of 15 and 70 with malignant melanoma. Patients with Stage I (level IV or V) or Stage II disease who have been or can be surgically rendered free of clinical disease are candidates for this protocol. Initial evaluation includes clinical and laboratory staging as well as assessment of each patient's immune status. Patients are randomly assigned to treatment with adjuvant immunotherapy, chemotherapy, or no further treatment. During follow-up they are monitored for evidence of antibody and cell mediated immune responses to melanoma cells, in parallel with clinical and laboratory monitoring for evidence of tumor recurrence. In addition, the nature of the immunologic response of patients to selected tumors other than melanoma is under investigation.

MEDICINE BRANCH

Chief: Robert C. Young, M.D.

Breast Carcinoma—With the exception of candidates for hormonal therapy (see below), patients for the breast cancer treatment programs must be under 65 years of age. There should be no other major complicating illnesses.

Patients with disseminated breast cancer who are candidates for chemotherapy must have measurable and evaluable disease and must not have received chemotherapy.

Candidates for hormonal therapy must be under 70 years of age. All must have measurable and evaluable disease. In addition, the Medicine Branch is particularly interested in male patients with breast carcinoma.

Endometrial Carcinoma—Patients under 65 years of age with metastatic disease who are candidates for either hormonal therapy or chemotherapy are eligible provided they have had no previous therapy with these modalities.

Hodgkin Disease and Other Lymphomas—Patients with all stages of disease are admitted for a series of studies using combination chemotherapy, irradiation therapy and combined modality approaches. Only patients with no prior chemotherapy are eligible. All histological types are of interest.

Melanoma—Patients under the age of 65 with no other complicating illnesses are eligible provided they have had no previous chemotherapy or immunotherapy. Stage I patients must have had level 4 or 5 invasion and Stage II patients must have had surgery with biopsy-proven positive nodes within 4 months of referral. Selected patients with metastatic disease may be accepted if they live locally or within a short drive of the NIH campus.

Ovarian Carcinoma—Patients under 65 years of age with no other major illnesses who have epithelial or granulosa cell tumors of the ovary are eligible for admission to the program. Patients at all states of disease are eligible provided they have had no prior chemotherapy or radiotherapy.

Osteogenic Sarcoma—For admission patients must be under 65 years of age with no other major complicating illnesses and have completed resection of the primary tumor within one month of referral. Patients with metastatic disease and without prior adriamycin treatment are eligible for other intensive chemotherapy trials.

Testicular Carcinoma—Patients under the age of 65 with no other complicating illnesses are eligible if they have non-seminomatous testicular cancer and have not received previous radiotherapy or chemotherapy.

METABOLISM BRANCH

Chief: Thomas A. Waldmann, M.D.

Agammaglobulinemia—Selected patients with X-linked agammaglobulinemia, thymoma and agammaglobulinemia are being studied.

Ataxia-Telangiectasia—Patients with ataxia-telangiectasia are admitted for thorough evaluation as well as intensive study of immunologic function. Selected patients with this syndrome and demonstrable T-cell deficiency will receive thymosin therapy.

Calcium Disorders—Selected patients with idiopathic osteoporosis, myositis ossificans progressiva, and calcinosis universalis are admitted for studies of calcium metabolism. Individuals should be between the ages of 21 and 51, ambulatory, and willing to remain in the Clinical Center 3 to 4 weeks for studies.

DiGeorge Syndrome—Selected patients with the DiGeorge syndrome are being admitted for study and therapy.

Gastrointestinal Disorders—Selected patients with gluten-sensitive enteropathy (celiac sprue) will be admitted for study of gastrointestinal and immunologic function. Selected patients with inflammatory bowel disease will be considered for study.

Growth Hormone Deficiency—Selected patients 4 to 20 years of age with isolated growth hormone deficiency or growth hormone deficiency as part of panhypopituitarism are being studied.

Isolated IgA Deficiency—Selected patients with isolated IgA deficiency or IgA deficiency associated with autoimmune disorders are being studied.

Serum Protein Abnormalities—Protein metabolism is being studied in patients with congenital and acquired disorders of the serum proteins, including subjects with idiopathic hypoproteinemia, gastrointestinal protein loss, intestinal lymphangiectasia, allergic gastroenteropathy, and analbuminemia.

Severe Combined Immunodeficiency—Patients with the severe combined immunodeficiency syndrome are being admitted for study and therapy.

Sézary Syndrome—Selected patients with cutaneous T-cell lymphomas and high circulating neoplastic cell counts are being admitted for study, and when indicated, chemotherapy will be given in collaboration with the Division of Cancer Treatment.

Wiskott-Aldrich Syndrome—Patients are admitted for extensive evaluation of their immunodeficiency state. Selected patients are being evaluated in terms of their response to transfer factor therapy.

NCI-VA MEDICAL ONCOLOGY BRANCH

Chief: John D. Minna, M.D.

Veteran and non-veteran patients with various unresectable neoplastic diseases may be referred to this branch for primary treatment protocols. Various clinical and basic research programs are conducted. Combination chemotherapy, radiation therapy, and immunotherapy are under clinical investigation. In addition, basic research in tumor cell virology, genetics, cytogenetics, and immunology is conducted on clinically available material.

Patients with the following neoplastic diseases are of particular interest: lung cancer (particularly small cell carcinoma), prostatic cancer, myeloma and macroglobulinemia, mycosis fungoides, Sézary syndrome, hepatocellular carcinoma, stomach cancer, and patients with a strong family history of malignancy. Preference is given to patients who have not had prior chemotherapy or radiotherapy.

Patients accepted for study and treatment in these programs will be admitted to the NCI-VA Medical Oncology Branch research ward at the Veterans Administration Hospital in the hospital center complex in northwest Washington, D.C.

PEDIATRIC ONCOLOGY BRANCH

Chief: Arthur S. Levine, M.D.

All patients accepted for admission to this Branch may be enrolled in studies of optimal supportive care techniques (e.g., HL-A matched platelet and granulocyte transfusion and laminar air flow protective isolation). Selected patients are considered for bone marrow transplantation, with emphasis on autologous marrow rescue after high-dose chemotherapy. Clinically available materials are employed in basic studies of tumor virology, kinetics, biology, biochemistry, immunology, and genetics.

Acute Leukemia—Untreated patients usually under 30 years of age will be considered for admission. The therapeutic emphasis is on the evaluation of drug combinations and new agents, cranial irradiation, and immunotherapy.

Neuroblastoma—Previously treated or untreated patients of any age over 2 years with metastatic neuroblastoma are being sought for treatment with high dose combination chemotherapy. Studies of cultured tumor cells and biological markers are carried out.

Ewing's Sarcoma—Previously untreated patients of any age with a biopsy-proven diagnosis are eligible for admission and treatment with radiation, chemotherapy, and immunotherapy. Patients who have had resection of the primary tumor are not eligible for these trials.

Non-Hodgkin Malignant Lymphoma (especially Burkitt's Lymphoma)—Patients under 30 years of age with a suspected or proven diagnosis of non-Hodgkin lymphoma are being sought. Patients with a specific diagnosis of Burkitt's lymphoma are considered for admission at any age. While untreated patients are preferred, selected treated patients will be accepted. The treatment emphasis is on combined modality therapy including surgery, radiation, and chemotherapy.

Osteogenic Sarcoma—Previously untreated patients with non-metastatic disease are offered surgical-adjuvant therapy in conjunction with the Surgery Branch. Patients with metastatic disease, with or without previous treatment, are considered for admission at any age. The emphasis is on high dose combination chemotherapy.

Rhabdomyosarcoma and Undifferentiated Sarcomas—Previously treated or untreated patients, usually under 30 years of age and with any stage of the disease, are considered for admission. Combined modality therapy will be evaluated.

RADIATION ONCOLOGY BRANCH

Chief: Eli Glatstein, M.D.

Carcinoma of the Esophagus—Patients with disease confined to the mediastinum will undergo intensive combined modality treatment.

Hodgkin Disease—Patients with previously untreated disease are eligible for full staging and therapy with radiation and/or combination chemotherapy.

Unresectable Chrondosarcoma or Osteogenic Sarcoma—Patients with locally unresectable tumors will receive radiation therapy and radiosensitizers.

Lung Cancer—Patients with biopsy-proven oat cell carcinoma of the lung are eligible for admission and treatment.

Malignant Lymphoma of Non-Hodgkin Type—Patients with a biopsy-proven diagnosis of lymphoma are eligible for admission and treatment if they have had no prior treatment.

SURGERY BRANCH

Chief: Steven A. Rosenberg, M.D., Ph.D.

Melanoma—Patients with malignant melanoma are eligible for admission under several new therapeutic protocols. There is special interest in patients with primary, unoperated, malignant melanomas *or* skin lesions suspected of being malignant melanoma. Patients who have had their primary surgery but do not have disseminated disease are also eligible for admission under several chemotherapeutic and immunotherapeutic adjuvant protocols.

Sarcomas of Bone and Soft Tissues—Patients with these tumors *either* unoperated, biopsied, or having had definitive surgical therapy are eligible for admission for treatment with new chemotherapeutic and immunotherapeutic adjuvant combined modality protocols.

Colorectal Neoplasms—Patients with Dirkes B2 and C malignancies of the colon. All patients with rectal lesions are accepted.

Breast Cancer—Patients with untreated, operable malignancies of the breast diagnosed clinically or by biopsy and patients with breast masses which require biopsy to exclude malignancy will be considered.

Malignancies of the Pancreas—Patients with these malignancies will be considered for admission to new combined therapeutic protocols.

Urinary Tract Tumors—Selected patients with testicular malignancies are considered for treatment. Data derived from investigations of various immunologic factors in these patients are being used to develop improved methods of treatment of testicular malignancies.

Where is the National Cancer Institute supporting rehabilitation research projects?

NCI rehabilitation research projects include studies of methods for assisting patients following surgery for head and neck cancer, psychosocial supports, and nutritional support. Your doctor may consult the principal investigator to get information or to inquire about entering a patient in a study.

HEAD AND NECK CANCERS

Dr. Salvatore Esposito, Principal Investigator
Case Western Reserve University School of Medicine
2040 Adelbert Road
Cleveland, Ohio 44106
(Reconstruction of facial defects in cancer patients)

Dr. Douglas A. Atwood, Principal Investigator
Department of Prosthetic Dentistry
Harvard School of Dental Medicine
188 Longwood Avenue
Boston, Mass. 02115
(Maxillofacial prosthetic rehabilitation for cancer)

Dr. Jerilyn A. Logemann, Principal Investigator
Northwestern University Medical School
303 East Chicago Avenue
Chicago, Ill. 60611
(Prosthetic rehabilitation or oropharyngeal cancer and evaluation of rehabilitation of oropharyngeal cancer)

Dr. Hans R. Lehmeis, Principal Investigator
New York University
New York, N.Y. 10016
(Advanced prosthetics/orthodontics in cancer management)

HEAD AND NECK CANCERS (continued)

Dr. Frank Clippinger, Principal Investigator
Duke University Medical Center
Department of Surgery
P.O. Box 2919
Durham, N.C. 27710
(Sensory feedback leg prosthesis for cancer patients)

Dr. Byron Bailey, Principal Investigator
University of Texas Medical Branch
Department of Otolaryngology
Galveston, Texas 77550
(Electronic laryngeal prosthesis)

Dr. Raymond H. Colton, Principal Investigator
SUNY, Upstate Medical Center
Weiskotten Hall, Room 89
750 East Adams Street
Syracuse, N.Y. 13210
(Investigation of voice change after radiotherapy)

Dr. George A. Gates, Principal Investigator
University of Texas Health Science Center at San Antonio
7730 Floyd Curl Drive
San Antonio, Texas 78284
(Comprehensive rehabilitation of the laryngectomee)

NUTRITIONAL SUPPORT

Dr. Thomas Nealon, Jr., Principal Investigator
St. Vincent's Hospital and Medical Center of New York
153 West 11th Street
New York, N.Y. 10011
(Nutritional component of cancer therapy)

Dr. C.E. Butterworth, Jr., Principal Investigator
University of Alabama at Birmingham School of Medicine
University Station
Birmingham, Ala. 35294
(Nutritional support rehabilitation for cancer patients)

PSYCHOSOCIAL REHABILITATION

University of Kansas Medical Center
Mid-America Cancer Center Program
39th and Rainbow Boulevards
Kansas City, Kans. 66103
(Childhood cancer: psychosocial rehabilitation)

Dr. Ida M. Martinson, Principal Investigator
University of Minnesota School of Nursing
3313 Powell Hall
Minneapolis, Minn. 55455
(Home care for child with cancer)

Dr. George W. Marten, Principal Investigator
St. Jude Children's Research Hospital
332 North Lauderdale
Memphis, Tenn. 38101
(Psychological adaptions to childhood leukemia)

Dr. Jerome Schulman, Principal Investigator
Children's Memorial Hospital
2300 Children's Plaza
Chicago, Ill. 60614
(Coping in families with a leukemic child)

PSYCHOSOCIAL REHABILITATION (continued)

Dr. Joseph R. Castro, Principal Investigator
Mt. Zion Hospital and Medical Center
Zellerback Saroni Tumor Institute
P.O. Box 7921
San Francisco, Calif. 94120
(Exploratory studies for rehabilitation of cancer patients)

Dr. Allen Enelow, Principal Officer
West Coast Cancer Foundation
P.O. Box 7999
San Francisco, Calif. 94120
(Psychosocial aspects of cancer rehabilitation)

Dr. Raphael Good, Principal Investigator
University of Miami School of Medicine
Miami, Fla. 33152
(Psychosocial rehabilitation of oncologic patients)

Dr. Jimmie Holland, Principal Investigator
Montefiore Hospital and Medical Center
Bronx, N.Y. 10467
(Psychological adjustment of radiotherapy)

Dr. Richard S. Lazarus, Principal Investigator
University of California
Berkeley, Calif. 94720
(Coping and cancer: a process-oriented approach)

Dr. Margaret W. Linn, Principal Investigator
Veterans Administration Hospital
1201 N.W. 16th Street
Miami, Fla. 33125
(Humanistic oncology—the omega experience)

Dr. Leo Reeder, Principal Investigator
University of California School of Public Health
Los Angeles, Calif. 90024
(Processes of health behavior and cancer control)

Dr. Arthur Schmale, Principal Investigator
University of Rochester Medical Center
601 Elmwood Avenue
Rochester, N.Y. 14642
(Psychological collaborative group for cancer control)

Drs. Avery D. Weisman and J. William Worden, Principal Investigators
Massachusetts General Hospital
Fruit Street
Boston, Mass. 02114
(Psychosocial interventions in cancer care and suicide and other coping behaviors of cancer patients)

Dr. Charles W. Halbrook, Principal Investigator
Cancer Research Center
Ellis Fischel State Cancer Hospital
Business Loop 70 and Garth Avenue
Columbia, Mo. 65201
(Clerical counseling of the cancer patient)

OTHER

Dr. Jerome Yates, Principal Investigator
Medical Center Hospital
Burgess Residence, Room 122
Burlington, Vt. 05401
(Cancer care and rehabilitation in a rural setting)

What programs are the National Cancer Institute supporting in bone-marrow transplantation?

The National Cancer Institute is supporting programs in bone-marrow transplantation projects in several institutions.

University of California at Los Angeles
School of Medicine
Los Angeles, Calif.
Dr. Martin J. Cline
Dr. Robert F. Gale

Baylor College of Medicine
Houston, Texas
Dr. John J. Trentin

Mercy Catholic Medical Center
Darby, Penn.
Dr. Isaac D'Jerassi

University of Minnesota
Minneapolis, Minn.
Dr. Philip R. Craddock

Johns Hopkins University
Baltimore, Md.
Dr. George W. Santos

University of Pennsylvania
Philadelphia, Penn.
Dr. Richard A. Cooper

Fred Hutchinson Cancer Research
Center
Seattle, Wash.
Dr. Edward D. Thomas
Dr. Rainer F. Storb

University of Washington
Seattle, Wash.
Dr. E. Donnall Thomas

Children's Hospital
Boston, Mass.
Dr. David G. Nathan

Memorial Sloan-Kettering Cancer
Center
New York, N.Y.
Dr. Joseph Burchenal
Dr. Richard O'Reilly

Where is the National Cancer Institute supporting studies on hyperthermia?

The National Cancer Institute is supporting hyperthermia programs in several institutions as well as conducting studies itself. The National Cancer Institute contact is Joan Bull, M.D.

MICROWAVE HYPERTHERMIA:

Dr. Richard Johnson
Roswell Park
Buffalo, N.Y.

Dr. Jane Marmor
Stanford University
Palo Alto, Calif.

Radiation Oncology Groups at University of California (San Francisco, Calif.), Washington University, St. Louis, Mo., Thomas Jefferson University, Philadelphia, Penn.

WHOLE-BODY HYPERTHERMIA

Dr. Sacki
University of New Mexico
Albuquerque, N.M.
505-227-4951

There are a number of other physicians studying hyperthermia. In the field of radio-frequency therapy, a leader is Harry H. LeVeen, M.D., Chief of Surgery at the Veterans Administration Hospital, Fort Hamilton, Brooklyn, N.Y.

Can I get a list of pain clinics?

For a directory of pain clinics, write Committee on Pain Therapy and Acupuncture, American Society of Anesthesiologists, 515 Busse Highway, Park Ridge, Ill. 60068.

Is the National Cancer Institute supporting studies on pain control?

Yes, there are several research programs funded by the National Cancer Institute on the nature of pain and ways to cope with it.

Effect of Biofeedback and
 Hypnosis on Cancer Pain

Dr. Charles Graham
Principal Investigator
Midwest Research Institute
Behavioral Sciences Laboratory
425 Volker Laboratory
Kansas City, Kan. 64110

Pain Control Through
 Hypnosis in Children

Dr. Ernest Hilgard
Principal Investigator
Stanford University
Department of Psychology
Stanford, Calif. 94305

The Comparative Use of
 Supportive Drugs in
 Cancer Patients

Dr. William Regelson
Principal Investigator
MCV Station, Box 273
Medical College of Virginia
Richmond, Va. 23928

Cancer Rehabilitation Through
 Pain Control

Dr. Hubert Rosomoff
Principal Investigator
Department of Neurological Surgery
University of Miami School of Medicine
P.O. Box 520875, Biscayne Annex
Miami, Fla. 33152

Evaluation and Control of Chronic Pain in Cancer	Dr. Berthold Wolff Principal Investigator New York University Medical Center 550 First Avenue New York, N.Y. 10016
Electrical Analgesia for Intractable Pain	Dr. Ronald Ignelzi Department of Psychiatry University of California at San Diego La Jolla, Calif. 92093
Pain Control in Cancer Patients	Dr. Wolff Kirsch University of Colorado Medical Center 4200 East Ninth Avenue Denver, Colo. 80220

How can I find people working on biofeedback in my area?

To locate those in your area working on biofeedback, write: Biofeedback Research Society, University of Colorado, Medical Center, Denver, Colo. 80262.

What are the cancer programs approved by the American College of Surgeons?

The American College of Surgeons maintains a certification program relating to the quality of cancer care in hospitals in the United States. Cancer programs are surveyed at the request of their administrators or their medical staffs or both. The approved status is based on the level of excellence in relation to established standards established by the College of Surgeons. In order to be certified, the hospital must have a cancer committee, a cancer registry, a clinical education program, and means for evaluating the quality of care in the hospital. Hospitals listed in the directory, published annually and updated twice during the year, have been approved for cancer treatment by the College. Directory (*Cancer Programs Approved by the American College of Surgeons*) is available from the Assistant Director, Professional Activities (Cancer), American College of Surgeons, 55 East Erie Street, Chicago, Ill. 60611. Inquiries about current status of an institution's cancer program should be sent to the same address.

Listed are those hospitals which have been approved as of 1980. Approval is given for three years (* indicates provisional approval subject to correction of certain deficiencies).

ALABAMA

Birmingham
*University of Alabama Medical Center
Veterans Administration Hospital

Mobile
*University of South Alabama Medical Center

Tuskegee
*Veterans Administration Hospital

ALASKA

Anchorage
Alaska Hospital and Medical Center
Providence Hospital
USPHS Alaska Native Medical Center

Fairbanks
Fairbanks Memorial Hospital

ARIZONA

Mesa
Desert Samaritan Hospital & Health Center and Mesa Lutheran Hospital

Phoenix
Good Samaritan Hospital
Maricopa County General Hospital
Memorial Hospital
Veterans Administration Hospital

Scottsdale
Scottsdale Memorial Hospital

Tucson
Tucson Medical Center
University Hospital
Veterans Administration Hospital

ARKANSAS

Fayetteville
Washington Regional Medical Center

ARKANSAS (continued)

Little Rock
University Hospital
Veterans Administration Hospital

Texarkana
St. Michael Hospital

CALIFORNIA

Alhambra
Alhambra Community Hospital

Anaheim
Anaheim Memorial Hospital
Martin Luther Hospital

Arcadia
Methodist Hospital of Southern California

Bakersfield
Kern Medical Center

Bellflower
Bellwood General Hospital
Kaiser Foundation Hospital

Berkeley
Alta Bates Hospital
Herrick Memorial Hospital

Burbank
St. Joseph Medical Center

Canoga Park
West Hills Medical Center

Concord
Mount Diablo Hospital Medical Center

Covina
Inter-Community Hospital

Culver City
Dr. David Brotman Memorial Hospital

Duarte
City of Hope Medical Center

Fontana
Kaiser Foundation Hospital

Fountain City
Fountain City Community Hospital

CALIFORNIA (continued)

Fresno
Veterans Administration Hospital

Glendale
Glendale Adventist Medical Center

Granada Hills
°Granada Hills Community Hospital

Harbor City
Kaiser Foundation Hospital

Imola
°Napa State Hospital

Inglewood
Centinela Hospital
°Daniel Freeman Memorial Hospital

La Jolla
Green Hospital of Scripps Clinic
Scripps Memorial Hospital

La Mesa
°Grossmont District Hospital

Livermore
Veterans Administration Medical Center

Loma Linda
Loma Linda University Medical Center

Long Beach
Long Beach Community Hospital
Los Altos Hospital
Memorial Hospital Medical Center of Long Beach
Naval Regional Medical Center
St. Mary Medical Center

Los Angeles
California Hospital Medical Center
Children's Hospital of Los Angeles
Hollywood Presbyterian Medical Center
Hospital of the Good Samaritan
Kaiser Foundation Hospital—Cadillac
Kaiser Foundation Hospital—Sunset
Los Angeles County, USC Medical Center
Martin Luther King, Jr. General Hospital
Orthopaedic Hospital
°Queen of Angels Hospital
St. Vincent's Medical Center
UCLA Hospital
White Memorial Medical Center

CALIFORNIA (continued)

Lynwood
St. Francis Hospital of Lynwood

Montebello
Beverly Hospital

Monterey Park
Garfield Medical Center

Newport Beach
Hoag Memorial Hospital—Presbyterian

Oakland
Naval Medical Center
Samuel Merritt Hospital

Orange
St. Joseph Hospital
University of California
    Irvine Medical Center

Oxnard
St. John's Hospital

Palm Springs
Desert Hospital

Panorama City
Kaiser Foundation Hospital

Pasadena
Huntington Memorial Hospital
St. Luke Hospital of Pasadena

Pomona
Pomona Valley Community Hospital

Redlands
Redlands Community Hospital

Redondo Beach
South Bay Hospital

Redwood City
Sequoia Hospital

Riverside
Parkview Community Hospital
Riverside General Hospital—University Medical Center

Sacramento
*Mercy General Hospital
Sacramento Medical Center
Sutter Community Hospital of Sacramento

CALIFORNIA (continued)

San Bernardino
St. Bernadine Hospital
°San Bernardino County Medical Center

San Diego
Children's Hospital & Health Center
Donald Sharp Memorial Community Hospital
Kaiser Foundation Hospital
°Mercy Hospital and Medical Center
°Naval Regional Medical Center
University Hospital

San Dimas
Tri-Hospital Cancer Program
   Foothill Presbyterian Hospital, *Glendora*
   Glendora Community Hospital, *Glendora*
   San Dimas Community Hospital, *San Dimas*
   West Covina Hospital, *West Covina*

San Francisco
French Hospital
Letterman Army Medical Center
Mount Zion Hospital and Medical Center
St. Francis Memorial Hospital
St. Joseph's Hospital
St. Mary's Hospital and Medical Center
°San Francisco General Hospital Medical Center
USPHS Hospital
University of California Hospitals and Clinics
Veterans Administration Medical Center

San Gabriel
Community Hospital

San Jose
O'Connor Hospital
Santa Clara Valley Medical Center

San Pablo
Brookside Hospital

San Pedro
San Pedro and Peninsula Hospital

Santa Ana
Santa Ana—Tustin Community Hospital

Santa Barbara
Santa Barbara College Hospital

CALIFORNIA (continued)

Santa Monica
St. John's Hospital and Health Center
The Santa Monica Hospital Medical Center

Torrance
°Los Angeles County Harbor General Hospital

Travis AFB
°David Grant USAF Medical Center

Van Nuys
Valley Presbyterian Hospital

Visalia
Kaweah Delta District Hospital

Walnut Creek
John Muir Memorial Hospital

Whittier
Presbyterian Intercommunity Hospital

COLORADO

Colorado Springs
Penrose Hospital

Denver
American Cancer Research Center and Hospital, *Lakewood*
Fitzsimons Army Medical Center
Porter/Swedish Cancer Program
   Porter Memorial Hospital
   Swedish Medical Center
Presbyterian Medical Center
Rose Medical Center
St. Anthony Hospital Systems
St. Joseph Hospital
°St. Luke's Hospital
University of Colorado Medical Center
Veterans Administration Hospital

Fort Carson
US Army Hospital

Fort Collins
Poudre Valley Memorial Hospital

Greeley
Weld County General Hospital

COLORADO (continued)

Longmont
Longmont United Hospital

Montrose
Montrose Memorial Hospital

Pueblo
St. Mary-Corwin Hospital

USAF Academy
USAF Academy Hospital

CONNECTICUT

Bridgeport
Bridgeport Hospital
Park City Hospital
°St. Vincent's Medical Center

Danbury
°Danbury Hospital

Derby
Griffin Hospital

Farmington
University of Connecticut Health Center—
    John Dempsey Hospital

Greenwich
Greenwich Hospital Association

Groton
Naval Submarine Medical Center

Hartford
Mount Sinai Hospital
St. Francis Hospital and Medical Center

Meriden
°Meriden-Wallingford Hospital

New Haven
Hospital of St. Raphael
Yale-New Haven Hospital

Norwalk
°Norwalk Hospital

Stamford
St. Joseph Hospital

CONNECTICUT (continued)

Torrington
Charlotte Hungerford Hospital

Waterbury
St. Mary's Hospital
Waterbury Hospital

DELAWARE

Lewes
Beebe Hospital of Sussex County

Wilmington
Veterans Administration Center
Wilmington Medical Center, Inc.

DISTRICT OF COLUMBIA

Washington
°Children's Hospital National Medical Center
Doctors Hospital
°Georgetown University Hospital
Greater Southeast Community Hospital
Howard University Hospital
Malcom Grow USAF Medical Center
Walter Reed Army Medical Center

FLORIDA

Daytona Beach
Halifax Hospital Medical Center

Gainesville
°Shands Teaching Hospital and Clinic

Jacksonville
Memorial Hospital
Naval Regional Medical Center
St. Vincent's Medical Center
University Hospital of Jacksonville

Miami
James M. Jackson Memorial Hospital

Pensacola
Naval Aerospace and Regional Medical Center
West Florida Hospital

Tallahassee
Tallahassee Memorial Hospital

FLORIDA (continued)

Tampa
°Tampa General Hospital

GEORGIA

Albany
°Phoebe Putney Memorial Hospital

Americus
Americus and Sumter County Hospital

Atlanta
Crawford W. Long Memorial Hospital
   of Emory University
Emory University Hospital
Georgia Baptist Hospital
Grady Memorial Hospital
Piedmont Hospital, Inc.
St. Joseph's Hospital

Augusta
Eugene Talmedge Memorial Hospital
University Hospital

Columbus
Medical Center

Dalton
Hamilton Memorial Hospital

Decatur
De Kalb General Hospital
Veterans Administration Hospital, Atlanta

East Point
South Fulton Hospital

Fort Benning
Martin Army Hospital

Fort Gordon
Dwight D. Eisenhower Army Medical Center

Gainesville
°Northeast Georgia Medical Center

La Grange
West Georgia Medical Center

Macon
Medical Center of Central Georgia

GEORGIA (continued)

Savannah
°Memorial Medical Center

Tifton
Tift General Hospital

HAWAII

Honolulu
Kaiser Foundation Hospital
Kapiolani Hospital
Kuakini Medical Center
Queen's Medical Center
St. Francis Hospital
Tripler Army Medical Center

IDAHO

Boise
St. Luke's Hospital & Mountain States Tumor Institute

Lewiston
St. Joseph's Hospital

Nampa
Mercy Medical Center

Twin Falls
Magic Valley Memorial Hospital

ILLINOIS

Arlington Heights
Northwest Community Hospital

Aurora
Copley Memorial Hospital

Carbondale
°Memorial Hospital of Carbondale

Chicago
Central Community Hospital
Children's Memorial Hospital
Columbus Hospital
Cook County Hospital
Franklin Boulevard Community Hospital
Holy Cross Hospital
Illinois Masonic Medical Center
Louis A. Weiss Memorial Hospital

ILLINOIS (continued)

Mercy Hospital and Medical Center
Mount Sinai Hospital Medical Center
Northwestern Memorial Hospital
Ravenswood Hospital Medical Center
Rush-Presbyterian-St. Luke's Medical Center
St. Elizabeth's Hospital
°St. Joseph Hospital
St. Mary of Nazareth Hospital Center
Swedish Covenant Hospital
University of Chicago Hospitals and Clinics
°University of Illinois Hospital
Veterans Administration West Side Hospital

Chicago Heights
St. James Hospital

Danville
Lake View Medical Center
St. Elizabeth Hospital

Decatur
Decatur Memorial Hospital

Elgin
St. Joseph Hospital

Elk Grove Village
Alexian Brothers Medical Center

Elmhurst
Memorial Hospital of DuPage County

Evanston
Evanston Hospital
St. Francis Hospital of Evanston

Great Lakes
Naval Regional Medical Center

Harvey
Ingalls Memorial Hospital

Hines
Veterans Administration Hospital

Hinsdale
°Hinsdale Sanitarium and Hospital

Kankakee
St. Mary's Hospital

McHenry
McHenry Hospital

ILLINOIS (continued)

Mendota
Mendota Community Hospital

Oak Lawn
Christ Hospital

Oak Park
West Suburban Hospital

Park Ridge
Lutheran General Hospital, Inc.

Peoria
Methodist Medical Center of Central Illinois
St. Francis Hospital and Medical Center

Quincy
*Blessing Hospital
St. Mary Hospital

Rockford
Rockford Memorial Hospital
St. Anthony Hospital
Swedish-American Hospital

Sterling
Community General Hospital

Streator
St. Mary's Hospital

Urbana
Carle Foundation Hospital

INDIANA

Bluffton
Caylor-Nickel Hospital, Inc.

Evansville
Deaconess Hospital
Welbourn Memorial Baptist Hospital

Gary
Methodist Hospital of Gary

Hammond
St. Margaret Hospital

Indianapolis
Community Hospital of Indianapolis
*Methodist Hospital of Indiana, Inc.
St. Vincent Hospital and Health Care Center

INDIANA (continued)

Lafayette
°St. Elizabeth Hospital Medical Center

Terre Haute
Terre Haute Regional Hospital
Union Hospital

Vincennes
Good Samaritan Hospital

IOWA

Des Moines
Iowa Methodist Medical Center
Mercy Hospital
Veterans Administration Hospital

Dubuque
Finley Hospital
Mercy Health Center—St. Joseph's Unit
Xavier Hospital

Iowa City
University of Iowa Hospitals and Clinics

KANSAS

Fort Riley
Irwin Army Hospital

Hays
Hadley Regional Medical Center
St. Anthony Hospital

Kansas City
Bethany Medical Center
University of Kansas Medical Center

Manhattan
°The St. Mary Hospital

Wichita
St. Francis Hospital
St. Joseph Medical Center
°Veterans Administration Center

KENTUCKY

Fort Campbell
United States Army Hospital

Lexington
Good Samaritan Hospital
University Hospital

KENTUCKY (continued)

Louisville
Highlands Baptist Hospital
Louisville General Hospital
Norton Children's Hospitals, Inc.
  Children's Hospital
  Norton Memorial Infirmary Unit
Veterans Administration Hospital

Madisonville
Hopkins County Hospital

LOUISIANA

Alexandria
Alexandria Tumor Registry Program
  Rapides General Hospital
  St. Frances Cabrini Hospital

Eunice
Moosa Memorial Hospital

Lake Charles
St. Patrick's Hospital

New Orleans
Charity Hospital of Louisiana
  Louisiana State University Cancer Service
  Tulane University Cancer Service
*Touro Infirmary
USPHS Hospital
Veterans Administration Hospital

Shreveport
Confederate Memorial Medical Center
Veterans Administration Hospital

MAINE

Augusta
Augusta General Hospital

Bangor
Eastern Maine Medical Center

Lewiston
Central Maine General Hospital
St. Mary's General Hospital

Norway
Stephens Memorial Hospital

MAINE (continued)

Portland
°Maine Medical Center

Presque Isle
Arthur Gould Memorial Hospital

Rockland
Penobscot Bay Medical Center

Togus
Veterans Administration Center

Waterville
Mid-Maine Medical Center

MARYLAND

Baltimore
Franklin Square Hospital
°Greater Baltimore Medical Center
Johns Hopkins Hospital
Sinai Hospital of Baltimore
South Baltimore General Hospital
USPHS Hospital
University of Maryland Hospital

Bethesda
National Naval Medical Center

Leonardtown
St. Mary's Hospital

Salisbury
Peninsula General Hospital

Towson
St. Joseph Hospital

MASSACHUSETTS

Boston
Beth Israel Hospital
°Boston City Hospital
Faulkner Hospital, *Jamaica Plain*
Lahey Clinic Foundation
New England Deaconess Hospital
°Peter Bent Brigham Hospital
St. Elizabeth's Hospital of Boston, *Brighton*
USPHS Hospital, *Brighton*
University Hospital
Veterans Administration Hospital, *Jamaica Plain*

Brockton
Brockton Hospital
Cardinal Cushing General Hospital

MASSACHUSETTS (continued)

Cambridge
Mount Auburn Hospital

Chelsea
Lawrence F. Quigley Memorial Hospital
  Soldier's Home in Massachusetts

Concord
Emerson Hospital

Denvers
°Hunt Memorial Hospital

Framingham
Framingham Union Hospital

Holyoke
Holyoke Hospital
Providence Hospital

Hyannis
Cape Cod Hospital

Lynn
Lynn Hospital

Medford
Lawrence Memorial Hospital

Newton Lower Falls
Newton-Wellesley Hospital

North Adams
North Adams Regional Hospital

Northampton
Cooley Dickenson Hospital

Norwood
Norwood Hospital

Pittsfield
Berkshire Medical Center

Salem
Salem Hospital

Springfield
Baystate Medical Center
Mercy Hospital

Stoughton
Goddard Memorial Hospital

Walpole
°Pondville Hospital

MASSACHUSETTS (continued)

Waltham
Waltham Hospital

Winchester
Winchester Hospital

Worcester
St. Vincent Hospital
The Memorial Hospital
*Worcester City Hospital

MICHIGAN

Allen Park
Veterans Administration Hospital

Ann Arbor
St. Joseph Mercy Hospital
University Hospital

Battle Creek
Calhoun County Medical Society Cancer Program
   Battle Creek Sanitarium Hospital
   Community Hospital Association
   Leila Y. Post Montgomery Hospital

Dearborn
Oakwood Hospital

Detroit
Detroit General Hospital
*Detroit-Macomb Hospital Association
Harper-Grace Hospitals
Henry Ford Hospital

Flint
Hurley Medical Center

Grand Rapids
Blodget Memorial Medical Center
Butterworth Hospital
Ferguson-Droste-Ferguson Hospital
St. Mary's Hospital

Menominee
Menominee County-Lloyd Hospital

Muskegon
Hackley Hospital and Medical Center

Rochester
Crittenton Hospital

MICHIGAN (continued)

Royal Oak
William Beaumont Hospital

Southfield
Providence Hospital

MINNESOTA

Crookston
Riverview Hospital

Fergus Falls
•Lake Region Hospital

Grand Rapids
Itasca Memorial Hospital

Hibbing
•Hibbing General Hospital

Minneapolis
Abbot-Northwestern Hospital
Children's Health Center & Hospital S
Metropolitan Medical Center
St. Mary's Hospital
Veterans Administration Hospital

Moorhead
St. Ansgar Hospital

Rochester
Mayo Clinic

St. Louis Park
Methodist Hospital

MISSISSIPPI

Biloxi
Howard Memorial Hospital
Veterans Administration Hospital

Hattiesburg
Forrest County General Hospital

Jackson
University Hospital
Veterans Administration Center

Keesler
USAF Medical Center

Vicksburg
Mercy Regional Medical Center

MISSOURI

Cape Girardeau
°St. Francis Hospital
Southeast Missouri Hospital

Columbia
Ellis Fischel State Cancer Hospital

Kansas City
Baptist Memorial Hospital
St. Luke's Hospital
Trinity Lutheran Hospital
Truman Medical Center

St. Louis
Deaconess Hospital
Jewish Hospital of St. Louis
°St. Anthony's Medical Center
St. Louis Children's Hospital
St. Mary's Health Center

Sikeston
Missouri Delta Community Hospital

MONTANA

Butte
°St. James Community Hospital
   Mary Swift Memorial Tumor Clinic

NEBRASKA

Lincoln
Lincoln General Hospital
Veterans Administration Hospital

Omaha
Archbishop Bergan Mercy Hospital
Bishop Clarkson Memorial Hospital
Immanuel Medical Center
Nebraska Methodist Hospital
St. Joseph Hospital
University of Nebraska Medical Center

NEW HAMPSHIRE

Exeter
°Exeter Hospital

Hanover
Mary Hitchcock Memorial Hospital

NEW HAMPSHIRE (continued)

Keene
Cheshire Hospital

Manchester
Catholic Medical Center
Elliot Hospital

Portsmouth
Portsmouth Hospital

Rochester
Frisbie Memorial Hospital

NEW JERSEY

Atlantic City
Atlantic City Medical Center

Belleville
Clara Maass Memorial Hospital

Camden
West Jersey Hospital System

Denville
St. Clare's Hospital

East Orange
Veterans Administration Hospital

Elizabeth
Elizabeth General Hospital and Dispensary
   Wuester Clinic

Englewood
*Englewood Hospital

Green Brook
Raritan Valley Hospital

Hackensack
Hackensack Hospital

Hackettstown
Hackettstown Community Hospital

Livingston
St. Barnabas Medical Center

Montclair
Mountainside Hospital

Morristown
Morristown Memorial Hospital

Mount Holly
Burlington County Memorial Hospital

NEW JERSEY (continued)

Neptune
*Jersey Shore Medical Center
  Fitkin Hospital

Newark
Martland Hospital of the College of Medicine & Dentistry of New Jersey
Newark Beth Israel Medical Center

Newton
Newton Memorial Hospital

Paterson
St. Joseph's Hospital and Medical Center

Phillipsburg
Warren Hospital

Plainfield
Muhlenberg Hospital

Princeton
The Medical Center of Princeton

Somerville
*The Somerset Hospital

Trenton
St. Francis Medical Center

Woodbury
Underwood Memorial Hospital

NEW MEXICO

Albuquerque
Bernalillo County Medical Center
Lovelace-Bataan Medical Center
St. Joseph Hospital
Veterans Administration Hospital

NEW YORK

Albany
Veterans Administration Hospital

Amityville
Brunswick Hospital Center

Binghampton
Our Lady of Lourdes Hospital

Buffalo
Children's Hospital of Buffalo
Deaconess Hospital of Buffalo
Edward J. Meyer Memorial Hospital
Roswell Park Memorial Institute
*Veterans Administration Hospital

NEW YORK (continued)

Castle Point
Veterans Administration Hospital

Cobleskill
Community Hospital of Schoharie County

Cooperstown
Mary Imogene Bassett Hospital

East Meadow
Nassau County Medical Center

Elmira
Arnot-Ogden Memorial Hospital

Glen Cove
°Community Hospital at Glen Cove

Johnson City
Charles S. Wilson Memorial Hospital

Kenmore
Kenmore Mercy Hospital

Manhasset
North Shore University Hospital

Mineola
Nassau Hospital

Mount Kisco
°Northern Westchester Hospital Center

Mount Vernon
Mount Vernon Hospital

New Hyde Park
°Long Island Jewish Medical Center

New Rochelle
New Rochelle Hospital Medical Center

New York City
Bronx (*Mailing address: Bronx*)
  °Bronx-Lebanon Hospital Center
  Misericordia Hospital Medical Center
  Montefiore Hospital and Medical Center
  °Veterans Administration Hospital
Brooklyn (*Mailing address: Brooklyn*)
  Brooklyn-Cumberland Medical Center
  °Jewish Hospital & Medical Center of Brooklyn
  Long Island College Hospital
  Lutheran Medical Center
  Methodist Hospital of Brooklyn

NEW YORK (continued)

St. John's Episcopal Hospital
State University Hospital, Downstate Medical Center
   Kings County Hospital Center
Wyckoff Heights Hospital
Manhattan *(Mailing address: New York)*
   Beekman-Downtown Hospital
   Bellevue Hospital Center
   Beth Israel Medical Center
   Cabrini Health Center
   Harlem Hospital Center
   Manhattan Eye, Ear and Throat Hospital
   Memorial Sloan-Kettering Cancer Center
   New York Hospital
   New York Infirmary
   New York University Medical Center
      University Hospital
   *St. Luke's Hospital Center
   St. Vincent's Hospital and Medical Center of New York
   *Veterans Administration Hospital
Queens *(Mailing addresses: Astoria,*
      Edgemere, Elmhurst, Far Rockaway, Flushing, Forest Hills, Glen Oaks,
      Hollis, Jackson Heights, Jamaica, Kew Gardens, Little Neck, Long Island
      City, Queens Village, St. Albans, and Whitestone)
   Booth Memorial Medical Center, *Flushing*
   Flushing Hospital and Medical Center, *Flushing*
   Jamaica Hospital, *Jamaica*
   LaGuardia Hospital, *Forest Hills*
   Mary Immaculate Hospital, Division of the Catholic Medical Center of
      Brooklyn and Queens, *Jamaica*
   Queens Hospital Center Inc., *Jamaica*
   St. John's Queens Hospital, Division of the Catholic Medical Center
      of Brooklyn & Queens, Inc., *Elmhurst*
Richmond *(Mailing address: Staten Island)*
   Doctors' Hospital of Staten Island
   St. Vincent's Medical Center of Richmond
   Staten Island Hospital
   USPHS Hospital

Nyack
Nyack Hospital

Oceanside
*South Nassau Communities Hospital

Port Jefferson
John T. Mather Memorial Hospital and St. Charles Hospital

Port Jervis
St. Francis Hospital of Port Jervis

NEW YORK (continued)

Poughkeepsie
Vassar Brothers Hospital

Rochester
Highland Hospital of Rochester
Park Ridge Hospital
St. Mary's Hospital of the Sisters of Charity

Rockville Centre
Mercy Hospital

Suffern
*Good Samaritan Hospital

Syracuse
St. Joseph's Hospital Health Center
University Hospital of Upstate Medical Center

Walton
Delaware Valley Hospital

White Plains
*White Plains Hospital

NORTH CAROLINA

Asheville
Veterans Administration Hospital

Camp Le Jeune
Naval Regional Medical Center

Chapel Hill
North Carolina Memorial Hospital

Durham
Duke University Medical Center
Veterans Administration Hospital

Shelby
Cleveland Memorial Hospital

Winston-Salem
North Carolina Baptist Hospital

NORTH DAKOTA

Fargo
St. John's Hospital
St. Luke's Hospital-Fargo Clinic

Grand Forks
The United Hospital

NORTH DAKOTA (continued)

Rugby
Good Samaritan Hospital Association

Williston
Mercy Hospital

OHIO

Akron
Akron City Hospital
Akron General Medical Center

Cincinnati
Children's Hospital Medical Center
°Cincinnati General Hospital
Good Samaritan Hospital
Jewish Hospital of Cincinnati

Cleveland
Cleveland Clinic Hospital
Deaconess Hospital of Cleveland
°Huron Road Hospital
Lutheran Medical Center
°St. Alexis Hospital

Columbus
Children's Hospital
Mount Carmel Medical Center
Ohio State University Hospitals

Dayton
Miami Valley Hospital
Good Samaritan Hospital and Health Center
St. Elizabeth Medical Center
Veterans Administration Hospital

Dover
Union Hospital Association

Kettering
Kettering Medical Center

Mayfield Heights
Hillcrest Hospital

Sandusky
°Good Samaritan Hospital

Springfield
Community Hospital of Springfield and Clark County
Mercy Medical Center
Springfield-Urbana Cancer Program—
    Mercy Memorial Hospital

OHIO (continued)

Sylvania
Flower Hospital

Toledo
Medical College of Ohio Hospital
Toledo Hospital

Wright-Patterson AFB
°USAF Medical Center

Youngstown
Youngstown Hospital Association

OKLAHOMA

Ada
Valley View Hospital

Ardmore
Memorial Hospital of Southern Oklahoma

Bartlesville
Jane Phillips Episcopal Memorial
   Medical Center

Chickasha
Grady Memorial Hospital

Oklahoma City
Baptist Medical Center of Oklahoma
Mercy Health Center
Oklahoma Children's Memorial Hospital
Presbyterian Hospital
St. Anthony's Hospital
University Hospitals & Clinics

Okmulgee
Okmulgee Memorial Hospital Authority

Shattuck
Newman Memorial Hospital

Shawnee
Shawnee Medical Center Hospital

Tulsa
Hillcrest Medical Center
°St. Francis Hospital
St. John's Hospital Medical Center

OREGON

Bend
St. Charles Medical Center

OREGON (continued)

Coos Bay
Bay Area Hospital

Corvallis
Good Samaritan Hospital

Eugene
Sacred Heart General Hospital

Grants Pass
Josephine General Hospital

Medford
Medford Tumor Clinic
　°Providence Hospital
　°Rogue Valley Memorial Hospital

Oregon City
Williamette Falls Community Hospital

Pendleton
°St. Anthony Hospital

Portland
Emanuel Hospital
Good Samaritan Hospital and Medical Center
Kaiser Foundation Hospitals, Oregon Region
Physicians and Surgeons Hospital
Portland Adventist Medical Center
Providence Medical Center
°St. Vincent Hospital and Medical Center
University of Oregon Health Sciences
　Center Hospital & Clinics
Veterans Administration Hospital

Roseburg
Veterans Administration Hospital

Salem
Salem Hospital

Tualafin
°Meridian Park Hospital

PENNSYLVANIA

Allentown
°Allentown Hospital Association
Sacred Heart Hospital

Altoona
Altoona Hospital
Mercy Hospital

PENNSYLVANIA (continued)

Bethlehem
St. Luke's Hospital

Bryn Mawr
°Bryn Mawr Hospital

Danville
Geisinger Medical Center

Easton
Easton Hospital

Erie
Hamot Medical Center

Greensburg
Westmoreland Hospital

Johnstown
°Conemaugh Valley Memorial Hospital

Lancaster
°Lancaster General Hospital
St. Joseph Hospital

Latrobe
Latrobe Area Hospital

Lewistown
Lewistown Hospital

McKeesport
McKeesport Hospital

Natrona Heights
Allegheny Valley Hospital

Norristown
Montgomery Hospital
Sacred Heart Hospital

Paoli
Paoli Memorial Hospital

Philadelphia
°Albert Einstein Medical Center—Northern Division
°American Oncologic/Jeanes Cancer Program
   American Oncologic Hospital
   Jeanes Hospital
Children's Hospital of Philadelphia
Episcopal Hospital
Graduate Hospital of the University of Pennsylvania
Hahnemann Medical College and Hospital
°Hospital of the University of Pennsylvania

PENNSYLVANIA (continued)

Lankenau Hospital
°Medical College of Pennsylvania and Hospital
Mercy Catholic Medical Center
Naval Regional Medical Center
Presbyterian-University of Pennsylvania Medical Center
Temple University Hospital
Thomas Jefferson University Hospital

Pittsburgh
Allegheny General Hospital
Children's Hospital of Pittsburgh
Magee-Women's Hospital
°Mercy Hospital of Pittsburgh
St. Francis General Hospital
°St. Margaret Memorial Hospital

Pottsville
Pottsville Hospital and Warne Clinic

Reading
Community General Hospital

Sayre
Robert Packer Hospital

State College
Center Community Hospital

West Chester
Chester County Hospital

Wilkes-Barre
Veterans Administration Hospital
°Wilkes-Barre General Hospital

York
York Hospital

RHODE ISLAND

Newport
°Naval Hospital

SOUTH CAROLINA

Anderson
Anderson Memorial Hospital

Beaufort
Naval Hospital

Charleston
°Medical University of South Carolina Hospital

SOUTH CAROLINA (continued)

Columbia
Richland Memorial Hospital
South Carolina Baptist Hospital
Veterans Administration Hospital

Florence
McLeod Memorial Hospital

Fort Jackson
Moncrief Army Hospital

Greenwood
Self Memorial Hospital

Spartanburg
Spartanburg General Hospital

SOUTH DAKOTA

Aberdeen
St. Luke's Hospital

Watertown
Watertown Memorial Medical Center

Yankton
Sacred Heart Hospital

TENNESSEE

Bristol
Bristol Memorial Hospital

Johnson City
Veterans Administration Center

Memphis
Baptist Memorial Hospital
Methodist Hospital
St. Jude Children's Research Hospital
University of Memphis/City of Memphis Hospitals

Millington
Naval Hospital Memphis

Nashville
George W. Hubbard Hospital of Meharry Medical College
Nashville Metropolitan General Hospital
Vanderbilt University Hospital

TEXAS

Amarillo
Panhandle Regional Tumor Clinic and Registry
   High Plains Baptist Hospital
   Northwest Texas Hospital
   St. Anthony's Hospital
   Deaf Smith General Hospital, *Hereford*

Big Spring
Malone-Hogan Hospitals, Inc.
Veterans Administration Hospital

Corpus Christi
Memorial Medical Center
Naval Regional Medical Center
Spohn Hospital

Dallas
Baylor University Medical Center
Methodist Hospitals of Dallas
Parkland Memorial Hospital
St. Paul Hospital

El Paso
R.E. Thomason General Hospital
William Beaumont Army Medical Center

Fort Sam Houston
Brooke Army Medical Center

Fort Worth
John Peter Smith Hospital

Galveston
University of Texas Medical Branch Hospitals

Houston
Ben Taub General Hospital
Park Plaza Hospital
Rosewood General Hospital
St. Elizabeth Hospital
St. Joseph Hospital
Texas Children's Hospital
The University of Texas, M.D. Anderson Hospital and Tumor Institute

Jacksonville
°Nan Travis Memorial Hospital

Kerrville
°Veterans Administration Hospital

Lubbock
Highland Hospital
Methodist Hospital

TEXAS (continued)

Plainview
°Central Plains General Hospital

San Antonio
Bexar County Teaching Hospital
Santa Rosa Medical Center

Stephenville
Stephenville Hospital

Temple
King's Daughters Hospital
Scott and White Memorial Hospital
Veterans Administration Center

Texarkana
St. Michael Hospital

Waco
Hillcrest Baptist Hospital
Providence Hospital

Wharton
Gulf Coast Medical Center

UTAH

Salt Lake City
°Holy Cross Hospital
Latter-Day Saints Hospital
University of Utah Medical Center
Veterans Administration Hospital

VERMONT

Burlington
Medical Center Hospital of Vermont

Randolph
°Gifford Memorial Hospital, Inc.

VIRGINIA

Big Stone Gap
Lonesome Pine Hospital

Charlottesville
University of Virginia Hospital

Clifton Forge
Emmett Memorial Hospital

Danville
Memorial Hospital

VIRGINIA (continued)

Falls Church
Fairfax Hospital

Hampton
°Veterans Administration Center

Harrisonburg
Rockingham Memorial Hospital

Leesburg
Loudoun Memorial Hospital

Lynchburg
Lynchburg General-Marshall Lodge Hospitals
Virginia Baptist Hospital

Norfolk
DePaul Hospital
°Norfolk General Hospital

Portsmouth
Naval Regional Medical Center

Richmond
Medical College of Virginia Hospitals
St. Luke's Hospital
St. Mary's Hospital

Roanoke
Community Hospital of Roanoke Valley
Roanoke Memorial Hospital

Salem
Lewis-Gale Hospital
Veterans Administration Hospital

Winchester
Winchester Memorial Hospital

WASHINGTON

Aberdeen
Aberdeen Cancer Program
 Grays Harbor Community Hospital
 St. Joseph Hospital

Bellevue
Overlake Memorial Hospital

Bellingham
St. Joseph Hospital
St. Luke's General Hospital

WASHINGTON (continued)

Bremerton
Naval Regional Medical Center

Everett
General Hospital and Providence Hospital

Kirkland
Evergreen General Hospital

Mount Vernon
Skagit Valley Hospital

Olympia
St. Peter Hospital

Seattle
Children's Orthopedic Hospital & Medical Center
°Group Health Hospital
Northwest Hospital
Providence Medical Center
°Swedish Hospital Medical Center
University Hospital
Virginia Mason Hospital

Sedro Woolley
United General Hospital

Spokane
Deaconess Hospital
Sacred Heart Medical Center

Tacoma
Madigan Army Medical Center
Tacoma General Hospital

Wenatchee
Wenatchee Valley Clinic

WEST VIRGINIA

Beckley
Appalachian Regional Hospital
Beckley Hospital, Inc.

Charleston
Charleston Area Medical Center, Inc.
    General Division
    Memorial Division

Clarksburg
Veterans Administration Hospital

WEST VIRGINIA (continued)

Elkins
Davis Memorial Hospital
Memorial General Hospital

Huntington
°Cabell Huntington Hospital
St. Mary's Hospital
Veterans Administration Hospital

Kingwood
Preston Memorial Hospital

Man
Man Appalachian Regional Hospital

Montgomery
Montgomery General Hospital

Morgantown
West Virginia University Hospital

Philippi
Broaddus Hospital

Wheeling
Ohio Valley Medical Center

WISCONSIN

Appleton
St. Elizabeth Hospital

Cudahy
Trinity Memorial Hospital

Eau Claire
Luther Memorial Hospital
Sacred Heart Hospital

Green Bay
St. Vincent Hospital

Janesville
Mercy Hospital of Janesville

La Crosse
La Crosse Lutheran Hospital
St. Francis Hospital

Madison
Madison General Hospital
Methodist Hospital
St. Mary's Hospital Medical Center
°University of Wisconsin Hospitals

WISCONSIN (continued)

Manitowoc
Holy Family Hospital

Marinette
Marinette General Hospital

Marshfield
Marshfield Clinic

Milwaukee
Columbia Hospital
Deaconess Hospital
Milwaukee County General Hospital
Mount Sinai Medical Center
St. Francis Hospital
St. Joseph's Hospital
St. Luke's Hospital
St. Mary's Hospital

Oshkosh
Mercy Medical Center

Watertown
Watertown Memorial Hospital

Wausau
Wausau Hospital

Wood
Veterans Administration Center

WYOMING

Cheyenne
De Paul Hospital
Memorial Hospital of Laramie County

PUERTO RICO

Ponce
Clinica Oncológica Andrés Grilasca
Hospital de Damas

San Germán
Hospital de la Concepcion

San Juan
I. Gonzales Martinez Oncologic Hospital
University District Hospital
Veterans Administration Center

°Provisional Approval

Where can I get articles on cancer subjects?

Articles which appear in the most popular nontechnical magazines and journals are listed in the *Readers' Guide to Periodical Literature* or in the *Public Affairs Information Service.* These are usually available in most public libraries. Look in the index under the subject you are interested in, or if you know it, under the author's name.

Where can I find articles which are in health-science journals?

The *Index Medicus,* which is found in medical libraries, most university and college libraries, and some public libraries, lists articles appearing in over 2,400 health-sciences journals. The National Library of Medicine's MEDLARS program, a computerized system, can provide lists of articles. Individuals can request searches through their Regional Medical Library. A fee may be charged for the service, which is sponsored by the International Cancer Research Data Bank Program of the National Cancer Institute. The programs include:

- CANCERLIT: 160,000 citations and abstracts of articles from technical literature since 1963 on all aspects of cancer.
- CANCERPROJ: Summaries of over 18,000 ongoing cancer research projects federally and privately funded during the most recent three fiscal years; foreign and domestic studies listed.
- CLINPROT: Small, highly specialized file. Primarily designed for the clinical oncologist engaged in development and testing of clinical protocols. Data base is over 1,000 descriptions of clinical investigations of new agents. Includes patient-entry criteria, therapy regimens, special study parameters.
- MEDLINE: Computerized counterpart to *Index Medicus.* Citations to biomedical literature published since 1969.

What are the addresses of the public information offices of the various governmental institutions concerned with cancer or cancer-related subjects?

Office of Cancer Communications
National Cancer Institute
Building 31, Room 10 A 30
Bethesda, Md. 20014
301-496-6631

(Information on National Cancer Institute programs—research and patient services, public information and education materials)

Food and Drug Administration
Office of Consumer Inquiries
Room 15B-32
5600 Fishers Lane
Rockville, Md. 20857

(Federal regulations on drugs, food additives, polyvinyl-chloride food containers, etc.)

Consumer Products Safety Commission
5401 Westbard Avenue
Washington, D.C. 20207
Toll-free: 800-638-2666 (in Maryland, 900-492-2938)

(Questions about potential hazards of commercial products)

Office of Information
Department of Labor
Occupational Safety and Health Administration
Washington, D.C. 20210

(Work-related hazards)

Public Information Center, PM-215
Environmental Protection Agency
401 M Street, S.W.
Washington, D.C. 20460

(Hazards in the environment, outside of industry)

National Clearinghouse for Smoking and Health
Center for Disease Control
Atlanta, Ga. 30333

Industrial Union of Metal Trades Department of AFL-CIO
815 16th Street, N.W.
Washington, D.C. 20006

(Asbestos control, insurance matters)

chapter 24

Update

This chapter, written as *Choices: Realistic Alternatives in Cancer Treatment* is ready to go to press, covers developments in cancer treatment and research since our manuscript was turned over to the publisher. Much of this material is discussed in other parts of the book and is updated here.

What conclusions came out of the Mayo study on the use of vitamin C for treating cancer patients?

In an article in the *New England Journal of Medicine* (September 26, 1979) a team of researchers from the Mayo Clinic concluded that large amounts of Vitamin C showed no therapeutic benefit to a group of 150 Mayo Clinic patients with advanced cancer. Headed by Edward T. Creagan, M.D., the Mayo team noted that it could detect "no appreciable difference in changes of symptoms"—weight, appetite or survival benefits between two groups of patients. (The patients volunteered to be treated each day with 10 grams of Vitamin C or a placebo—a sugar pill.) The Mayo group conducted a randomized scientifically-controlled study in which the groups were similar in age, sex, type of cancer, ability to swallow medicine and other medically important factors. All were patients who were considered unsuitable for treatment with chemotherapy, either because their disease had progressed despite prior treatment with standard drugs or because the drugs could not be used because of their condition.

Some of the results of the Mayo study:

- 63 percent of those given Vitamin C reported some improvement in symptoms in treatment. 58 percent of the patients given the placebo also reported improvement.
- Mild nausea and vomiting were the most frequent toxic reactions reported. About 40 percent of the patients were affected with no statistically significant difference between the two groups.
- Median survival was about seven weeks. The longest survivor (still alive 63 weeks after entering the study) received the placebo.
- Only nine of the patients had not previously received chemotherapy or radiation therapy. Because of this, the Mayo team felt it was "impossible to draw any conclusions about the possible effectiveness of Vitamin C in previously untreated patients."

It seems safe to conclude from this report that there is no final evidence of the value of Vitamin C in treating patients who have not been treated with chemotherapy or radiation therapy. Dr. Linus Pauling, when confronted with the results of the study, felt strongly that better studies are needed to determine the value of Vitamin C for treating cancer.

Is less radical breast surgery now considered acceptable by cancer specialists?

According to a blue-ribbon panel of experts at a consensus development conference sponsored by the National Cancer Institute in June, 1979 on the treatment of primary breast cancer, less radical surgery is being considered as a standard treatment. The conference to discuss alternative treatments to radical mastectomy brought together practicing physicians, biomedical research scientists, consumers and others to reach a general agreement. Among the recommendations of the panel:

- For women with Stage I or Stage II disease (cancers confined to the breast and detected while very tiny or microscopic), a total mastectomy with axillary dissection (complete removal of the breast and of the nodes in the armpit) should be recognized as the current standard treatment.
- The two-step procedure should be done in most cases, with the biopsy performed separately from the mastectomy.

- The panel decided that the question of the effectiveness of postoperative radiotherapy could not be answered without further results from ongoing clinical trials.
- The panel felt that segmental mastectomy poses problems because of remaining residual breast tissue. However, early data presented from the National Cancer Institute of Milan, Italy, indicates that the breast tissue that remains after segmental resection and postoperative radiation does not appear to harbor clinically important breast cancer cells. The length of patient follow-up in this trial is approximately four years.
- In discussing radiation, the panel noted radiation can be used in addition to a minimal surgical procedure or as a single method of treatment. The research involving primary radiation and that dealing with segmental mastectomy are not advanced enough to determine survival benefits. However, control of local recurrence appears to be similar to that achieved with current surgical procedures.
- The panel agreed that trials involving lesser surgical procedures, or treatment other than surgery, warrant further follow-up observation and enthusiastic support.

National Cancer Institute, *NIH Consensus Development Conference Summary,* "The Treatment of Primary Breast Cancer: Management of Local Disease," June, 1979, Volume 2, Number 5.

Can a change in diet make cystic breast lumps disappear?

Dr. John Minton of Ohio State University in an article published in *Surgery* (Vol. 86) reported a study on forty-seven patients with confirmed, clearly benign fibrocystic disease. He asked patients to give up coffee, tea, cola drinks and chocolate (all contain a compound classified as methylxanthine). Twenty of the forty-seven patients abstained—all had symptoms of methylxanthine withdrawal, a headache which lasted from one to seven days. Of these twenty women, thirteen experienced complete disappearance of all breast nodules, both by physical examination and on the mammogram, within one to six months. Of the patients who continued eating and drinking the items, only one experienced disappearance of the breast lumps. Doctors are calling for further studies in this area.

Minton, John P., M.D.; Foecking, M.K, M.S.; Webster, D.J.E., Ch. B.; F.R.C.S. and Matthews, R.H., Ph.D.; *Cancer Update,* Ohio State University Comprehensive Cancer Center, Vol. 3, Number 2, 1979.

What is the latest evidence on the use of estrogen receptors in managing breast cancer?

A consensus development conference on estrogen receptors in breast cancer was sponsored by the National Cancer Institute in June, 1979. Among the conclusions of the group of biomedical research scientists, practicing physicians, and consumers:

- It was recommended that each primary tumor be analyzed at the time of the first biopsy for estrogen receptor so that the information will be available when needed. For most early breast cancer patients, there should be enough of the primary tumor available to conduct such a test, since if the tumor recurs, tissue from the metastasis may be more difficult or impossible to obtain.

- Studies in the five years since the original NCI-sponsored meeting on estrogen receptors in 1974 have confirmed the use of estrogen receptor tests in managing advanced breast cancer. It is clear that more than half the patients whose tumors contain estrogen receptors respond to hormonal treatment, while few persons whose breast cancers do not contain clear estrogen receptors respond to hormonal treatment.

- In general, persons with tumors containing higher concentrations of estrogen receptors are more likely to respond to hormonal therapy. In addition, knowing whether the tumor contains progestin receptors seems to add to the ability to predict whether the patient will respond.

- At present, there does not seem to be any histopathologic features that can predict the estrogen receptor status of cancer, but it appears that more highly differentiated tumors have a higher proportion containing estrogen receptors than do the more poorly differentiated tumors.

- There is presently no evidence of any correlation between response to chemotherapy and the presence or absence of estrogen receptors.

- Persons with Stage II tumors which do not have estrogen receptors seem to recur earlier than those with estrogen receptor positive tumors, despite the size of the tumor or nodal involvements. There was agreement that further data must be accumulated on Stage I patients before any statement regarding length of survival or prognosis for recurrence could be made for these patients.

- Getting the proper tissue sample is of extreme importance in insuring the reliability of the test. This requires the cooperation of the surgeon, pathologist and assay laboratory. The consensus panel recommended five procedures for persons performing steroid receptor assays.
- The panel felt that there is a need for quality control of steroid receptor assays and recommended a quality control resource be developed in order to properly support the conduct of clinical trials in breast cancer.

National Cancer Institute, *NIH Consensus Development Conference Summary,* "Steroid Receptors in Breast Cancer," Volume 2, Number 5, June 27-29, 1979.

Is there any information on the effectiveness of using an ice-filled tourniquet on the head to reduce hair loss during chemotherapy?

Some doctors have found that some hair loss from intravenously delivered chemotherapy drugs can be reduced by cooling the scalp. One of our friends, Gloria Apisdorf, heard of this development through a newspaper story, and brought crushed ice, a plastic cap, turban and towels with her to her chemotherapy treatments. She happily reports that her hair loss has been minimal. According to a study reported at the meeting of the American Society of Clinical Oncology in May, 1979, cooling of the skin among a group of patients resulted in local constriction of the blood vessels in the scalp, thereby decreasing the delivery of drugs and hair loss. Mrs. Apisdorf has passed along information on a new Chemo Cap, distributed by M & M Medical Company, 241 Gemini Avenue, Brea, California, 92621, which employs a specially developed freezing gel which is pliable enough to be shaped to a patient's head. This device is placed on the patient twenty minutes prior to treatment and should remain in place for thirty minutes after treatment is completed. Though not tested by Mrs. Apisdorf, it seems to be a breakthrough.

Where is further testing being done on various forms of hyperthermia?

In addition to those listed in Chapter 23, new techniques for generating and fine-tuning high temperatures on and in the human body in treating cancer are being studied at various hospitals.

Memorial Sloan-Kettering Cancer Center, New York City
Jae Ho Kim, M.D., director of clinical hyperthermia research unit

(212) 794-6823

Type: Local hyperthemia by conductive heating using radio-frequency device at 13.56 MHz or inductive heating at 27.12 MHz

For: Patients with superficial cancers, including malignant melanoma and recurrent or metastatic tumors, for prospective randomized trial of local hyperthermia with or without x-ray; patients with advanced lung tumors confined to chest for inductive heating with or without x-rays

University of Mississippi School of Medicine, Jackson
Leon C. Parks, M.D., assistant professor of surgery

(601) 968-4675

Type: Systemic (whole-body) hyperthermia by extracorporeal heat exchanger (thermal regulating device)

For: Highly motivated late-stage patients with solid tumors not amenable to conventional treatment

Indiana University School of Medicine, Indianapolis
Ned B. Hornback, M.D., radiation-oncology chairman

(317) 264-2524

Type: Microwave hyperthermia at 433.92 MHz as adjunct to radiation therapy

For: Patients who have undergone conventional medical therapy unsuccessfully, especially those with carcinoma of the pancreas, adenocarcinoma of the bowel, and advanced carcinoma of the cervix.

University of Arizona Health Sciences Center, Tucson
Michael R. Manning, M.D., radiation-oncology division

(602) 626-6723

Type: Local hyperthermia, surface and interstitial, by a range of radio frequency heating sources

For: Patients with local accessible malignant tumors who have had unsuccessful standard treatment and are willing to try experimental hyperthermia

St. *Joseph Hospital, Houston*
John S. Stehlin Jr., M.D., Stehlin Foundation director

(713) 652-3161

Type: Regional hyperthermia by extracorporeal perfusion plus chemotherapy

For: Patients with malignant melanoma or soft-tissue sarcoma of extremities

David N. Leff, "Hyperthermia, Hottest News in Cancer Treatment," *Medical World News*: 52-55, May 14, 1979.

Should I see a dentist before I start having radiation treatment in the head and neck area?

Dentists have become more aware of the effects of radiation on the teeth and recommend that if there is to be radiation in the head and neck area (and remember that even though your primary disease may be in one area, your radiation may extend to another), you should be taking special care of your teeth and mouth before, during, and after treatment. You should visit your dentist or a dentist who has had experience in treating persons who have had head and neck radiation. Before your treatment starts, the dentist will probably take x-rays and examine your teeth. He will try to do any major work which he feels is necessary or will become necessary within the next year. He will explain the special care you should take to protect your teeth and mouth.

- Brush your teeth several times a day with a soft toothbrush, using a fluoride toothpaste which is not abrasive.
- Floss twice a day.
- Rinse your mouth well with a water, baking soda and salt solution.
- Apply fluoride (your dentist will show you how this is done) at least once a day to prevent tooth decay and decrease sensitivity.
- Do not use commercial mouthwashes which contain alcohol.
- Arrange follow-up visits more frequently than normal, both during and after treatment.

Is there any new information on the use of estrogens for relieving menopausal symptoms?

There was a consensus development conference on estrogen use and postmenopausal women, sponsored by the National Institute of Aging in September, 1979. The conference brought together biomedical research scientists, practicing physicians, consumers and others in an effort to reach general agreement on the risks and benefits of estrogen use.

Among the agreements of the panel:

- Estrogens are more effective than a placebo (sugar pill) in decreasing the severity and frequency of hot flashes and sweating. The decision of whether or not to use estrogens should depend on how severe the symptoms are and the patient's perceived need for relief. The lowest effective dose should be used. Since hot flashes naturally decline over time, treatment should not be prolonged unnecessarily.

- Estrogens are effective in overcoming vaginal dryness, burning, itching and pain in intercourse. However, there is evidence that the estrogens in the creams used to relieve these problems may be absorbed rapidly into the bloodstream; further study is needed on this effect.

- There is no evidence that estrogens relieve any emotional or mental problems that may be associated with menopause.

- Trials have shown that estrogens can retard bone loss if given around the time of menopause. However, discontinuance of the estrogen results in bone loss at an accelerated pace.

- The risk of endometrial cancer is increased several fold by estrogen replacement therapy—beginning after about 2-4 years of use with the risk increasing with the length of use and decreasing after the treatment stops. The panel felt that even in the absence of bleeding, the endometrium should be sampled yearly before and during estrogen therapy.

- There is presently no sufficient evidence that the risk of breast cancer is increased by the use of menopausal estrogens; however, further study is needed.

- Concern was expressed about women who have undergone menopause many years in advance of the normally expected age; support was voiced for conserving the ovaries of young women when possible, along with studies to determine the proper use of estrogens in young women having undergone oopherectomies ten years or more before the natural time of menopause.

- Patients should be given as much information as possible about the evidence for the effectiveness of estrogens in treating specific menopausal conditions and the risks that their use may entail. Given the current state of knowledge, no general recommendation which applies to all women can be made. Each individual patient must base her decision on the relative values that she assigns to relief of symptoms, to expectations for optimizing health and well-being and to various risks sustained in the process.

National Institutes of Health, *NIH Consensus Development Conference Summary,* "Estrogen Use and Postmenopausal Women." September, 1979, Vol. 2, No. 8.

Is research being done on the relationship of diet and nutrition to cancer?

According to reports delivered at the Cancer Nutrition Research Hearings in October 1979, before the Nutrition Subcommittee of the Senate Agriculture, Nutrition and Forestry Committee, there is considerable research being done which suggests that dietary habits play a role in causing cancer. A high fat intake may be associated with an increased risk of cancer. Fiber in the daily diet appears to protect against diseases of the bowel, including cancer. Presently under study are the roles of: total caloric balance, vitamins (especially A, C and E), minerals (especially selenium and zinc), naturally occurring carcinogens (such as cycasin, saffrole, mycotoxins, flavonoids), and man-made carcinogens (such as pesticides, preservatives, dyes, flavoring agents, packaging materials, etc.).

Dr. Arthur C. Upton, statement before the Subcommittee on Nutrition, Senate Committee on Agriculture, Nutrition and Forestry, October 2, 1979.

Is there any new information on rehabilitation exercises for cancer patients?

An excellent revised book, *Up and Around* details exercise programs developed in conjunction with the Physical and Occupational Therapy Departments of Mount Zion Hospital and Medical Center, San Francisco, California. It is published by *Life, Mind and Body,* San Francisco, California. The rehabilitation program initiates exercise at the earliest possible moment in the recovery period and is divided into three graduated levels. Stage I, for the bedridden and postsurgery patient, consists of simple range-of-motion exercises requiring low energy expenditure.

Stage II consists of moderate resistive exercises for the sitting and ambulatory patient. Stage III is a full-activity and maintenance program. The booklet is but one part of the exercise program that also utilizes videotape, recorded exercise instructions and a simple gym equipment package. The exercises are demonstrated by Jack LaLanne.

Are attempts being made to use the holistic approach in cancer treatment?

Many hospitals and doctors are awakening to the need for a comprehensive approach which uses the mind and body as well as the latest medical treatments to fight cancer. Some hospitals have instituted programs in nutrition and exercise for patients with cancer; others are exploring group sessions with oncologist, psychologist, nutritionist, patient and family to help acquaint everyone with the services the team can provide. "A Patient's Perspective on Cancer" by Fiore, in the February 8, 1979, *New England Journal of Medicine* advocates the need for "cancer-therapy teams that could provide patient-support groups or individual psychotherapy to assist patients during at least six stages of cancer therapy. At the time of diagnosis, to help them accept and understand the diagnosis of cancer, to make decisions about treatment alternatives and to deal with reactions from the family. In the preoperative period, to help prepare patients for the consequences of surgical procedures and to lessen anxiety about them. After the operation, to assist in recovery, in adjustment to loss of physical functioning or parts, and in preparation for subsequent cancer therapy. During postoperative cancer therapy, to prevent premature termination of treatment, to lower anxiety and tension about tests and side effects and to help with physical and psychological depression from setbacks and side effects. At termination of cancer therapy to assist with rehabilitation and to aid in the transition from dependence on medication and doctors to a return of faith in the ability of the patient's body to maintain health. And, in the five-year survival period, to help patients cope with the fear of recurrence and with long-term side effects. A holistic approach to the patient with cancer uses a team of experts, including the patients, as experts on their own feelings and the reactions of their bodies, and as the ones ultimately responsible for their lives."

Where can I find someone trained in hypnotism to help me?

For lists of trained medical, psychological and dental personnel who use hypnotism write:

Society for Clinical and Experimental Hypnosis
129A Kings Park Drive
Liverpool, N.Y. 13088

The American Society of Clinical Hypnosis
2400 East Devon Avenue, Suite 218
Des Plaines, Illinois 60018

What devices are available for patients who suffer impotence as a result of surgery?

Some relatively simple prosthetic devices are available to help correct the problem. Perhaps the best available at this time is the Flexirod. It uses two very flexible rods surgically inserted in the corpora cavenosa which can be straightened for intercourse and directed downward after intercourse. Another device, the forerunner of the Flexirod, called the Small-Carrion prosthesis, uses surgically implanted rods of much less flexibility and patients using this type have reported complications, including infections and the embarassment of a permanent erection. Another device, the Brantley-Scott prosthesis, an inflatable device which uses mechanical tubing, requires more complicated surgery.

"Sexual Prostheses Give Hope to Male Ostomates," *North Carolina Cancergram*, Duke Comprehensive Cancer Center, Durham, N.C.

Is it true that there are cancer-causing agents in beer and Scotch whisky?

Traces of cancer-causing nitrosamine substances were found in some domestic beers and the Food and Drug Administration has said that it will take regulatory action against any domestic beer made after January 1, 1980 which contains more than five parts per billion of cancer-causing nitrosamine substances. In October, the agency reported that more than half of American brewers had altered their brewing process to reduce formation of nitrosamines and that more than 80 percent will have done so in the next months. Test results on a check of Scotch whiskies found very low trace levels. The agency does not consider findings below five parts per billion to be scientifically reliable. "On the basis of the report from the Brewers Association and of its findings on Scotch, F.D.A. reiterates its previous position that there is no reason for consumers to alter their consumption of these products," the agency reported.

What rights do cancer patients have when faced with job discrimination?

Job discrimination is a serious problem which affects many cancer patients—but the rights of cancer patients are being reinforced through recent court decisions. Many patients try to conceal their condition, thereby running the risk of being fired if they are discovered. The 1973 Vocational Rehabilitation Act prohibits employers from discrimination against qualified handicapped individuals. A 1972 study, conducted by the Metropolitan Life Insurance Company, of employees with a history of cancer concluded that the hiring of persons treated for cancer is sound management policy. The study found no difference in turnover rates of cancer patients compared to other employees. The employment records for the groups were good, absenteeism was average and work performance was adequate. It is a good idea to discuss the question with your doctor and ask his advice on how to cope with any questions that might arise concerning your health condition. He can give you a statement that your condition will not interfere with your ability to fulfill your responsibilities. Information and assistance concerning discrimination complaints are available from a number of sources including the U.S. Department of Labor, your U.S. senator or representative, state representatives, Rehabilitation Services Administration, Equal Opportunities Commission, National Labor Relations Board and American Civil Liberties Union.

Johnson, Sharon, "Job Discrimination: The Special Case of Cancer Patients," *The New York Times*, August 26, 1979.

Wheatley, George M., William R. Cumnick, Barbara P. Wright, and Donald van Keuren. "The Employment of Persons with a History of Treatment for Cancer," *Cancer* 33 (No. 2): 441-45, February 1974.

References

ABRAMS, RUTH. *Not Alone with Cancer.* Springfield, Ill.: Charles C. Thomas, 1974.

AMERICAN CANCER SOCIETY. *A Cancer Source Book for Nurses.* American Cancer Society, 1975.

A Manual for Practitioners. Boston: American Cancer Society, 1968.

A variety of public education and professional education materials, 1970-78.

AMERICAN JOINT COMMITTEE. *Manual for Staging of Cancer.* Chicago: American Cancer Society, American Joint Committee, 1977.

AMERICAN JOURNAL OF NURSING COMPANY. *Nursing and the Cancer Patient.* New York: American Journal of Nursing Company—Education Services Division, 1973.

BAKER, LYNN S. *You and Leukemia—A Day at a Time.* Rochester, Minn.: Mayo Comprehensive Cancer Center, 1976.

BELSKY, MARVIN S., AND GROSS, LEONARD, *How to Choose and Use Your Doctor.* Greenwich, Conn.: Fawcett Publications, 1975.

CAMERON, CHARLES S. *The Truth About Cancer.* New York: Macmillan, 1971.

CHANEY, PATRICIA S. *Dealing with Death and Dying.* Horsham, Pa.: Eugene W. Jackson, 1976.

CHISARI, FRANCIS, AND NAKAMURA, ROBERT. *The Consumer's Guide to Health Care.* Boston: Little, Brown, 1976.

CLARK, LEE R., AND HOWE, CLIFTON D., EDS. *Cancer Patient Care at M.D. Anderson Hospital and Tumor Institute.* Chicago: Yearbook Medical Publishers, 1976.

COPE, OLIVER. *The Breast: Its Problems—Benign and Malignant and How to Deal with Them.* Boston: Houghton Mifflin, 1977.

COWLES, JANE. *Informed Consent.* New York: Coward, McCann and Geoghegan, 1976.

DEVESA, SUSAN S.; GODWIN, DAVID J., II; LEVIN, DAVID L.; AND SILVERMAN, DEBRA T. *Cancer Rates and Risks.* Washington, D.C.: U.S. Department of Health, Education and Welfare, 1974.

EISENBERG, HOWARD, AND SEHNERT, KEITH W. *How to Be Your Own Doctor—Sometimes.* New York: Grosset and Dunlap, 1975.

FREDERICKS, CARLTON. *Breast Cancer: A Nutritional Approach.* New York: Grosset and Dunlap, 1977.

FREESE, ARTHUR S., AND GLABMAN, SHELDON. *Your Kidneys, Their Care and Their Cure, A Modern Miracle of Medicine.* New York: E.P. Dutton, 1976.

GARFIELD, CHARLES A., ed. *Psychosocial Care of the Dying Patient.* New York: McGraw-Hill, 1978.

GUTTERMAN, JORDAN U. *Frontiers of Clinical Cancer, Research with Chemotherapy and Immunotherapy.* Houston: M.D. Anderson Hospital and Tumor Institute, 1978.

HOLLAND, JAMES F., AND FREI, EMIL III. *Cancer Medicine.* Philadelphia: Lea and Febiger, 1973.

HOLVEY, DAVID N., ed. *The Merck Manual of Diagnosis and Therapy.* Rahway, N.J.: Merck Sharp & Dohme Research Laboratories, 1972.

JOHNSON, TIMOTHY G. *What You Should Know About Health Care Before You Call a Doctor.* New York: McGraw-Hill, 1975.

JONES, GIFFORD W. *What Every Woman Should Know About Hysterectomy.* New York: Funk and Wagnalls, 1977.

KUSHNER, ROSE. *Breast Cancer: An Investigative Report.* New York. Harcourt Brace Jovanovich, 1975. (Paperback: *Why Me?*, New York: Signet Books, 1977.)

KUBLER-ROSS, ELISABETH. *On Death and Dying.* New York: Macmillan, 1969.

———. *Questions and Answers on Death and Dying.* New York: Macmillan, 1974.

LAWRENCE, WALTER, JR., AND TERZ, JOSE J. *Cancer Management.* New York; Grune & Stratton, 1977.

LAWS, PRISCILLA W. *X-Rays: More Harm than Good?* Emmaus, Pa.: Rodale, 1977.

LEVIN, ARTHUR. *Talk Back to Your Doctor: How to Demand High Quality Health Care.* Garden City, N.Y.: Doubleday, 1975.

MEMORIAL SLOAN-KETTERING CANCER CENTER. *Guidelines for Comprehensive Nursing Care in Cancer.* New York, N.Y.: Springer, 1973.

MILLMAN, MARCIA. *The Unkindest Cut—Life in the Backrooms of Medicine.* New York: Morrow, 1977.

NACHTIGALL, LILA, WITH HEILMAN, JOAN LILA. *Nachtigall Report.* New York: Putnam, 1977.

NATIONAL CANCER INSTITUTE. A variety of public information pamphlets and materials. Washington D.C.: The National Cancer Institute, Department of Health, Education and Welfare, 1975-1979.

ROTHENBERG, ROBERT E., ED. *Understanding Surgery.* New York: Trident, 1969.

RUBIN, PHILIP, ED. *Clinical Oncology for Medical Students and Physicians.* Rochester, N.Y.: American Cancer Society, 1978.

SEAMAN, BARBARA, AND SEAMAN, GILDEON. *Women and the Crisis in Sex Hormones.* New York: Rawson, 1977.

SHIMKIN, MICHAEL B. *Science and Cancer.* New York: U.S. Department of Health, Education and Welfare, 1973.

U.S. DEPARTMENT OF HEALTH, EDUCATION AND WELFARE. *Cancer Patient Survival,* Report No. 5. Bethesda, Md.: Public Health Service, 1976.
Compilation of Clinical Protocol Summaries. Bethesda, Md.: Public Health Service, 1977.

WINKLER, ANN. *Post Mastectomy: A Personal Guide to Physical and Emotional Recovery.* New York: Hawthorn, 1976.

ZALON, JEAN. *I Am Whole Again: The Case for Breast Reconstruction After Mastectomy.* New York: Random House, 1978.

In the process of reading and using this book, questions which are not included in it may come to your mind. The authors would be most pleased if you would share your thoughts with them.

Kindly send any comments to:

Eve Potts, Marion Morra
c/o Avon Books
959 Eighth Avenue
New York, New York 10019

Index